Patient Encounters

The Inpatient Pediatrics Work-Up

Patient Encounters

The Inpatient Pediatrics Work-Up

Samir S. Shah, MD, MSCE

Assistant Professor of Pediatrics and Epidemiology
University of Pennsylvania School of Medicine
Attending Physician in Infectious Diseases and General Pediatrics
The Children's Hospital of Philadelphia
Philadelphia, Pennsylvania

Gary Frank, MD, MSEM

Pediatric Hospitalist
Scottish Rite Children's Hospital
Medical Director, Quality
Children's Healthcare of Atlanta, Atlanta, Georgia

Series Editor

Alfa O. Diallo, MD, MPH

Department of Emergency Medicine
Johns Hopkins Hospital, Baltimore, Maryland

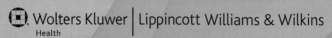

Wolters Kluwer | Lippincott Williams & Wilkins
Health

Philadelphia · Baltimore · New York · London
Buenos Aires · Hong Kong · Sydney · Tokyo

Acquisitions Editor: Susan Rhyner
Product Manager: Stacey L. Sebring
Marketing Manager: Christen Melcher
Compositor: Aptara, Inc.

Printed in the United States of America

Library of Congress Cataloging-in-Publication Data

Shah, Samir S.
  Patient encounters. The inpatient pediatrics work-up / Samir S. Shah, Gary Frank.
     p. ; cm.
  Includes bibliographical references and index.
  ISBN 978-0-7817-9400-8 (alk. paper)
  1. Pediatrics—Handbooks, manuals, etc. 2.   Clinical clerkship—Handbooks, manuals, etc.
I. Frank, Gary, 1971-   II. Title.   III. Title: Inpatient pediatrics work-up.
  [DNLM: 1. Pediatrics—methods—Handbooks. 2.   Child. 3.   Diagnostic
Techniques and Procedures—Handbooks. 4.   Infant. 5.   Inpatients—Handbooks.
WS 39 S525p 2010]
  RJ48.S535 2010
  618.92—dc22

                                                                                    2009035928

To our families—for providing love and support.

To our mentors—for sharing their wisdom and knowledge.

*To our patients—for teaching us and to their families
for trusting us.*

Contributors

Brian Alverson, MD
Assistant Professor of Pediatrics
Department of Pediatrics
The Warren Alpert School of Medicine
at Brown University
Head, Section of Pediatric Hospitalist
Medicine
Department of Pediatrics
Hasbro Children's Hospital
Providence, Rhode Island

Sandra Amaral, MD, MHS
Assistant Professor
Department of Pediatrics
Division of Nephrology
Emory University
Attending Physician
Department of Pediatrics
Division of Nephrology
Children's Healthcare of Atlanta
Atlanta, Georgia

Deborah J. Andresen, MD
Pediatric Hospitalist
Department of General Pediatrics
Children's Healthcare of Atlanta
Atlanta, Georgia

Mercedes M. Blackstone, MD
Assistant Professor of Clinical
Pediatrics
University of Pennsylvania School of
Medicine
Attending Physician in Emergency
Medicine
The Children's Hospital of
Philadelphia
Philadelphia, Pennsylvania

Christopher P. Bonafide, MD
Instructor
Department of Pediatrics
University of Pennsylvania
Chief Resident
Department of Pediatrics
The Children's Hospital of Philadelphia
Philadelphia, Pennsylvania

Laura K. Brennan, MD
Instructor
Department of Pediatrics
University of Pennsylvania
Attending Physician
Division of General Pediatrics
The Children's Hospital of Philadelphia
Philadelphia, Pennsylvania

Lindsay H. Chase, MD
Associate Professor
Department of Pediatrics
Baylor College of Medicine
Texas Children's Hospital
Houston, Texas

Tony Cooley, MD
Assistant Professor
Division of General Pediatric Hospitalists
Department of Pediatrics
Emory University School of Medicine
Atlanta, Georgia

Diva D. De León, MD
Assistant Professor
Department of Pediatrics
University of Pennsylvania School of
Medicine
Attending Physician
Department of Pediatrics
Division of Endocrinology/Diabetes
Philadelphia, Pennsylvania

Stephen C. Eppes, MD
Professor
Department of Pediatrics
Thomas Jefferson University
Philadelphia, Pennsylvania
Chief, Division of Infectious Disease
Department of Pediatrics
Alfred I. duPont Hospital for Children
Wilmington, Delaware

Gary Frank, MD, MS
Clinical Assistant Professor
Department of Pediatrics
Emory University School of Medicine
Pediatric Hospitalist
Scottish Rite Pediatric and Adolescent
  Consultants
Children's Healthcare of Atlanta
Atlanta, Georgia

Patricio A. Frias, MD
Associate Professor
Department of Pediatrics
Emory University
Director, Outpatient Operations
Sibley Heart Center Cardiology
Children's Healthcare of Atlanta
Atlanta, Georgia

Sher Lynn Gardner, MD
Assistant Professor
Department of Pediatrics
Emory University
Department of Pediatrics
Children's Healthcare of Atlanta
Atlanta, Georgia

Christopher L. Gaydos, MD
Pediatric Hospitalist
Department of Pediatrics
Children's Healthcare of Atlanta at
  Scottish Rite
Atlanta, Georgia

Susan K. Goldberg, MD
Assistant Professor
Department of Pediatrics
Emory University
Physician
Department of Emergency Medicine
Children's Healthcare of Atlanta
Atlanta, Georgia

Dafina M. Good, MD
Pediatric Emergency Medicine Fellow
Department of Pediatrics
Emory University School of Medicine
Children's Healthcare of Atlanta
Atlanta, Georgia

Larry A. Greenbaum, MD, PhD
Division Director and Marcus Chair
Pediatric Nephrology
Emory University
Children's Healthcare of Atlanta
Atlanta, Georgia

Adda Grimberg, MD, FAAP
Assistant Professor
Department of Pediatrics
University of Pennsylvania School of
  Medicine
Attending Physician
Division of Endocrinology
The Children's Hospital of Philadelphia
Philadelphia, Pennsylvania

Andrew B. Grossman, MD
Clinical Assistant Professor
Department of Pediatrics
University of Pennsylvania School of
  Medicine
Attending Physician
Division of Gastroenterology,
  Heptology, and Nutrition
The Children's Hospital of Philadelphia
Philadelphia, Pennsylvania

David E. Hall, MD
Clinical Associate Professor
Department of Pediatrics
Emory University School of Medicine
Director of Medical Affairs
Children's Healthcare of Atlanta at
    Scottish Rite
Atlanta, Georgia

Jessica Hart, MD
Division of General Pediatrics
The Children's Hospital of Philadelphia
Philadelphia, Pennsylvania

Joseph A. Hilinski, MD
Assistant Professor
Department of Pediatrics
Division of Infectious Diseases
Emory University
Attending Physician
Children's Healthcare of Atlanta
Atlanta, Georgia

David A. Hsu, MD, PhD
Assistant Professor
Department of Neurology
University of Wisconsin
Madison, Wisconsin

Lisa Humphrey, MD
Clinical Instructor
Department of Pediatrics
Stanford University School of Medicine
Hospitalist
Division of General Pediatrics
Lucile Packard Children's Hospital
Palo Alto, California

Jennifer A. Jackson, MD
Fellow
Division of Pediatric Nephrology
Emory University
Children's Healthcare of Atlanta
Atlanta, Georgia

Sarah D. Keene, MD
Clinical Fellow
Department of Pediatrics
Division of Neonatology
The University of Pennsylvania
Fellow Physician
Department of Pediatrics
Division of Neonatology
The Children's Hospital of Philadelphia
Philadelphia, Pennsylvania

**Naghma S. Khan, MD, FAAP,
FACEP**
Assistant Professor
Departments of Pediatrics and
    Emergency Medicine
Emory University School of Medicine
Children's Healthcare of Atlanta
Atlanta, Georgia

David Kotzbauer, MD
Attending Physician
Scottish Rite Pediatric and Adolescent
    Consultants
Children's Hospital of Atlanta at
    Scottish Rite
Atlanta, Georgia

Carmen M. Lebrón, MD
Fellow
Division of Pediatric Emergency
    Medicine
Department of Pediatrics
Emory University School of Medicine
Atlanta, Georgia

Grace E. Lee, MD
Clinical Associate in Pediatrics
Department of Pediatrics
University of Pennsylvania
Attending Physician
Department of General Pediatrics
The Children's Hospital of Philadelphia
Philadelphia, Pennsylvania

Glen Lew, MD
Assistant Professor
Department of Pediatrics
Emory University
Staff Physician
Aflac Cancer Center and Blood
  Disorders Service
Children's Healthcare of Atlanta
Atlanta, Georgia

Jeffrey F. Linzer, Sr., MD
Associate Professor
Department of Pediatrics and
  Emergency Medicine
Emory University School of Medicine
Associate Medical Director for
  Compliance
Department of Emergency Services
Children's Healthcare of Atlanta at
  Egleston and Hughes Spalding
Atlanta, Georgia

Wendalyn K. Little, MD, MPH
Assistant Professor
Department of Pediatrics and
  Emergency Medicine
Emory University
Children's Healthcare of Atlanta
Atlanta, Georgia

Petar Mamula, MD
Associate Professor
Department of Pediatrics
University of Pennsylvania School
  of Medicine
Director, Endoscopy
Division of Gastroenterology,
  Hepatology and Nutrition
The Children's Hospital of Philadelphia
Philadelphia, Pennsylvania

Brian McAlvin, MD
Chief Resident
Department of Pediatrics
Emory University
Children's Healthcare of Atlanta at
  Egleston
Atlanta, Georgia

Stephanie McGee Jernigan, MD
Clinical Professor
Department of Pediatric Nephrology
Emory University
Vice Section Chief
Department of Pediatric Nephrology
Children's Healthcare of Atlanta at
  Scottish Rite
Atlanta, Georgia

Tracy Ann Merrill, MD
Assistant Professor
Department of Pediatrics
Emory University School of Medicine
Professional Staff
Pediatric Emergency/Urgent Care
Children's Healthcare of Atlanta
Atlanta, Georgia

Darryl R. Morris, MD, FAAP
Pediatric Hospitalist
Scottish Rite Pediatric and Adolescent
  Consultants
Children's Healthcare of Atlanta
Atlanta, Georgia

David A. Munson, MD
Attending Neonatologist
Associate Medical Director
Newborn/Infant Intensive Care Unit
The Children's Hospital of Philadelphia
Philadelphia, Pennsylvania

Thao M. Nguyen, MD
Pediatric Emergency Fellow
Department of Pediatrics
Division of Emergency Medicine
Emory University
Children's Healthcare of Atlanta
Atlanta, Georgia

Kalpesh N. Patel, MD
Pediatric Emergency Medicine Fellow
Department of Pediatrics
Emory University
Atlanta, Georgia

Melinda Penn, MD
Fellow
Division of Endocrinology
Children's Hospital of Philadelphia
Philadelphia, Pennsylvania

Jack Percelay, MD, MPH, FAAP, FHM
E. L. M. O. Pediatrics
New York, New York

Sara E. Pinney, MD
Fellow
Division of Endocrinology/Diabetes
The Children's Hospital of Philadelphia
Philadelphia, Pennsylvania

Jonathan Popler, MD
Fellow
Department of Pediatric Pulmonary
  Medicine
University of Colorado School of
  Medicine
The Children's Hospital, Denver
Denver, Colorado

James J. Reese, Jr., MD, MPH
Child Neurology Resident
Department of Neurology
LSU Health Sciences Center
New Orleans, Louisiana

Stacey R. Rose, MD
Attending Physician
Department of Pediatrics
The Children's Hospital of
  Philadelphia
Philadelphia, Pennsylvania

Michele Saysana, MD, FAAP
Clinical Assistant Professor
Department of Pediatrics
Indiana University School of Medicine
Pediatric Hospitalist
Riley Hospital for Children
Indianapolis, Indiana

Lekha Shah, MD
Division of Emergency Medicine
Children's Healthcare of Atlanta at
  Egleston
Emory University
Atlanta, Georgia

Samir S. Shah, MD, MSCE
Assistant Professor
Departments of Pediatrics and
  Biostatistics and Epidemiology
University of Pennsylvania School of
  Medicine
Attending Physician
Division of Infectious Diseases and
  General Pediatrics
The Children's Hospital of
  Philadelphia
Philadelphia, Pennsylvania

Samuel J. Spizman, MD
Assistant Professor
Department of Pediatrics
Emory University
Emergency Room Attending
  Physician
Department of Pediatrics
Children's Healthcare of Atlanta
Atlanta, Georgia

Jesse J. Sturm, MD, MPH
Assistant Professor
Department of Pediatrics
Emory University
Children's Healthcare of Atlanta
Atlanta, Georgia

Nicholas Tsarouhas, MD
Associate Professor of Clinical
  Pediatrics
Department of Pediatrics
University of Pennsylvania School of
  Medicine
Medical Director, Emergency
  Transport
Division of Emergency Medicine
The Children's Hospital of
  Philadelphia
Philadelphia, Pennsylvania

Pamela F. Weiss, MD
Assistant Professor
Department of Pediatrics
Division of Rheumatology
Children's Hospital of Philadelphia
Philadelphia, Pennsylvania

Deborah W. Young, MD
Assistant Professor of Pediatrics
Division of Pediatric Emergency
  Medicine
Emory University School of Medicine
Atlanta, Georgia

Megan K. Yunghans, MD
Hospitalist
Hospital-based Specialties
Children's National Medical Center
Washington, D.C.

Reviewers

Aswin Chandrakantan
New Jersey Medical School

Emery H. Chang, MD
University of California Los Angeles

Silvia Chiang
Case Western Reserve University
of Medicine

Erica M. Fallon, MD
Harvard Medical School
Beth Israel Deaconess Medical
Center

Ashlee Goldsmith
University of Illinois College of
Medicine at Chicago

Ashima Gupta, MD
Loyola University Medical Center

Shreevidya V. Menon, BA, DO
Midwestern University
Cook County Hospital

Shilpa Shah, DO
University of Texas Medical Branch at
Galveston

Shiwan K. Shah, DO
University of Texas Medical Branch
at Galveston

Stephanie L. Siehr, MD
Stanford University
Lucille Packard Children's Hospital

Anouar Teriaky
University of Ottawa Faculty of
Medicine

Meghan D. Treitz, MD
The Children's Hospital

Ian Turkstra
University of Western Ontario

Kerry Wilkins
University of Arkansas for Medical
Sciences College of Medicine

Preface

The *Patient Encounters series* has been developed to provide a concise review of patient assessment and management. Each book in this series is organized logically and provides medical students with specialty-specific steps for managing patient care. The goal of this series is to remove the focus from "acing the shelf" to a focus on helping medical students become good doctors.

The books in this series provide a specialty-specific, step-by-step guide for managing a patient by candidly addressing, in a very practical fashion, a new clinical clerk's anxiety as well as hunger for learning. Each title within this series is a companion guide that candidly cuts to need-to-know information, directing medical students to what they need to do in each step of the patient encounter.

The books in this series discuss patient care from an overview of the disease or disorder, with brief pathophysiology information presented as necessary to support optimal patient assessment and care. It includes specific information that will help medical students from the point of reviewing the patient's chart to walking into the room and assessing the stability of the patient, including potential life threats. Each book then addresses acute management and workup, directing the student through the diagnosis, treatment, extended inhospital management, and discharge goals and outpatient care.

Each title provides students with the rationale for ordering appropriate diagnostic studies and allows clinical decision making that is consistent with the patient's disposition. The books provide an extended view of patient care so that the medical student can propose a well-informed choice of diagnostic studies and interventions when presenting his or her case to house staff and faculty.

The books use algorithms, tables, figures, icons, and a stylized design to support concise and easy-to-find patient management information. They also provide diagnosis-based, evidence-based information that includes peer-reviewed journal references.

Feedback from student reviewers gives high praise to this new series. Each of these new books was developed to provide practical information and to address the basics needed during a particular clinical rotation:

Patient Encounters: The Neurology and Psychiatry Work-Up
Patient Encounters: The Obstetrics and Gynecology Work-Up
Patient Encounters: The Internal Medicine Work-Up

How to Use This Book

Patient Encounters: The Inpatient Pediatrics Work-Up provides you with a concise, organized review of the most important patient assessment and management in pediatrics. This book is designed for you to quickly and efficiently review and enhance the knowledge you need to effectively manage patient care.

This book can help you ease the transition from the basic sciences to clinical medicine by providing you with a practical "how-to" guide for approaching a patient, including:

- Identifying pertinent positives and negatives in the patient history and physical exam
- Determining how to work up a patient by addressing pertinent diagnostic studies and procedures
- Explaining the rationale for clinical decision making

Each of the 44 chapters feature essential information related to patient assessment and management, supplemented with patient case studies that provide you with the opportunity to apply patient care principles and management goals to patient cases that are specific to each chapter's topic.

This book, as with all the books in the series, includes common features that will allow you to glean necessary information quickly and easily:

- **The Patient Encounter:** Each chapter begins with a patient case study that is followed up on at several intervals throughout the chapter. The patient encounter allows you the opportunity to see some of the common signs and symptoms with which a patient may present.
- **Overview:** This section provides an introduction to the chapter topic and includes the definition, epidemiology, and etiology of the disease or disorder. Brief pathophysiology information is included to support optimal patient assessment and care.
- **Acute Management and Workup:** This section includes the key information that you need to obtain in order to provide excellent patient care, addressing first what you need to do within the first 15 minutes through the first few hours. Topics include the initial assessment, admission and level of care criteria, the patient history, the physical examination, labs and imaging to consider, and key treatment information.
- **Extended Inhospital Management:** This section provides information that you need to know when a patient needs extended inhospital management.

- **Disposition:** In this section, you will find the key discharge goals and out-patient care related to a patient with the specific condition or disorder addressed in the chapter.
- **What You Need to Remember:** This feature is a bulleted list of key points that are most helpful to remember about the chapter topic.
- **Suggested Readings:** Each chapter provides diagnosis- and evidence-based peer-reviewed journal references.
- **Clinical Pearl:** This feature presents clinical tips, statistics, or findings that will help you understand the patient's clinical presentation or help you better address diagnosis and management.

In addition to the features noted above, this text contains tables, line drawings, and photographs to supplement your learning.

We hope this text improves your knowledge of pediatrics, allowing you to feel confident that you're providing quality patient care. The ultimate goal of this book is to better prepare you to provide effective care to patients who you will encounter in your medical career.

Samir S. Shah, MD, MSCE
Assistant Professor of Pediatrics and Epidemiology
University of Pennsylvania School of Medicine
Attending Physician in Infectious Diseases and General Pediatrics
The Children's Hospital of Philadelphia
Philadelphia, Pennsylvania

Gary Frank, MD, MSEM
Pediatric Hospitalist
Scottish Rite Children's Hospital
Medical Director, Quality
Children's Healthcare of Atlanta
Atlanta, Georgia

Contents

Acute Renal Failure

STEPHANIE MCGEE JERNIGAN

THE PATIENT ENCOUNTER

A 10-year-old boy presents to the local emergency room with a 2-day history of tea-colored urine. His urine output has been below normal and his parents have noticed some puffiness around his eyes. On physical exam, vital signs are stable with the exception of his blood pressure (BP), which is elevated at 150/100 mm Hg. He has periorbital edema and fullness of his abdomen with a positive fluid wave. The patient's urine is grossly bloody.

OVERVIEW

Definition

Acute renal failure (ARF) is defined as a rapid decline in glomerular filtration rate, resulting in the impairment of renal functions, including the impairment of waste product excretion, acid–base regulation, and electrolyte and water balance. This chapter focuses on the identification, diagnosis, and acute management of ARF, particularly as it relates to acute glomerulonephritis.

Pathophysiology

The pathophysiology of ARF can be divided into three categories: prerenal disease, intrinsic renal disease, and postrenal disease. Prerenal causes of ARF result from loss of circulatory volume from bleeding or volume losses from the urinary tract, gastrointestinal tract, or skin. ARF may also result from the loss of effective intravascular pressure or volume secondary to shock, heart failure, or the loss of oncotic pressure, as seen in hypoalbuminemic states such as cirrhosis or nephrotic syndrome. If not corrected, prerenal failure may progress to acute tubular necrosis (ATN).

Intrinsic renal disease can be categorized as vascular, glomerular, or tubulointerstitial disease. Intrinsic renal disease results from direct injury to the kidney from thrombosis, hypertension, immune-mediated injury, or toxic/ischemic injury. ATN is also a cause of intrinsic renal disease.

Postrenal ARF results from obstruction of the urinary tract. Postrenal disease is typically bilateral, although it is possible for a solitary kidney to be involved.

Epidemiology

The incidence of ARF in children is difficult to determine. From a retrospective study in Great Britain, it has been estimated to be 0.8 per 100,000 population. This is approximately one-fifth that seen in the adult population. With advances in medical technology—including bone marrow and solid organ transplantation, surgical correction of congenital heart disease, and the care of premature infants—the increasing incidence of ARF in children has been more clearly reported.

Etiology

Some of the more common etiologies of ARF are listed by pathophysiology in Table 1-1.

ACUTE MANAGEMENT AND WORKUP

The initial assessment of a patient with renal disease is directed toward deciding which patients need inpatient care, including intensive care, versus those who may have their workup started during the initial visit but are then followed on an outpatient basis.

The First 15 Minutes

The initial assessment of the patient should include vital signs, with particular attention to the patient's BP. In fact, unless they present with gross urinary findings, many patients with ARF often have only vague complaints, with hypertension being the first indicator that there is a renal problem. Hypertension is a primary reason for admission in renal disease and can be a true emergency if symptomatic. The case patient would need admission for control of his BP. The topic of hypertension is more thoroughly discussed in Chapter 18.

Second, physical finding of edema should be addressed. Rarely, edema may be severe enough to impinge on respiratory status because of pulmonary effusions or edema or secondary to restriction of respiratory excursion from increased abdominal girth.

Finally, although electrolytes may be abnormal in ARF, it is rare to find symptomatic abnormalities unless there is a prolonged course, a significant decrease in urine output, or oliguria. Acidosis can lead to compensatory tachypnea; hypocalcemia can lead to tingling in the extremities and cramping; and hyperkalemia can result in electrocardiographic (ECG) changes. Rarely, uremia will lead to seizures as well as to pleural and pericardial effusions.

The First Few Hours

Following the initial assessment, a directed history and thorough physical exam as well as appropriate lab and radiographic evaluation can begin the process of diagnosing and then managing the patient with acute renal failure.

TABLE 1-1
Common Etiologies of Acute Renal Failure in Childhood

Prerenal Disease	Intrinsic Renal Disease	Postrenal Disease
Intravascular depletion	Acute tubular necrosis	Urethral obstruction (posterior urethral valves)
Bleeding	Hypoxic–ischemic injury	
Dehydration	Drug/toxin-induced	
Gastrointestinal losses	Rhabdomyolysis/ myoglobinuria	
Cutaneous losses/burns	Hemoglobinuria	Unilateral obstruction of solitary kidney
Third-spacing	Tumor lysis syndrome	
Capillary leak syndrome	Acute GN	
Nephrotic syndrome	Postinfectious	Bilateral ureteral obstruction
Sepsis	IgA nephropathy	
Cirrhosis	Systemic SLE	
Diabetes insipidus	MPGN	
Salt wasting (renal or adrenal)	HSP	
	ANCA GN	
	Goodpasture's syndrome	
	Anti-GBM nephritis	
Decreased effective intravascular volume	Rapidly progressive GN	
	Acute interstitial nephritis, drug-induced	
Congestive heart failure	Vascular injury/thrombosis	
	HUS	
Cardiac tamponade	Renal artery thrombosis	
	Hypertension	
Shock	Pyelonephritis	
	Congenital disease	
	Dysplasia	
	Cystic kidney disease	

ANCA, antineutrophil cytoplasmic antibody; Anti-GBM, anti–glomerular basement membrane; GN, glomerulonephritis; HSP, Henoch–Schönlein purpura; HUS, hemolytic uremic syndrome; MPGN, membranoproliferative glomerulonephritis; SLE, systemic lupus erythematosus.

History

In approaching the patient with ARF, a thorough but directed history should be taken. Questions about the patient's hydration status should include asking about oral intake, vomiting, diarrhea, and urine output or the number of wet diapers. The presence of bloody diarrhea should also be noted. Decreased urine output or poor urinary stream in newborns is suggestive of anatomic abnormalities.

Fever may be present in infections and some types of vasculitis. In addition, the patient's history should include questions about previous urinary tract infections or unexplained fevers. These may be seen in undiagnosed vesicoureteral reflux. The patient should be asked about painful urination and/or costovertebral angle (CVA) tenderness, especially in the presence of grossly bloody urine. Also, with gross hematuria, it is helpful to ask about the presence of preceding or concurrent illness. Special note should be made of a history of past pharyngitis or impetigo.

You should ask the patient about present or past episodes of swelling. Hemoptysis may also be associated with some types of ARF. Joint pain or unusual rashes should be documented. A history of fatigue and malaise may suggest how long the process has been going on. A history of headaches and/or nosebleeds may be secondary to hypertension. Finally, a history of recent medications should be taken. This includes over-the-counter (OTC) medications, especially nonsteroidal anti-inflammatory drugs (NSAIDs).

Physical Examination

The physical exam should include careful attention to BP. Edema of the eyelids, abdomen, and lower extremities should be noted. A careful lung exam can help determine the presence of pulmonary edema with rales or pleural effusions with decreased lung sounds, particularly in the lung bases. Several types of kidney disease are associated with rashes. Purpura, especially of the lower extremities, is seen in Henoch–Schönlein purpura (HSP), a malar rash in systemic lupus erythematosus (SLE), and petechiae in SLE or hemolytic uremic syndrome (HUS). Joints should be carefully examined.

Labs and Tests to Consider

Lab and imaging studies in the patient with renal failure not only identify the need for urgent intervention but also assist with diagnosis and determining the time frame of the illness, helping to distinguish acute from chronic illness. A renal biopsy is warranted when less invasive tests are unable to suggest a diagnosis. Another indication for renal biopsy is rapidly progressing glomerulonephritis, in which urgent and accurate diagnosis is required in order to start appropriate therapy.

Key Diagnostic Labs and Tests

The most important first tests are a urinalysis and complete metabolic panel. A urinalysis reveals the presence of hematuria or proteinuria. On microscopic exam, urinary red blood cell (RBC) casts are suggestive of glomerulonephritis. Hematuria without RBCs may lead one to look for hemoglobin or myoglobin as a source of renal injury. White blood cells (WBCs) can be seen in infection or interstitial nephritis. Specific gravity testing helps to identify dehydration or the inability to concentrate the urine, as is often seen in structural abnormalities.

The complete metabolic panel identifies the creatinine level and thus the degree of renal insufficiency. It will also identify electrolyte abnormalities such as hyperkalemia, acidosis, and hypocalcemia. Hyperphosphatemia develops over time in ARF, and a normal phosphorus level suggests acute onset. Hypoalbuminemia is a worrisome finding in the face of glomerulonephritis and will often herald the need for more aggressive treatment.

CLINICAL PEARL

The blood urea nitrogen (BUN):creatinine (Cr) ratio can be helpful in identifying the cause of renal failure. BUN:Cr ratios of 10 to 20:1 are considered normal and may also be seen in postrenal disease (i.e., within the ureter). BUN:Cr ratios >20:1 are concerning for prerenal disease as well as dehydration. BUN:Cr ratios <10:1 may be seen with intrarenal disease.

A complete blood count (CBC) may help identify renal illness as well. Evidence of hemolytic anemia with thrombocytopenia suggests HUS. Thrombocytopenia is also seen in SLE. The degree of anemia can help to determine the time line of renal disease. More anemic patients are likely to have had prolonged ARF with diminished erythropoietin production.

Some lab tests may prove more diagnostic but also take more time. Complement C3 and often also C4 is lowered in membranoproliferative glomerulonephritis (MPGN), SLE, nephritis related to hepatitis B and C, as well as bacterial endocarditis or shunt nephritis. C3 is lowered but C4 is normal in postinfectious glomerulonephritis. Many forms of rapidly progressive glomerulonephritis are positive for antinuclear cytoplasmic antibodies (ANCA). C–ANCA is often positive in Wegener's glomerulonephritis. If the pulmonary system is involved, the presence of antiglomerular basement membrane (anti-GBM) antibodies suggests anti-GBM or Goodpasture's disease.

In our patient, labs revealed a BUN of 67 mg/dL and a creatinine of 3.2 mg/dL. Chemistries revealed normal electrolytes with the exception of a serum bicarbonate of 16. His albumin is low at 2.2 g/dL.

Imaging

A noninvasive renal ultrasound can reveal the presence of one or two kidneys, evaluate renal size, and evaluate renal parenchyma both in quality and quantity. Obstructive disease that results in ARF may cause large kidneys but very little healthy parenchyma. The size of the kidneys gives some prognostic information as well. Kidneys in ARF that remain large have greater potential for reversal of the disease process than kidneys that have already shrunken to smaller-than-normal size because of irreversible scarring. Especially in the infant with ARF, a voiding cystourethrogram is needed to rule out posterior urethral valves and also evaluate for vesicoureteral reflux. Computed tomography (CT) scans and nuclear studies are useful but rarely needed in the acute setting. It is also important to remember that in the setting of ARF, intravenous (IV) contrast for CT scan is contraindicated and may worsen renal injury.

Treatment

The treatment of ARF varies by etiology. Prerenal ARF requires fluid resuscitation and resolution of the source of fluid losses. Postrenal failure requires placement of a Foley catheter to correct obstruction beyond the bladder; then further urologic evaluation is needed to determine additional interventions. Following the correction of urinary obstruction, caretakers should remain aware of the possibility of a brisk postobstructive diuresis. Fluids must be adjusted accordingly by closely following input and output.

The treatment of acute glomerulonephritis is more complex. For patients with ARF due to immune-mediated glomerulonephritis or biopsies that reveal significant inflammation or cellular crescents, more urgent medical therapy is needed. The first line of therapy is "pulse" intravenous steroids at very large doses given either daily or every other day. Dosing may vary but steroids are often given as three doses of 30 mg/kg per dose. Lower doses of oral steroids should follow intravenous dosing. Cytoxan is another commonly used medication in acute glomerulonephritis. It is often used in patients with SLE and ANCA-positive diseases such as pauci-immune glomerulonephritis and Wegener's glomerulonephritis. Finally, on some occasions, plasmapheresis is used to deplete serum levels of offending antibodies. This is particularly true in anti-GBM or Goodpasture's disease. It may also be used in some atypical forms of HUS.

Admission Criteria

In general, the treatment of ARF requires an inpatient stay. Patients with ARF and an altered fluid status, either dehydration or fluid overload, should be admitted. Infants with ARF should be admitted, as the likelihood of obstructive disease is high. Finally, patients with progressive renal failure and metabolic or hematologic abnormalities – such as severe anemia, acidosis, hyperkalemia, or hypocalcemia – need admission to correct these abnormalities.

Hypertension is another frequent indication for admission and may require admission to the intensive care unit (ICU) if symptomatic. ICU admission is also warranted for symptomatic electrolyte abnormalities or if urgent dialysis is needed.

EXTENDED IN-HOSPITAL MANAGEMENT

In order to avoid fluid overload, attention to fluid management is important in the extended care of the patient admitted with renal failure. Insensible losses as well as urinary and gastrointestinal losses should be taken into careful consideration. A patient may be kept euvolemic by replacing insensible losses and also by replacing output. Fluid status should be assessed daily by utilizing laboratory data and performing a clinical exam.

In our initial patient case study, fluid overload is suggested by edema. Clinicians are often quick to think of using diuretics in renal patients with fluid overload, and this can be helpful, especially in the face of pulmonary edema or congestive heart disease. Diuretics can also do harm, as they may lower intravascular volume but have little effect on total body water in patients with third spacing from nephrotic syndrome or capillary leak. The treatment of hypertension that may stem from fluid overload or intrinsic renal pathology is discussed in Chapter 18.

Potassium is always of concern in the patient with poor renal function. IV fluids should contain little or no potassium. Serum bicarbonate is often altered in patients with renal failure because the ability to regulate acid–base excretion is diminished. Remember that potassium and $H+$ shift in opposite directions across the cell. Hyperkalemia may be correctable by simply correcting the acidosis; acidosis is correctable with IV or oral bicarbonate in most cases. Hypocalcemia is corrected with oral or IV doses of calcium, although IV calcium is not recommended unless central IV access is available.

When medical management fails to control fluid overload, electrolyte abnormalities, or uremia, dialysis should be considered. In children, three modalities for acute dialysis exist:

- Hemodialysis allows for rapid fluid and electrolyte removal across a filter membrane but requires a stable patient with adequate BP and heart function. In very small children, this is problematic from an access standpoint, and many small children are too sick to tolerate this procedure well.
- An alternative is continuous venovenous hemofiltration (CVVH). This form of dialysis also calls for central access and a filter for removal of

wastes from the blood, but it requires less cardiovascular stability, as the blood-flow and fluid-removal rates are slower and less demanding on the sick patient. The continuous nature of this procedure for fluid removal allows for better nutrition as well as the administration of blood products and medications, all of which contribute to a positive fluid balance in patients with ARF.

• Finally, peritoneal dialysis (PD) is also a good option, especially in the very small child or infant in whom central access may be difficult. It does require surgical intervention to place an intraperitoneal catheter. PD relies on the exchange of waste products and fluid across the peritoneal membrane. It is not a good option for ill children with significant pulmonary disease or intra-abdominal pathology.

The patient in the initial case study was admitted for BP control. His C3 was depressed at 19, his C4 was normal at 16, and his antistreptolysin-O (ASO) titer was elevated at 1,024. A diagnosis of poststreptococcal glomerulonephritis was made. A low-salt diet was prescribed in order to avoid worsening of the edema. His levels of BUN and Cr remained stable, and once his BP was controlled, he was ready for discharge and outpatient care.

DISPOSITION
Discharge Goals

Prior to discharge, renal function should be stable or improving. Electrolyte and fluid status should be well managed by medications and diet. Hypertension must be resolved or controlled by medications. This is especially true in young children and infants, for whom outpatient monitoring is difficult owing to the need for small cuff sizes and automated machines. Renal biopsy, if needed, should be completed or scheduled on an outpatient basis. Treatment of the primary disease should be started if immunosuppressive medications are needed and then continued on an outpatient basis.

OUTPATIENT CARE

Outpatient follow-up includes clinic visits, outpatient labs, and, if needed, BP monitoring. Our case patient was seen in the office 1 week later for the evaluation of renal function and edema. His gross hematuria cleared in 7 days with concurrent improvement in hypertension and renal function. In patients with poststreptococcal glomerulonephritis, proteinuria usually clears within 2 months and the C3 returns to normal by 3 months from presentation. Microscopic hematuria may be present for months following resolution of this disease.

WHAT YOU NEED TO REMEMBER

- ARF is defined by a rapid decline in glomerular function, resulting in a decreased ability to eliminate waste products as well as to regulate fluid, electrolyte, and acid–base balance.
- Hypertension, gross hematuria, and/or edema may be the only objective findings suggesting kidney disease. Symptoms are often vague; a high index of suspicion is needed.
- The clinician should pay close attention to the patient's hydration status in his or her history and physical in order to calculate fluid needs accurately.
- A urinalysis is a noninvasive and useful screening tool for kidney disease.
- A kidney/bladder ultrasound is the most useful first imaging study in the patient with ARF.
- Worrisome findings in kidney disease include associated renal insufficiency, proteinuria with hypoalbuminemia, and hypertension.

SUGGESTED READINGS

Andrioli SP. Acute renal failure. *Curr Opin Pediatr* 2002;14(2):183–188.

Andrioli SP. Clinical evaluation and management (acute renal failure). In Avner ED, Harmon WE, Niaudet P, eds. *Pediatric Nephrology*, 5th ed. Philadelphia: Lippincott Williams & Wilkins; 2004:1233–1251.

Barletta G-M, Bunchman T. Acute renal failure in children and infants. *Curr Opin Crit Care* 2004;10(6):499–504.

Benfield MR, Bunchman TE. Management of acute renal failure. In Avner ED, Harmon WE, Niaudet P, eds. *Pediatric Nephrology*, 5th ed. Philadelphia: Lippincott Williams & Wilkins; 2004:1253–1266.

Williams DM, Sreedhar SS, Mickell JJ, Chan JC. Acute kidney failure: a pediatric experience over 20 years. *Arch Pediatr Adolesc Med* 2002;156(9):893–900.

Anemia

DAVID KOTZBAUER

PATIENT ENCOUNTER

A 4-year-old African American male presents to the ER with a 4-day history of fever up to 38.9°C (102°F), fatigue, and a sore throat. His mother has also noticed that his urine has been dark in color. He denies any headache, diarrhea, vomiting, dark stools, shortness of breath, or dysuria. His past medical history is significant only for jaundice in the newborn period; it is otherwise unremarkable. His mother has been giving him acetaminophen for fever but no other medications. On examination, his temperature is 39°C (102.2°F), heart rate 132, blood pressure 110/70 mm Hg, and respiratory rate 34. His height and weight are at the 50th percentile for age. The sclerae are icteric and the mucous membranes pale. His heart exam reveals a regular rate and rhythm with a II/VI vibratory systolic ejection murmur at the lower left sternal border. There is no hepatomegaly or splenomegaly. The extremities have good peripheral pulses but there is pallor at the nail beds.

OVERVIEW

Definition

Anemia is present when a patient's hemoglobin and/or hematocrit is ≥ 2 standard deviations below the normal level for age. The lower limits of normal (LLN) for hemoglobin and hematocrit vary with age, as do the normal red blood cell indices. Infants reach a physiologic nadir at age 2 months, and the LLN for hemoglobin at this age is 9 g/dL. The mean corpuscular volume (MCV) declines from birth, when the LLN for the MCV is 98 fL, to age 12 months, when the LLN for the MCV is 70 fL. After 1 year of age, the LLN for the MCV is 70 + the patient's age in years. Patients considered to have mild anemia are just slightly below the LLN for their age. Moderate anemia is present when the hemoglobin is 6 to 8 g/dL; severe anemia is present at a hemoglobin level <6 g/dL.

Pathophysiology

Anemia results from blood loss, a decreased production of red blood cells (RBCs), an increased destruction of RBCs, or splenic sequestration. In the absence of traumatic injury, blood loss in children is almost always from the GI tract and rarely from the nasopharynx (as in patients with coagulopathies), lungs (as in pulmonary hemosiderosis), or the urinary tract (as in renal tumors or cystic disease). Blood cells are produced primarily in the bone marrow. This process requires a normal marrow environment with sufficient growth factors such as erythropoietin, cofactors such as folate and vitamin B12, and iron. Destruction of RBCs can be from intrinsic abnormalities of the RBC, such as hemoglobin and membrane abnormalities, or from antibody-mediated destruction or microangiopathy.

Epidemiology

Abnormalities of RBC hemoglobin, membranes, and enzymes are more common in certain ethnicities. Thalassemias are most common in African Americans, southeast Asians, and people of Mediterranean descent. Glucose-6-phosphate dehydrogenase (G6PD) deficiency is most common in African Americans and Asians. Membrane defects, such as spherocytosis, are more common in people of northern European descent. Iron deficiency is rare in the first few months of life but more common in toddlers, who no longer receive iron-fortified formula and may be picky eaters. Iron deficiency can also occur in children with chronic GI blood loss, as from inflammatory bowel disease or Meckel's diverticulum. People who are strict vegans are at risk for B12 deficiency. The rare infant who is fed goat's milk exclusively is at risk for folate deficiency.

Etiology

In considering a patient's differential diagnosis, it is extremely helpful to first classify the anemia as microcytic, normocytic, or macrocytic (Table 2-1).

The most common causes of microcytic anemia are iron deficiency and thalassemia trait or disease; these two conditions can usually be distinguished by the red cell indices. Iron deficiency anemia presents with a low MCV together with a high red blood cell (RBC) distribution width (RDW) and a low RBC count. Thalassemia trait or disease, however, presents with a low MCV together with a normal RDW and a high RBC count. If available, the hemoglobin electrophoresis at birth is very helpful. Bart's hemoglobin is present on the newborn electrophoresis in patients with alpha thalassemia trait or disease, whereas hemoglobins F and A2 are elevated in beta thalassemia trait or disease.

Normocytic anemias are common, especially with acute or chronic infection. These anemias, which are likely due to bone marrow suppression from inflammation and decreased production of erythropoietin, are diagnoses of exclusion. The physical exam is important to rule out splenomegaly and sequestration.

Macrocytic anemias are less common in children. Vitamin B12 and folate deficiencies cause macrocytic anemia with a high lactate dehydrogenase (LDH), hypersegmented neutrophils on the peripheral blood smear, and megaloblasts in the bone marrow. These deficiencies can sometimes result

TABLE 2-1
Differential Diagnosis of Anemia

Microcytic Anemia	Normocytic Anemia	Macrocytic Anemia
• Iron deficiency • Thalassemia disease or trait • Anemia of chronic disease – kidney failure, inflammatory bowel disease, juvenile idiopathic arthritis • Hemoglobin E • Sideroblastic anemia – congenital or acquired (lead poisoning, alcohol, isoniazid)	• Acute blood loss • Marrow infiltration (leukemia, neuroblastoma) • Splenic sequestration • Anemia of chronic disease (can also be microcytic) • RBC enzyme defects (G6PD deficiency, pyruvate kinase deficiency) • RBC membrane defects (hereditary spherocytosis, elliptocytosis) • Autoimmune hemolytic anemia • Microangiopathic hemolysis (DIC, HUS, TTP) • Intraerythrocytic infections (malaria, babesiosis, bartonellosis) • TEC • Anemia of any acute infection • Wilson's disease	• B12 deficiency • Folate deficiency • Diamond–Blackfan anemia or other congenital bone marrow failure • Hypothyroidism • Liver disease • Hereditary orotic aciduria • Congenital dyserythropoietic anemias

DIC, disseminated intravascular coagulation; G6PD, glucose-6-phosphate dehydrogenase; HUS, hemolytic uremic syndrome; RBC, red blood cell; TEC, transient erythroblastopenia of childhood; TTP, thrombotic thrombocytopenic purpura.

in pancytopenia and may be confused with acute leukemias because of the megaloblastic changes in the marrow. Congenital aplastic anemias, such as Diamond–Blackfan anemia, usually present in the first year of life and are typically macrocytic.

The history and physical exam can be very helpful in evaluating patients for the hemolytic anemias. Jaundice in the newborn period, episodes of splenic enlargement, and a family history of splenectomies and cholecystectomies can be present in patients with membrane defects, which are autosomal dominant. Antibody-mediated hemolytic anemias can be idiopathic but are sometimes associated with autoimmune disorders such as lupus, mycoplasmal infection, and Epstein–Barr virus (EBV) infection. G6PD is a very common enzyme deficiency and is X-linked. Patients with this disorder are typically male and have episodic anemia with hemolysis and dark urine. These episodes are precipitated by any oxidative stress, such as infection or medications. The most common medications are sulfa drugs, nitrofurantoin, dapsone, and antimalarials. In addition, numerous hemoglobinopathies can result in chronic hemolytic anemia.

The most important disorders to exclude in a sick child with anemia are the microangiopathies. Disseminated intravascular coagulation (DIC) is most commonly due to septicemia. Hemolytic uremic syndrome (HUS) often results from gastroenteritis due to *Escherichia coli* 0157:H7 or from pneumococcal sepsis/meningitis. These disorders cause inflammation of the small blood vessels and hemolysis due to shearing of RBCs. Intravascular hemolysis with dark-colored urine but no RBCs on microscopic urinalysis often occurs. Of note, intravascular hemolysis can also result from malaria, babesiosis, G6PD deficiency, and IgM-mediated autoimmune hemolytic anemia (AIHA).

ACUTE MANAGEMENT AND WORKUP

The acute management and workup should first focus on the airway, breathing, and circulation (the ABCs) and then on blood analysis.

The First 15 Minutes

The ABCs should first be assessed. IV access and normal saline boluses may be needed if the patient has signs of hypovolemia or hypotension. If a history of traumatic injury or GI blood loss is found in a severely anemic patient, a surgical consult should immediately be obtained to stop the blood loss.

The First Few Hours

A complete blood count (CBC) with differential and RBC morphology, reticulocyte count, complete metabolic panel, urinalysis, stool guaiac, and type and cross match for RBC transfusion should be obtained. In patients with severe blood loss who cannot wait hours for a cross match, type O-negative packed RBCs can be transfused. In sick patients with a history of fever, a DIC panel [prothrombin time (PT), partial thromboplastin time (PTT), fibrinogen, and D-dimer] and blood cultures should be obtained. If the patient has recently traveled to equatorial areas, order a thick smear of the blood to look for malaria. Consider lumbar puncture and empiric treatment with IV antibiotics in patients who appear septic, have signs of poor peripheral perfusion, an altered mental status, or a petechial rash.

History

Parents should be questioned about the onset of symptoms and whether symptoms have been present for just a few days or have been more chronic. Ask "Has there been trauma, fever, jaundice, dark-colored stools, dark urine, abdominal pain, epistaxis, cough, or shortness of breath?" "Has the patient ever been anemic before?" "Have you been told that results of the hemoglobin electrophoresis on newborn screening were abnormal?" "Has there been recent travel that would expose the patient to malaria or other infections?" "Have you been exposed to undercooked beef, ticks, mosquitoes, or other animals?" "Are you vegans or do you have any unique dietary habits?" "Is there a family history of anemia, bleeding disorders, jaundice, splenectomy, or cholecystectomy?"

Physical Examination

The patient's head and neck should be examined, especially for scleral icterus, signs of blood in the nose or oropharynx, the color of the mucous membranes (i.e., blood-tinged or pale), nuchal rigidity, or lymphadenopathy. The chest exam might reveal a hyperactive precordium, tachycardia, or systolic ejection murmurs. The abdomen should be assessed for tenderness, distention, and hepatosplenomegaly. Extremities and skin should be carefully examined for color and evidence of petechiae or other rash. Nail beds in particular should be assessed for color and splinter hemorrhages. A thorough neurologic exam should also be performed.

Labs and Tests to Consider

The results of initial laboratory testing are critical for diagnosis and the remainder of the diagnostic evaluation.

Key Diagnostic Labs and Tests

The results of the lab tests mentioned earlier (i.e., blood tests and cultures) should be obtained immediately. Assess all cell lines and their morphology on peripheral blood smear. A low WBC count or very high WBC count with blasts could indicate leukemia. Thrombocytopenia together with anemia could indicate marrow dysfunction from leukemia or microangiopathy. Knowing the reticulocyte count is also helpful because a low count is a strong indicator of marrow dysfunction. A high reticulocyte count together with unconjugated hyperbilirubinemia is characteristic of the hemolytic anemias. The RBC morphology can also provide excellent clues to diagnosis. Fragments of RBCs, such as schistocytes, are typical with hemolytic uremic syndrome (HUS) and disseminated intravascular coagulation (DIC). Target cells are most commonly found with hemoglobinopathies such as thalassemia. Spherocytes or elliptocytes are found with membrane defects. Spherocytes and sometimes Rouleaux formation (the clumping of RBCs) can be seen with autoimmune hemolytic anemia. Bite cells are often evident with G6PD deficiency. These dysmorphologies, together with RBC indices, can guide the decision to order other tests, such as a G6PD level, direct Coombs test, osmotic fragility, and hemoglobin electrophoresis. If multiple cell lines are abnormal on the CBC, strongly consider hematology consultation for bone marrow aspirate and biopsy.

The Mentzer index can be used to help differentiate iron deficiency anemia from beta thalassemia. This index is calculated by dividing the mean corpuscular volume by the RBC count. A Mentzer index <13 is more likely with thalassemia, whereas an index >14 may be seen in iron deficiency anemia.

The patient in this chapter's case study was found to have a WBC of 12,000/mm^3 with a normal differential, Hb of 6.5 g/dL, and platelet count of 225,000/mm^3. His reticulocyte count was 20%, and MCV was 60 fL with an RDW of 14.5. The morphology showed target cells and bite cells, which is suspicious for hemoglobinopathy and G6PD deficiency. The urine dipstick showed blood but microscopic urinalysis showed no RBCs, likely the result of hemoglobinuria from intravascular hemolysis.

Imaging

Computed tomography of the chest, abdomen, and pelvis may be needed in trauma patients. Imaging of the abdomen may be considered in patients with hepatomegaly or splenomegaly in order to rule out other abdominal masses, such as neuroblastoma or lymphoma. Patients with hematuria should have imaging of the kidneys and bladder to evaluate for Wilms' tumor or cystic kidney disease.

Treatment

Assessment of the patient's hemodynamic status is the most important first step. IV access, cardiorespiratory monitoring, and pulse oximetry should be obtained. Normal saline boluses should be administered initially. For the critically ill patient with severe anemia resulting from trauma or DIC, O-negative packed RBCs can be transfused if necessary. If the patient has severe anemia but appears stable, a type and cross match can be performed. Many clinicians may even choose to observe a patient with a hemoglobin level of 5 to 6 if the patient appears stable and there is no evidence of rapid blood loss. In these cases, serial CBCs may have to be checked every 8 to 12 hours while other testing is performed and treatments are given. When packed RBC transfusions are indicated, a volume of 10 to 15 mL/kg, up to 1 to 2 units, is typically used.

> ### CLINICAL PEARL
>
> *If the etiology of the anemia is unclear, consider saving a blood sample for further analysis prior to the transfusion.*

Admission Criteria and Level-of-Care Criteria

Patients with severe anemia (hemoglobin ≤6 g/dL) should likely be admitted and have an immediate workup performed. Patients with moderate anemia (hemoglobin of 7 to 9 g/dL) may be followed closely on an outpatient basis if no signs of severe illness, rapid blood loss, or rapid hemolysis are found. Mildly anemic patients (hemoglobin of 9 g/dL or higher) can be worked up as outpatients.

Regarding our case study, the patient's pediatrician was contacted and revealed that the newborn electrophoresis had 4% Bart's hemoglobin and that the baseline hemoglobin level was 9.5, consistent with alpha thalassemia trait. The G6PD level was checked and found to be low. Thus, this patient had two causes for his severe anemia. He recovered with just supportive care, and his mother was warned about possible triggers for hemolysis in G6PD deficiency.

EXTENDED IN-HOSPITAL MANAGEMENT

The specific cause of the anemia must be addressed. Patients with bacterial sepsis or malaria must be treated with appropriate antibiotics and supportive care. Causes of GI blood loss must be addressed surgically or perhaps endoscopically, as in a patient with esophageal varices or an intestinal polyp. Chronic diseases such as inflammatory bowel disease may call for steroid treatment or other immunosuppressants. Steroid therapy is also indicated for treatment of IgG-mediated autoimmune hemolytic anemia (AIHA). IgM-mediated AIHA may respond to steroids but is more likely to improve with plasmapheresis. Induction chemotherapy would be necessary for marrow-infiltrative disorders, such as leukemia or neuroblastoma. Treatment of HUS is supportive, with dialysis for patients who develop renal failure. Splenectomy is sometimes a last resort in sickle cell patients with sequestration crisis.

Iron deficiency anemia can be treated with oral ferrous sulfate (4 to 6 mg/kg of elemental iron per day divided three times daily for approximately 3 months). B12 and folate deficits can be replaced more quickly. Patients with G6PD deficiency need education and must be instructed to avoid oxidant medications. Parents should also be warned that hemolysis can occur with any febrile illness. For patients with RBC membrane defects, emergent splenectomy is rarely indicated but can be considered on an outpatient basis if the patient has a chronically large spleen and significant anemia. Cholecystectomy is often performed simultaneously to avoid the risk of future gallstones.

DISPOSITION

Discharge Goals

The cause of the anemia must be determined and the anemia must be stable or improving.

Outpatient Care

Chronic illnesses must be addressed by appropriate specialists. Syndromes of bone marrow failure or severe thalassemia often necessitate chronic RBC transfusions. Children with renal failure benefit from epoetin alfa (Epogen) therapy, which can help to limit the number of transfusions they will require. Patients with iron deficiency anemia should be checked 2 to 4 weeks after initiation of oral iron therapy; some improvement should be found in the anemia at this time. After 3 months of iron therapy, the anemia should be resolved. A multivitamin with iron can then be helpful in preventing the anemia from recurring. Children with thalassemia trait require no therapy other than genetic counseling. Patients with enlarged spleens should avoid contact sports if possible or wear protective devices.

 WHAT YOU NEED TO REMEMBER

- In patients with severe anemia, it is important to rule out blood loss, which most commonly occurs from the GI tract.
- The reticulocyte count is an excellent indicator of bone marrow function and should be checked in any patient with significant anemia.
- The RBC indices and morphology are always helpful.
- In children with microcytic anemias, the newborn hemoglobin electrophoresis is needed to rule out thalassemia disease or trait.

SUGGESTED READINGS

Hudson WR, Gussack CS. Otolaryngology: head and neck surgery. In: Davis JE, ed. *Major Ambulatory Surgery*, 2nd ed. Baltimore: Williams & Wilkins, 1986.

Kaplan NM. *Clinical Hypertension*, 4th ed. Baltimore: Williams & Wilkins, 1986:23.

Lee GR, Foerster J, Lukens J, et al, eds. *Wintrobe's Clinical Hematology*, 10th ed. Baltimore: Williams & Wilkins, 1999.

Nathan DG, Orkin SH, Ginsburg D, Look AT, eds. *Nathan and Oski's Hematology of Infancy and Childhood*, 6th ed. Philadelphia: Saunders, 2003.

Richardson M. Microcytic anemia. *Pediatr Rev* 2007;28:5–14.

Segel GB, Anemia. *Pediatr Rev*1988;10(3):77–88.

Apparent Life-Threatening Event

JACK PERCELAY

THE PATIENT ENCOUNTER

An 8-week-old boy is brought to the pediatrician's office because he "turned blue and stopped breathing." The event occurred while the infant was held in his mother's arms shortly after feeding. The infant spit up a small amount, gagged, and then turned blue around the lips. Afterwards, the infant appeared not to breathe for an undetermined period of time. No change in tone was noted, but his mother was too frightened to notice. She stimulated the infant, who recovered "in about a minute." He was delivered at term and his medical history is unremarkable. When seen in your office 75 minutes after the event, the patient is well appearing with a normal exam, but the family is very frightened and you refer the infant to the ER for further evaluation.

OVERVIEW

Definition

In 1986, a National Institutes of Health expert panel defined an apparent life-threatening event (ALTE) as *"an episode that is frightening to the observer and that is characterized by some combination of apnea* (central or occasionally obstructive), *color change* (usually cyanotic or pallid but occasionally erythematous or plethoric), *marked changed in muscle tone* (usually marked limpness), *choking or gagging."*[1] In this sense, ALTE is not a single disease entity but rather a presentation of symptoms that may be the result of a myriad of causes.

Sudden infant death syndrome (SIDS) is the sudden death of a child younger than 1 year of age that remains unexplained after a thorough investigation. The incidence of SIDS has decreased by more than half since the "Back to Sleep" campaign promoted placing babies on their backs for sleep. It is important to note that ALTEs are generally not precursors to SIDS.

Pathophysiology

Apnea may be central (no respiratory efforts), obstructive (respiratory efforts, but no exchange of air), or mixed. Infants have a relatively immature regulation of respiratory control, and brief pauses in breathing of up to

20 seconds are considered normal. This sinusoidal pattern of respiratory effort with brief pauses is called "periodic breathing" and is more pronounced in younger infants. Events lasting longer than 20 seconds and/or those associated with physiologic compromise are considered pathologic. *Color changes* result from changes in blood flow and/or oxygen saturation and are mediated by both cardiorespiratory and autonomic events. *Cyanosis* that is peripheral (acrocyanosis) or perioral is less significant than central cyanosis, which is best seen in the tongue or lips. Cyanosis is a result of oxygen desaturation. *Plethora* results from increased blood flow or vasodilatation, usually venous, and may be difficult to distinguish from cyanosis. *Pallor* can result from local vasoconstriction or from generalized vasodilatation as in vasovagal syncope. *Loss of tone* reflects some form of altered neurologic control and may result from a variety of insults to the nervous system, including, hypoxia, metabolic derangement (hypoglycemia), toxins, and seizures.

Epidemiology

The multitude of causes for ALTEs and the subjective nature of events that are "frightening to an observer" make it difficult to provide accurate information about the incidence and prevalence of ALTE. Lack of a uniform diagnostic code for ALTEs further complicates data collection. Estimates are that 1% of infants may have an ALTE. The most common age range for ALTEs is 6 to 10 weeks. Not all of these events require hospitalization or ER evaluation. Many can be managed in the pediatrician's office.

Etiology

ALTE, like failure to thrive, can be the presenting complaint for disorders in many different organ systems as well as a result of child abuse. An understanding of the wide range of potential causes allows the pediatrician to conduct a focused yet comprehensive history, physical, and laboratory evaluation of the child presenting with ALTE. The differential diagnosis for ALTE includes viral respiratory infections, such as respiratory syncytial virus, as well as serious bacterial infections, gastroesophageal reflux, periodic breathing of the newborn, cardiac arrhythmias, and seizures.

ACUTE MANAGEMENT AND WORKUP

The acute management and workup involves distinguishing patients who require immediate intervention from those who are now well appearing following an event that occurred several hours previously. Patients who require immediate attention may either present in extremis and require immediate stabilization and intervention or may present without physiologic compromise but with minimal residua that warrant immediate laboratory evaluation to assess the severity of the resolved or resolving event.

The First 15 Minutes

The ABCDs (airway, breathing, circulation, plus dextrose) of emergency resuscitation are appropriate for the acutely ill child. The acute management of seizures, respiratory arrest, sepsis, trauma, hypoglycemia, toxins, and arrhythmias is discussed elsewhere in this text. Therapy is directed to the underlying signs, symptoms, and likely causes. Interventions are made, responses are noted, the patient is reassessed, and further therapy is pursued. As a general rule, once an etiology is determined, further management and the ultimate prognosis are determined by the specific diagnosis. The remainder of this chapter will concentrate on children in whom no obvious etiology is identified for their presenting symptom(s).

For the child who presents soon after the event, who is afebrile with normal oxygen saturation and does not appear acutely ill but may be slightly sleepy with moderately decreased tone but no or minimal cardiorespiratory compromise (i.e., the typical ER patient), some immediate measures are helpful outside of the ABCs prior to gathering a thorough history and performing a physical evaluation. **First, order screening laboratory studies.** Studies of immediate value are a measure of serum glucose (by bedside glucometer) for immediate recognition of hypoglycemia and a basic metabolic panel and/or (venous) blood gas to look for evidence of an anion-gap metabolic acidosis or CO_2 retention. These laboratory abnormalities imply a more significant underlying event that warrants a more comprehensive evaluation. **Second, immediately place the child on a cardiorespiratory and oxygen saturation monitor.** This will help capture any repeat events that occur while the child is observed in the ER.

The First Few Hours

In the well-appearing child who presents hours after the event, no immediate interventions are necessary; therefore, the physician can conduct a thorough history and physical that will guide further diagnostic and therapeutic measures.

History

The art of obtaining a history in a child with an ALTE lies in accurately recreating the details of an extraordinarily stressful event, usually brief and unanticipated, from a layperson. Question one individual at a time to get each observer's perspective. Determine the observer's ability to report events reliably by asking about the lighting in the room, the observer's position relative to the infant, and any clothes or blankets that may have covered the infant. Use a calm, slow, stepwise approach to reproduce the events. Reports of time intervals are notoriously unreliable in these situations. Ask carefully about parts of the baby's body that changed color. To identify changes in tone, distinguish between a baby who is still and one who is limp. If parents report no respiratory efforts, try to recreate the time period during which the parents monitored the child before intervening and determine whether an assessment of chest movement was made.

> ## CLINICAL PEARL
>
> *Historical clues that suggest specific diagnoses include frequent emesis of feeds (gastroesophageal reflux), fever (bacterial or viral infection), diaphoresis or rapid heart rate (arrhythmia), and stiffening of body (reflux or seizure).*

Physical Examination

A low oxygen saturation is always concerning in an infant with an ALTE. Fever will drive therapy in infants younger than 2 to 3 months of age. Again, cardiorespiratory monitoring is key and should be sustained for the majority of most ER visits to reassure both physician and parent that the child's underlying cardiorespiratory status is normal. The physical exam of the child with an ALTE entails a comprehensive search for potential etiologies.

Labs and Tests to Consider

Based on the history and physical, one can pursue a judicious laboratory evaluation targeted to the potential causes suggested by the patient's presentation. For children who present well-appearing hours after an event, no laboratory studies may be necessary if no likely etiologies are suggested by the history and physical. Clearly, when a specific etiology is identified, testing should proceed related to that specific diagnosis, with the severity of the ALTE symptoms influencing the aggressiveness and immediacy of the workup.

The most common diagnostic dilemma relates to the child in whom an etiology is not obvious. Without a nationally published ALTE guideline, pediatricians divide into two camps of ALTE management. One group aggressively looks for an underlying etiology by pursuing any or all of the following studies: electroencephalogram, echocardiogram, barium swallow, computed tomography of the head, urine organic acids, full septic workup, pneumogram (with or without pH probe). The other school of thought promotes watchful waiting. Students will do well do understand the rationale for these different tests and to question advocates on both sides about their evidence rather than their anecdotes.

Certainly there is uniform agreement that severe and/or repeat episodes (i.e., complicated ALTEs) warrant a more complete workup; for an isolated "uncomplicated" event, however, this is probably not necessary. Under this categorization scheme, an uncomplicated event is isolated; brief (<20 seconds); not associated with any physiologic compromise, physical exam abnormalities, or abnormal (screening) labs; and requires no or minimal stimulation. A complicated ALTE is repeated; prolonged (>20 seconds); associated with physiologic compromise, physical exam abnormalities, and/or abnormal screening labs; and requires moderate or vigorous stimulation.

Treatment

The treatment of ALTE depends on the underlying diagnosis. When a specific underlying etiology is identified, specific therapy is instituted. Controversies regarding the use of home monitors as a treatment modality are discussed in the "Disposition" section.

Another area of controversy in the management of ALTEs relates to the role that gastroesophageal reflux plays in inducing apnea. Gastroesophageal reflux (see Chapter 16) is a normal phenomenon in infants but is pathologic when it results in failure to thrive, esophagitis, or apnea. In patients with clinically obvious reflux and apneic or cyanotic episodes, controversy exists as to whether pH probe testing will alter the proposed therapy. Given grossly evident reflux, many would institute routine therapies such as thickening of feeds, positioning, H2 blockers, and promotility agents without performing pH probe testing.

Admission Criteria and Level-of-Care Criteria

Not surprisingly, admission criteria vary depending on the severity of the presentation and the biases of the treating physician. Patients with complicated ALTEs that are recurrent or require significant intervention (bagging, vigorous stimulation) will need to be admitted to the intensive care unit, as will children who present with ALTE who turn out to have sepsis, head trauma, or other significant alterations in their physiology. In contrast, a child with a simple ALTE may be sent home from the ER after a complete history, physical, and judicious laboratory testing. It is often particularly reassuring to parents to have their child monitored for a 3- to 4-hour period in the ER that includes at least one feeding session before the family is sent home. Other parents will require an overnight stay to be reassured. Plans must be individualized based on the child's diagnosis or lack thereof and etiology in conjunction with the parents' comfort level, medical sophistication, and access to care as well as the preference of the primary care pediatrician.

The case patient presented to the ER, where a basic metabolic panel revealed normal serum electrolytes. Although he appeared well, his parents were very anxious about the event, and he was, therefore, admitted to an observation unit. He was placed on a cardiorespiratory monitor as well as pulse oximetry. He had no further concerning episodes, although he did spit up several times after feeds. His parents were instructed about reflux precautions, and he was discharged the following day.

EXTENDED IN-HOSPITAL MANAGEMENT

Prolonged hospital stays are generally reserved for patients in whom an underlying etiology is revealed that requires ongoing therapy or for those without a working diagnosis who require continued monitoring for repeat events.

A reasonable approach that can be helpful with uncomplicated ALTEs is to take advantage of the reassurance that comes from monitoring a child in the hospital overnight without automatically initiating a series of expensive and invasive tests. In these instances, if the infant does well with a 23-hour stay, the family can be sent home the next day with some additional instruction and teaching. If a 23-hour stay uncovers a worrisome respiratory pattern, significant GE reflux, or a suspicion of seizures, the hospital stay can be extended an additional 24 hours and a more detailed and targeted evaluation can be initiated at that time. Overall, this seems to provide appropriate reassurance and instruction to most families, and the additional hospital day required for those patients who do have abnormalities noted during their initial observation stay is balanced by the number of children who can be sent home, having been spared the iatrogenic, emotional, and financial consequences of unnecessary testing.

DISPOSITION

Discharge Goals

Patients are ready for discharge once appropriate diagnostic testing is completed, specific therapies are instituted when indicated, the patient's condition is stable (typically event-free for a 12- to 24-hour time period in uncomplicated ALTEs), and parents are educated about both infant cardiorespiratory resuscitation (CPR) and particular signs to watch for in their child. If home monitoring is planned, monitor training must be completed along with CPR training.

Outpatient Care

The most controversial therapies for ALTE involve the use of home monitors. The benefits of home monitoring for apnea of prematurity is increasingly questioned, as there is no evidence that home monitors protect fully against sudden infant death syndrome (SIDS). Home monitoring as a therapy in children with ALTEs of undetermined etiology is even less proven. Nonetheless, few parents, having just lived through a "near-death" experience with their infant, are prepared to forego the theoretical benefits of home monitoring and the comfort it initially provides when offered the option. Evidence-based or not, home monitoring does give parents reassurance. New monitors store data that can be downloaded to document the infant's status for the previous 30-day period and false alarms are frequent. In most instances, both the parents and the patient outgrow the monitor.

Some infants do have repeat episodes and also altered cardiorespiratory function. Their treatment requires expert pediatric pulmonary consultation, which is beyond the scope of this chapter. In either case, it is crucial that parents be appropriately instructed in infant CPR. Children rarely require rescue breaths and chest compressions, but the training empowers parents to remain calm when their child has a sputtering episode and turns blue. Thus, when a child has a brief respiratory pause, it gives parents the peace of mind to wait an additional 5 seconds and look for evidence of respiratory distress or cyanosis.

WHAT YOU NEED TO REMEMBER

- ALTE is a symptom complex that represents a variety of different disease presentations. It is not a diagnosis.
- A careful history and physical is the cornerstone of the management of ALTE. Laboratory testing is ancillary and is targeted toward concerns identified by the history and physical exam.
- For patients who present shortly after an episode, checking the serum glucose, electrolytes, and venous blood gas can help to identify a more significant episode.
- A period of monitoring in the ER or overnight in the hospital can help provide reassurance to a frightened family.
- Home monitors may reassure frightened parents, but they do not decrease the risk of SIDS.

REFERENCES

1. National Institutes of Health. Infantile apnea and home monitoring. NIH Consensus Statement 1986;6:1–10. Accessed November 8, 2008, at: http://consensus.nih.gov/1986/1986InfantApneaMonitoring058html.htm

SUGGESTED READINGS

Brand DA, Altman RL, Purtill K, et al. Yield of diagnostic testing in infants who have had an apparent life-threatening event. *Pediatrics* 2005;115:885–893.

Claudius I, Keens T. Do all infants with apparent life-threatening events need to be admitted? *Pediatrics* 2006;119:679–683.

DeWolfe CC, Chidekel AS. Apparent life-threatening event, infant apnea and pediatric obstructive sleep apnea syndrome. In Zaoutis LB, Chiang VW, eds. *Comprehensive Pediatric Hospital Medicine*. Philadelphia: Mosby, 2007.

Fu LY, Moon RY. Apparent life-threatening events and the role of home monitors. *Pediatr Rev* 2007;28:203–208.

Tieder JS, Cowan CA, Garrison MM, et al. Variation in inpatient resource utilization and management of apparent life-threatening events. *J Pediatr* 2008;152:629–635.

Appendicitis

KALPESH N. PATEL AND NAGHMA S. KHAN

THE PATIENT ENCOUNTER

A 9-year-old boy presents to the emergency department with abdominal pain in his lower right abdomen, which is worse when he walks and better when he lies still. He has not eaten much since yesterday and developed midabdominal pain yesterday evening. Overnight he had fever to 38.9°C (102°F) oral. He had two episodes of vomiting earlier today. He has no significant past medical history, family history, or allergies to any medications. Initial vital signs show a pulse of 122, respirations of 22, a temperature of 38.2°C (100.8°F) oral, blood pressure of 118/76 mm Hg, and a pain score of 6 out of 10. On physical exam, he has pain to his right lower quadrant (RLQ) on palpation with guarding.

OVERVIEW

Definition

Appendicitis refers to an obstruction of the appendiceal lumen that leads to inflammation of the appendix with subsequent bowel necrosis and perforation.

Pathophysiology

The anatomy of the appendix varies according to age and must be considered in the pathophysiology of appendicitis. The appendix arises from the cecum, which can vary in its position in the abdomen. In most children, the cecum resides in the right lower quadrant (RLQ) of the abdomen, but it may lie anywhere in the upper abdomen or even on the left side in children with congenital anomalies, such as intestinal malrotation. In the first year of life, the appendix is funnel-shaped, making obstruction less likely.

After the first year, the appendix assumes its tubular appearance. It begins as a thin-walled structure until it reaches maturity during adolescence. Concurrently, as the immune system develops, lymphoid follicles are interspersed in the colonic epithelium and reach their maximal size during adolescence. This lymphoid tissue may obstruct the appendix as it reacts to the inflammatory processes.

Last, the omentum is underdeveloped in young children and cannot contain the products of infection released after appendiceal perforation, leading to widespread dissemination in the abdominal cavity and more significant signs and symptoms of peritonitis compared with a self-contained abscess that develops in adolescents and adults.

Epidemiology

Appendicitis is the most common indication for emergent abdominal surgery in childhood. A delayed diagnosis is common, particularly in young children (up to 57% of cases <6 years of age). Perforation correlates strongly with delayed diagnosis.

Prevalence

Appendicitis is diagnosed in 1 of 8 children evaluated in urgent care centers for abdominal pain. Boys are more commonly affected than girls (lifetime risk of 9% and 7%, respectively).

Incidence

The incidence increases from an annual rate of 1 to 2 per 10,000 children between birth and 4 years of age to 19 to 28 per 10,000 children <14 years.

Etiology

When the appendix is obstructed, the patient develops poorly localized, colicky abdominal pain from stretching of the wall of the appendix. Sensory visceral nerve fibers cause referred abdominal pain in the periumbilical area. Within the appendix, bacterial overgrowth leads to breakdown of the mucosal barrier, causing fever, anorexia, nausea, and vomiting. Most infections are due to fecal flora, which include aerobic and anaerobic gram-negative rods. Invasion of these bacteria into the luminal wall leads to inflammation, ischemia, gangrene, and ultimately perforation of the appendiceal wall.

Once perforation occurs, there is classically a temporary relief from pain. However, as the inflammation progresses to perforation and peritonitis, the typical RLQ abdominal pain develops. Perforation is rare within the first 12 hours but is increasingly common thereafter, especially after 72 hours. Further progression leads to generalized peritonitis followed by sepsis, shock, and ultimately death if untreated.

This classic presentation of appendicitis is rare in pediatrics, especially with younger patients. Although rare in infancy, appendicitis nearly always presents with perforation because of the thin wall and an inherent delay in diagnosis in this nonverbal age group.

ACUTE MANAGEMENT AND WORKUP

Your initial goals are to ensure adequate pain control and hydration and to establish the correct diagnosis.

The First 15 Minutes

Pain should be addressed as soon as possible. Opioid analgesia is the preferred method, usually 0.1 to 0.2 mg/kg of morphine or the equivalent. The use of analgesics is proven not to mask the classic abdominal exam or to delay diagnosis, so there is no reason to delay pain control.

Appendicitis is a surgical disease and patients should not receive any liquids or food by mouth; instead, they should receive intravenous (IV) fluids. In most cases, these children have been anorexic and are at least mildly dehydrated, but advanced cases may show signs of shock. In either case, a fluid bolus of crystalloid, 20 mL/kg IV, is warranted. If the patient appears toxic or is in shock, rigorous IV hydration and early use of broad-spectrum antibiotics is warranted.

With a clinical presentation strongly suspicious for appendicitis, no further workup is required. Early involvement by a surgeon cannot be stressed enough, and labs and radiologic studies do not supersede the significance of clinical findings and history.

The First Few Hours

After initial fluid resuscitation has been given, the child should be hydrated with dextrose-containing IV fluids at a 1.5 maintenance rate. Repeat dosing of pain medication may also be required. If the presentation is not typical for appendicitis, supporting evidence can be elicited from laboratory and radiologic studies.

History

Symptoms vary with age from nonspecific vomiting, irritability, and fever in infants and young children to the more classic symptoms in adolescents.

CLINICAL PEARL

Classic features of appendicitis—such as fever, anorexia, nausea and vomiting, migration of abdominal pain from the periumbilical area to the RLQ, and rebound tenderness—are not consistently present in children with appendicitis.

Age-specific symptoms and signs are as follows:

- *Neonates (birth to 30 days.* Irritability, lethargy, abdominal distention, and vomiting.
- *Infants (<2 years of age).* Vomiting, pain, and fever.
- *Preschool (2 to 5 years of age).* Vomiting is the first symptom, followed by abdominal pain. Fever and anorexia also frequently occur. Children may have symptoms for at least 2 days prior to diagnosis.

- *School age (6 to 12 years of age).* Vomiting and abdominal pain occur but migration of pain may not. Fever, anorexia, and pain may also occur.
- *Adolescents (≥13 years of age).* Features are similar to those in adults, with anorexia, RLQ pain, and vomiting. Pain usually occurs before vomiting.

Physical Examination

The abdominal exam is key to the diagnosis of appendicitis. Examine the child in a position of comfort, as in the caretaker's lap, because this may assist in calming the child. It is also important to examine the abdomen before performing provocative maneuvers, such as looking at the ears, nose, or throat. Much like the history, many findings are age-specific:

- *Neonates (birth to 30 days).* Abdominal distention, a palpable abdominal mass, and abdominal wall cellulitis may be seen. Hypothermia, hypotension, and respiratory distress can also be present.
- *Infants (<2 years of age).* Fever and diffuse abdominal tenderness (often due to peritonitis) are common findings.
- *Preschool (2 to 5 years of age).* Fever and RLQ tenderness are noted.
- *School age (6 to 12 years of age).* Fever and RLQ tenderness are present. Involuntary guarding and rebound tenderness are seen with perforation.
- *Adolescents (≥13 years of age).* Features are similar to those in adults, showing the classic features of appendicitis.

Because diagnosis is often delayed in younger children, they typically appear sicker than older children. Peritoneal inflammation causes splinting; therefore, children prefer to lie still, in a position of comfort. The "jump test" is often employed to help identify these patients. This is performed by asking the child to jump in place several times. If pain is elicited, especially to the RLQ area, the diagnosis of appendicitis is likely. A rectal exam is not always warranted in children but may be useful in equivocal cases. When this is performed, pelvic tenderness on the right side is significant. Patients with a retrocecal appendix may have minimal abdominal tenderness to palpation but will have significant pain during the rectal examination.

The following signs may be noted on examination:

- *Rebound tenderness is* a reliable sign of peritoneal irritation when present, but testing in children is often unnecessary and painful because it is not present in up to 52% of cases.
- *Rovsing's sign* occurs when palpation of the left side of the abdomen elicits pain in the RLQ.
- The *obturator sign* indicates irritation to the obturator internus muscle. To elicit this sign, the patient lies supine with the right knee flexed. The examiner immobilizes the ankle and then rotates the hip externally and internally.
- The *psoas sign* indicates irritation to the iliopsoas group of hip flexors in the abdomen. To elicit this sign, the patient lies on his or her left side and the examiner passively extends the right hip.

Many of the classic physical exam maneuvers are difficult to elicit in young children and are often unreliable. In addition, their accuracy has not been well defined.

Labs and Tests to Consider

There are no laboratory tests that are specific for appendicitis, but laboratory and imaging studies may be helpful when the diagnosis of appendicitis is in question and other etiologies are being entertained.

Key Diagnostic Labs and Tests

An elevated white blood cell (WBC) count ($>10,000/mm^3$) and left shift may be seen with appendicitis. C-reactive protein (CRP) may be elevated, although CRP is less sensitive in patients presenting with symptoms for <12 hours. Urinalysis is performed to evaluate urinary conditions such as infection or nephrolithiasis. Up to 25% of patients with appendicitis may have pyuria, but bacteria are not typically present. A pregnancy test should be performed in postmenarchal females.

The following lab results were obtained in the case patient: the complete blood count (CBC) revealed elevated WBCs of $19,400/mm^3$ (6% band forms, 83% segmented neutrophils, 6% lymphocytes, and 5% monocytes). His hemoglobin was 14 and platelets were 227,000. His CRP was elevated at 2.3 mg/dL. Chemistry analysis revealed normal levels of electrolytes, blood urea nitrogen (BUN), creatinine, liver enzymes, amylase, and lipase. Urinalysis was normal.

Imaging

Common imaging includes plain abdominal x-rays, ultrasound, and computed tomography (CT) with contrast.

Plain Abdominal Films (Supine and Upright). The only definitive finding is an appendicolith (a radio-opaque fecal stone obstructing the appendix), which may be visible in the RLQ. Other findings may include a paucity of bowel gas in the RLQ, scoliosis away from the RLQ, and stacking of small bowel loops (Fig. 4-1). A negative abdominal film does not exclude appendicitis.

Ultrasound. In many pediatric centers, an abdominal ultrasound is performed routinely before an abdominal CT. The impetus for this was the recognition that children receive a high dose of ionizing radiation for their size compared with adults for abdominal and chest CTs. Positive findings on ultrasound include a noncompressible appendix with a wall thickness >2 mm and an overall appendiceal diameter of 6 mm. Free fluid and a thickened mesentery are frequently seen in the RLQ. A calcified fecalith may also be visible (Fig. 4-2). In order for appendicitis to be reliably excluded, a normal appendix must be visualized.

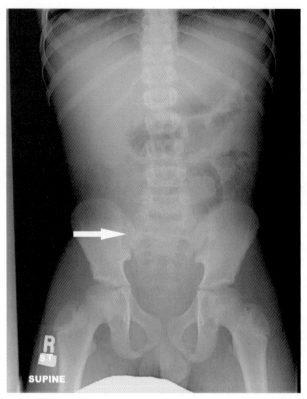

FIGURE 4-1: **Plain x-ray of the Abdomen.** An appendicolith is seen medial to the right iliac wing. Also note the paucity of bowel gas in the right lower quadrant and rectum and scoliosis away from the right lower quadrant.

CT with Contrast. Abdominal CT is the preferred imaging method in most institutions because it is less operator-dependent, more readily available, and more highly sensitive than other imaging modalities. Positive findings on CT may include an appendiceal wall thickness >2 mm, an appendicolith, concentric thickening of the appendiceal wall (target sign), phlegmon, abscess, free fluid, and thickening of the mesentery (fat stranding) (Fig. 4-3). To improve the accuracy of CT, a contrasted study is helpful. Although the preferred method of contrast administration is institution-dependent, most institutions recommend IV contrast. The use of GI contrast in children can be cumbersome and time consuming. In many instances, oral contrast is not tolerated because of nausea and vomiting. Similarly, rectal contrast may not be tolerated owing to diarrhea and discomfort with administration.

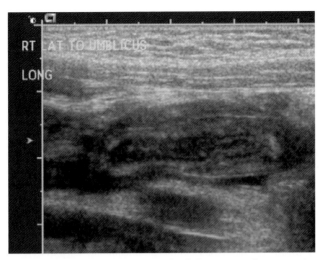

FIGURE 4-2: **Longitudinal Ultrasound of the Appendix.** Note the thickened appendiceal wall.

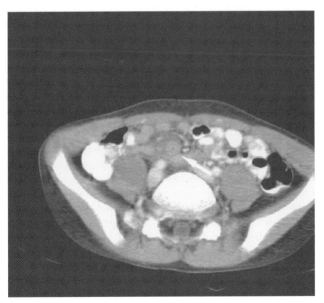

FIGURE 4-3: **CT of the Abdomen.** Note the target-shaped appendix.

Treatment

Remember that appendicitis is a surgical disease, so the goal of treatment is to provide IV fluid hydration, analgesia, antibiotic prophylaxis, and early surgery before gangrene and perforation of the appendix occur. Treatment is different for appendicitis before perforation (early appendicitis), perforated appendicitis, and appendiceal abscesses.

Early Appendicitis

The goal is to remove the appendix surgically prior to rupture and peritonitis. Preoperative care includes IV rehydration and pain control (typically with narcotic analgesics). Preoperative antibiotics help to reduce the incidence of wound infection and intra-abdominal abscess formation. Common choices are cefoxitin, cefotetan (second-generation cephalosporins), piperacillin/tazobactam (penicillin and beta-lactamase inhibitor), or a combination of gentamicin and either clindamycin or metronidazole. Traditionally ampicillin has been given to cover for *Enterococcus*, but this has fallen out of favor. Ideally antibiotics should be administered at least 30 to 60 minutes before the operative incision is made.

The classic method of surgical removal of the appendix is through an open appendectomy, but a laparoscopic approach is being used with greater frequency in uncomplicated cases. Children who receive laparoscopic surgeries tend to have shorter hospital stays and a lower risk of wound infection. During the operation, all purulent fluid should be removed and the base of the appendix should be ligated close to the cecum. The surgical specimen is always sent for pathology.

Postoperatively, IV narcotic analgesia is initiated immediately; this is replaced by oral agents when the child is drinking well. Oral fluids can be introduced as soon as the child is awake after surgery. Diet can be advanced to solid food as tolerated. Continued treatment with antibiotics is recommended if the appendix was gangrenous or perforated.

Appendicitis With Perforation

Once peritonitis has developed, there is no longer a need to rush to surgery. In these cases, prior to surgery, adequate fluid resuscitation, and correction of electrolyte and acid–base abnormalities is very important. Fluid resuscitation should continue until urine output is 1 to 2 mL/kg/hr as measured by a urethral catheter. In children with persistent vomiting, a nasogastric tube should be placed to low intermittent suction and the gastric contents should be replaced with normal saline in the IV fluids. Antibiotics should be started early. The choices are the same as for early appendicitis.

Limited data are available for the laparoscopic operative approach in cases of perforated appendicitis, but in experienced hands this has been successful. During the operation, a search for a fecalith should be made in the pelvis or periappendiceal area. The base of the appendix should be ligated close to the cecum. A drain should be placed if there is a well-formed abscess cavity.

Postoperatively, the use of IV antibiotics for a period of 7 days or longer is the common practice. Antibiotics are continued until the child is afebrile, has a normal CBC, and is tolerating a regular diet. CRP can also be followed serially until normal. Children who do not meet these criteria after 7 to 10 days should have imaging of the abdomen to look for an abdominal or pelvic abscess. Parenteral nutrition should be provided for children who are unable to eat after 1 week.

The case patient was given a bolus with normal saline of 20 mL/kg and a dose of cefoxitin in the ER. He was taken to the operating room by Pediatric Surgery, where he underwent a successful laparoscopic appendectomy. He was discharged home the following day.

Appendiceal Mass or Phlegmon

Patients who have an organized mass (usually children who present more than 5 to 7 days from the onset of illness) should be treated nonoperatively with parenteral antibiotics. A CT scan should be performed in all cases to identify large abscesses (>3 to 4 cm) that require image-guided percutaneous drainage. Children who do not have clinical improvement in 24 to 48 hours or who have continued fever, worsening abdominal tenderness, or increased abdominal mass size should be taken for surgical exploration. Otherwise an interval appendectomy may be performed in 6 to 12 weeks after treatment with IV antibiotics in the interim.

Admission Criteria and Level-of-Care Criteria

All patients with equivocal abdominal exams should be admitted for serial exams. Patients who have a concerning exam but normal laboratory or radiologic studies can be discharged home, with a recheck with their primary care physician in 8 to 12 hours to ensure lack of deterioration. All patients with appendicitis should be admitted to the hospital for IV antibiotics, pain management, and surgical removal or placement of a central venous catheter for long-term antibiotic administration. Most patients may be monitored on the general pediatric floor unless they experience shock or their clinical appearance has not improved after initial preoperative therapy. These children require early operative management.

EXTENDED IN-HOSPITAL MANAGEMENT

Hospital care should be extended for children who remain febrile or develop fever, are unable to tolerate their diet, or have a persistently abnormal CBC. Consider parenteral nutrition in these children and a nasogastric tube for persistent vomiting. Abdominal imaging may be required to seek other pathology or complications of appendicitis, such as abscess or fistula.

DISPOSITION

Discharge Goals

Patients are safe to discharge if they are tolerating a regular diet and have minimal abdominal pain that is controlled with oral pain medication as well as an absence of fever prior to discharge.

Outpatient Care

Children who have had an operation and are clear for discharge should be rechecked 5 to 7 days postoperatively. Patients who received nonoperative or delayed operative care should initially receive empiric antibiotics. These families should be instructed to return for immediate evaluation if their child develops escalating abdominal pain, fever, persistent vomiting, or a toxic appearance.

 WHAT YOU NEED TO REMEMBER

- Early diagnosis and surgical intervention lead to better outcomes.
- Once the diagnosis of appendicitis is suspected, consult your surgeon.
- If the diagnosis of appendicitis is clear, no laboratory work or imaging is necessary.
- Give antibiotics and IV fluid resuscitation early in cases of perforated appendicitis or sepsis.

SUGGESTED READINGS

Bundy DG, Byerley JS, Liles EA. Does this child have appendicitis? *JAMA* 2007;298:438–451.

Fleisher GR, Ludwig S, Henretig FM. *Textbook of Pediatric Emergency Medicine*, 5th Ed. Philadelphia: Lippincott Williams & Wilkins, 2006.

Kwok MY, Kim MK, Gorelick MH. Evidence-based approach to the diagnosis of appendicitis in children. *Pediatric Emergency Care* 2004;20:690–698.

McCollough M, Sharieff GQ. Abdominal pain in children. *Pediatr Clin North Am* 2006;53:107–137.

Taylor GA, Wesson DE. Diagnostic imaging for acute appendicitis in children. *UpToDate* [serial online]. January 22, 2008.

Wesson DE. Evaluation and diagnosis of appendicitis in children. *UpToDate* [serial online]. Febuary 11, 2008.

Wesson ED. Treatment of appendicitis in children. *UpToDate* [serial online]. February 12, 2008.

Bronchiolitis

BRIAN ALVERSON

THE PATIENT ENCOUNTER

An 8-month-old boy with no significant past medical history presents to the emergency department after a 2-day history of congestion, runny nose, and coughing. The mother notes that over the past day he has been having increasing difficulty with breathing, poor oral intake, and fewer wet diapers. On exam, he is sleepy but easily awakened and has significant nasal congestion and dry mucous membranes. His respiratory rate is 60 breaths per minute and both subcostal and supracostal retractions are noted. On auscultation, coarse rhonchi are noted throughout both lung fields.

OVERVIEW

Definition

Bronchiolitis is an infection of the small airways of the lung that affects infants and young children. It is the most common cause of pediatric hospitalizations in the United States but is only rarely associated with severe complications or death.

Pathophysiology

Bronchiolitis is predominantly of viral origin. Causative viruses are spread mostly by direct contact with infected individuals. Adults with mild upper respiratory infections may be vehicles for transmission of severe disease in infants. Additionally, contaminated surfaces may harbor viral particles.

Infections generally occur from viral pathogens inoculated into the eyes or inhaled into the upper respiratory tract; the primary pathology occurs in the lungs. Viruses directly invade cells lining the respiratory epithelium and thereby stimulate a cytotoxic response from the child's immune system, leading to a prolific production of mucous as well as necrosis and sloughing of dead respiratory cells. The degraded cells and mucous cause not only classic rhinorrhea but also, more significantly, obstruction of the small airways of the lungs. These obstructed bronchioles result in air trapping and atelectasis as well as general worsening of lung oxygenation and ventilation. As the viral illness proceeds, debris is cleared from the bronchioles by cilia in the respiratory tract; it then moves into the trachea, where the cough reflex assists in its elimination and clearing of the airway.

Epidemiology

Bronchiolitis is primarily a disease of young childhood. More than 20% of children suffer from bronchiolitis in their first year of life, and roughly 2% are hospitalized for the disease at some point in childhood. Most children who require hospitalization are <6 months of age. After age 2, hospitalization rates are much lower except in children with underlying pulmonary pathology, such as severe asthma or chronic lung disease of prematurity. Only about 100 infants and children die each year from viral bronchiolitis, and many of these have underlying conditions that render the disease more severe.

Because of the viral origin of the disease, bronchiolitis is seasonal and much more predominant in the winter months. It is often much more severe in infants with underlying cardiac or pulmonary disease, such as chronic lung disease of prematurity. Other risk factors for severe bronchiolitis include day care attendance, young infancy during the winter season, not being breast-fed, smoking in the home environment, school-age siblings, shared bedrooms, and lower socioeconomic status.

Etiology

Multiple viruses have been implicated in the cause of bronchiolitis. These include respiratory syncytial virus (RSV), influenza, adenovirus, parainfluenza, rhinovirus, coronavirus, and human metapneumovirus. Very rarely, *Chlamydia trachomatis*, usually from the mother's genitourinary tract, or *Mycoplasma pneumoniae* is implicated as the bacterial cause of an illness closely resembling viral bronchiolitis.

ACUTE MANAGEMENT AND WORKUP

The acute management of a patient with bronchiolitis is critical for determining which patients require observation in the hospital and which may be safely discharged home. However, bronchiolitis can fit a typical pattern of worsening over several days, followed by a period of gradual convalescence. Early in the course of disease, care should be taken to anticipate a child's potential deterioration.

The First 15 Minutes

As with all patients with respiratory disease, the initial assessment must focus on rapidly assessing and stabilizing the airway, especially in a critically ill patient. **First, assess airway patency and the adequacy of ventilation.** Generally, patients with severe intercostal and subcostal retractions, grunting, flaring, tachypnea >70 breaths per minute, profound hypoxia, or an altered mental status are at greatest risk of impending respiratory failure. If any of these findings are present, intervention may be warranted prior to eliciting a history or continuing on with the physical exam. In this situation:

- Notify the resident or attending immediately.
- Consider positive-pressure ventilation by an appropriately fitted bag-valve-mask.
- Administer supplemental oxygen as needed.

Second, assess hydration status. Patients with bronchiolitis may have poor oral intake. Additionally, both fever and tachypnea can increase insensible fluid losses. Acidosis from dehydration may worsen respiratory status because an infant's primary mechanism for correcting acute acidosis is through enhanced elimination of CO_2 from the respiratory tract. Any child with evidence of significant dehydration—such as dry mucous membranes, delayed capillary refill, or poor skin turgor—may need immediate fluid resuscitation.

The First Few Hours

Because bronchiolitis is primarily a diagnosis made by history and physical exam, routine laboratory study or radiologic imaging is not necessary for the early management of these infants. In children with severe respiratory distress, a chest radiograph may facilitate identifying an alternative cause for respiratory distress, such as pneumonia or pneumothorax. Efforts in the first few hours should focus on stabilizing the patient, obtaining a thorough history and physical exam, and triaging the patient to an inpatient bed or discharge home. Most patients do not respond significantly to therapeutic interventions in a way that will change the initial admission or discharge decision.

History

The history and physical exam are the mainstays in diagnosing and managing bronchiolitis. The average incubation period is about 5 days; a recent history of exposure to individuals with upper respiratory symptoms is common. Infants almost universally have a history of runny nose, congestion, and cough. Many children have fevers, posttussive emesis, and decreased fluid intake. Wheezing may be audible. The parents may note a child's use of accessory muscles during inspiration. Sometimes children have other hallmarks of viral disease, such as conjunctivitis. Very rarely, infants may exhibit extrapulmonary symptoms, such as cardiovascular failure.

You should also determine whether the child has comorbid conditions that increase the likelihood of severe illness. Important comorbid conditions include prematurity, asthma, congenital heart disease, and human immunodeficiency virus (HIV) infection.

Children with bronchiolitis have fevers, tachypnea, and poor fluid intake, all of which can lead to dehydration. However, elevated levels of antidiuretic hormone expressed by the pulmonary parenchyma can also rarely cause decreased urine output in bronchiolitis. A careful history of fluid intake and urine output is critical in these patients.

It is common for very young infants ill with bronchiolitis to present with apnea as a primary complaint. However, there is no evidence that well-appearing infants with bronchiolitis require observation to diagnose the presence of apnea.

Physical Examination

The presence of rhinorrhea and cough should be noted. Wheezing may be audible. On auscultation, localized or diffusely poor air entry, prolonged expirations, wheezing, rhonchi, rales, retractions, flaring, or grunting may be present. With an increasing severity of disease, supraclavicular retractions may be present. Children with severe disease may become cyanotic. Because fluid status is important, the presence of tears, moist mucous membranes, and brisk capillary refill are reassuring signs of adequate hydration.

Careful measurement of vital signs can identify impending respiratory failure. Severely ill patients may have a paradoxical improvement in their tachypnea as their disease progresses; such infants have impaired ventilation. Pulse oximetry may reveal poor oxygenation, but a pulse oximetry reading below 90% does not necessarily indicate distress. Likewise, good oxygen saturation does not preclude a child's developing respiratory failure.

Labs and Tests to Consider

The diagnosis of bronchiolitis is largely clinical. Blood tests, such as peripheral white blood cell counts, do not reliably distinguish between bacterial and viral causes of pulmonary infiltrates.

Key Diagnostic Labs and Tests

Many hospitals now offer rapid viral testing, typically for detection of RSV and influenza. These tests have been shown to be moderately useful for cohorting purposes, but they do not predict the outcome or suggest effective patient management except possibly to eliminate testing for alternative causes of fever in very young infants. Additional laboratory testing may be useful to identify bacterial coinfections in neonates with fever. Urinary tract infection is most common, occurring in about 2% of all infants with RSV. There is little utility for blood cultures in febrile but well-appearing, immunized children >3 months of age.

Imaging

Chest radiography is not necessary for most infants with clinically suspected bronchiolitis. In a child with severe respiratory distress, a chest x-ray is usually indicated to rule out bacterial illness or a respiratory complication such as pneumothorax or pneumomediastinum (Fig. 5-1). Typical radiographic findings include hyperinflation with flattening of the diaphragms, peribronchial cuffing, and patchy infiltrates (Fig. 5-2). The infiltrates are usually

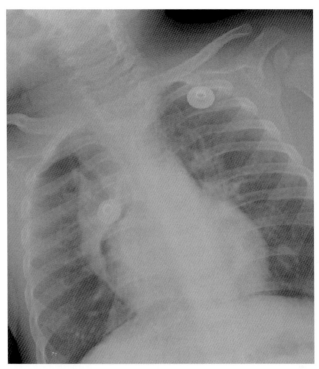

FIGURE 5-1: Chest x-ray of an 11-month-old boy with bronchiolitis who has pneumomediastinum. Note the air around the thymus and cardiac silhouette, as well as hyperinflation and areas of subsegmental atelectasis.

attributable to atelectasis and occur as a consequence of airway narrowing and mucous plugging. In isolation, such findings do not portend a worse clinical course.

Treatment

Bronchiolitis is a self-limited infection. Most treatment for bronchiolitis should focus on supportive care. Parents should be instructed in the proper technique of applying nasal saline drops and nasal bulb suctioning. Additionally, parents should be encouraged to carefully monitor urine output. Infants may often be effectively hydrated by syringe feeding, which can prevent the need for intravenous hydration and hospitalization in a child who otherwise appears well.

Although the benefits of administering bronchodilators such as nebulized albuterol or racemic epinephrine have not been established, these medications are often used in clinical practice. Bronchodilators should be considered

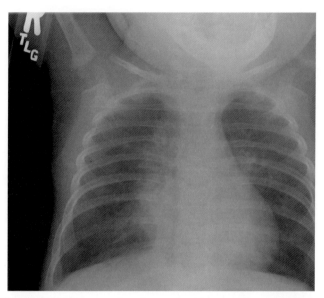

FIGURE 5-2: Chest x-ray of an 8-month-old boy with typical findings of bronchiolitis, including hyperinflation, peribronchial thickening, and scattered opacities representing areas of atelectasis.

in patients with severe respiratory distress, hypoxia, or impending respiratory failure. If no significant improvement occurs within 1 hour of administration, they should be discontinued. The role of corticosteroids is also controversial. A meta-analysis of placebo-controlled studies (1) demonstrated a small but statistically significant reduction in the duration of hospitalization; however, this difference was not significant when patients with a prior history of wheezing were excluded. These data suggest that a limited subgroup of children with bronchiolitis (e.g., older infants with recurrent wheezing episodes) may benefit from corticosteroid therapy.

Antibiotics may be necessary to treat children with concomitant bacterial pneumonia, which should be suspected in infants with pleural effusions or stable (rather than migratory) infiltrates and persistent fevers. Although bacterial coinfection is certainly possible, it is not common except in severely ill patients.

The case patient was admitted to the general pediatric service because of mild hypoxia (oxygen saturation of 88% on room air) and dehydration. His supportive care included IV fluids, oxygen via nasal cannula, and frequent nasal suction. After 2 days, he was able to maintain his oxygen saturation above 90% on room air and his oral intake improved; he was, therefore, discharged.

Admission Criteria and Level-of-Care Criteria

Any patient who has a significantly increased work of breathing, the need for supplemental oxygen, or an inability to maintain hydration should be admitted. A lower threshold for admission should be considered in children with underlying congenital heart disease, severe pulmonary disease such as cystic fibrosis, a history of prematurity, or a history of underlying immune deficiency.

Most patients can be effectively managed on the general pediatrics ward. However, some children will continue to experience a significant work of breathing or will start to tire from prolonged labored breathing. Others will require >2 L/min of oxygen via nasal cannula to achieve optimal oxygenation. These children should be transferred to the intensive care unit (ICU). In the pediatric ICU, patients may get increased ventilatory support, such as high-flow nasal cannula, continuous positive airway pressure (CPAP), or intubation and mechanical ventilation. In rare severe cases of RSV, ribavirin may be used as a virucidal agent.

EXTENDED IN-HOSPITAL MANAGEMENT

All children with bronchiolitis should be placed on strict contact precautions, including gowns and gloves. Caregivers should also routinely clean stethoscope heads and other surfaces. About 1 in 20 infants with RSV develops it as a consequence of transmission within the health care setting.

Children in distress will often respond to nasopharyngeal wall suctioning; however, this procedure can be painful and can cause nasal bleeding. Deep suctioning should therefore be reserved for children in significant distress from upper airway obstruction. Chest physiotherapy is contraindicated because it does not help with disease and can cause complications.

Infants with bronchiolitis should be tested for hypoxia. Most hospitals now accept a pulse oximetry reading >90% on room air.

CLINICAL PEARL

It should be noted that transient desaturations <90% commonly resolve on their own; moreover, there is little evidence that these predict a worsened outcome.

Some children may respond to nebulized therapy such as albuterol or racemic epinephrine. If this is attempted, care should be made to assess the patient objectively before and after therapy, as the majority of patients will have no significant improvement of symptoms. These drugs should be discontinued if they are not found to be of benefit after one trial.

DISPOSITION
Discharge Goals
Children generally have a 12-day length of illness, but the peak of severity occurs between the third and fifth day. Some children have symptoms that persist even 1 month after the onset of disease. Patients are generally considered safe for discharge when they have only mild subcostal retractions or no work of breathing, no longer have severe tachypnea, and have demonstrated an ability to maintain hydration. Care should be taken to note some improvement since admission in order to verify that patients are convalescing from their illness. Some hospitals, especially those at higher altitudes, will discharge patients with prolonged oxygen requirements on home oxygen if they demonstrate an improved work of breathing and adequate fluid intake.

Outpatient Care
Most patients with bronchiolitis do not require admission. However, among those who are discharged from hospitalization, close follow-up is necessary. The course of viral disease can be irregular, and it is not at all uncommon for infants with bronchiolitis to "bounce back." Also, remember to refer appropriate patients for RSV prophylaxis (palivizumab; trade name Synagis), which is indicated for premature patients and infants with congenital heart disease. Encourage families to stop smoking because infants in a smoke-free environment have a milder course of disease. Also, encourage breast-feeding, if appropriate, because it reduces disease severity. Finally, patients should be monitored over time because infantile bronchiolitis, particularly RSV, is an independent risk factor for the development of asthma.

WHAT YOU NEED TO REMEMBER

- Bronchiolitis is a clinical diagnosis: Most children do not require lab testing or chest x-rays.
- Check your patient before and after any nebulized therapy. If it does not work, discontinue it.
- Children with bronchiolitis can get dehydrated easily. Pay close attention to signs of dehydration and urine output.

REFERENCES

1. Garrison MM, Christakis DA, Harvey E, et al. Systemic corticosteroids in infant bronchiolitis: a meta-analysis. *Pediatrics* 2000;105(4):E44.

SUGGESTED READINGS

Bordley WC, Viswanathan M, King VJ, et al. Diagnosis and testing in bronchiolitis: a systematic review. *Arch Pediatr Adolesc Med* 2004;158(2):119–126.

Levine DA, Platt SL, Dayan PS, et al. Risk of serious bacterial infection in young febrile infants with respiratory syncytial virus infections. *Pediatrics* 2004;113(6): 1728–1734.

Schroeder AR, Marmor AK, Pantell RH, Newman TB. Impact of pulse oximetry and oxygen therapy on length of stay in bronchiolitis hospitalizations. *Arch Pediatr Adolesc Med* 2004;158(6):157–130.

Subcommittee on Diagnosis and Management of Bronchiolitis. Diagnosis and management of bronchiolitis. *Pediatrics* 2006;118(4):1774–1793.

Cervical Lymphadenitis

LEKHA SHAH AND SAMUEL J. SPIZMAN

THE PATIENT ENCOUNTER

A 5-year-old boy presents to the emergency department with 4 days of progressive neck swelling, pain, and malaise. Today he developed a fever up to 38.5°C (101.3°F) at home. There is no history of trauma. Vital signs are significant for a temperature of 38.9°C (102°F), a heart rate of 122 beats per minute, and a respiratory rate of 28 breaths per minute. On physical examination, he appears tired but nontoxic and is breathing easily. A 3.0- by 2.5-cm tender red mass without fluctuance is present in the right upper neck in the anterior triangle and he is unable to turn his head fully to the right. The rest of his examination is otherwise normal. Further questioning reveals no pets in the home, no known ill exposures, and no travel outside the United States.

OVERVIEW

Cervical lymphadenitis is a common childhood occurrence. Parents may seek medical attention for the evaluation of neck swelling, or it may be detected incidentally. Although the differential diagnosis is broad, it most commonly results from a viral upper respiratory infection (URI). Clinicians face the diagnostic challenge of detecting more serious underlying causes of cervical adenitis, both infectious and noninfectious.

Definition

Cervical lymphadenitis is defined by the presence of one or more enlarged, tender, inflamed lymph nodes in the neck. It may be unilateral or bilateral and may develop acutely over several days or follow a subacute/chronic course over weeks and months. While *lymphadenopathy* refers simply to the enlargement of lymph nodes, the terms are frequently interchanged.

Pathophysiology

Lymphadenitis may result from the following: drainage of a source of infection by lymph nodes (Fig. 6-1), the multiplication of cells within the node, or the infiltration of cells from outside the node. Infectious cervical lymphadenitis occurs when lymph nodes become inflamed as a result of lymphatic drainage from head or neck infections. The source of infection may be obvious or occult on physical examination; for example, the skin papule resulting from *Bartonella*

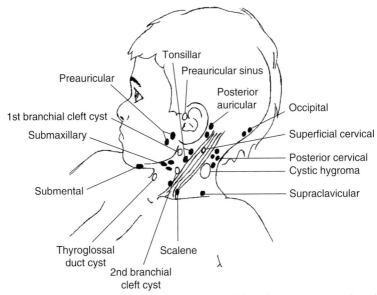

FIGURE 6-1: Typical locations of cystic and solid neck masses. Reproduced with permission from Frank G, Shah SS, Catallozzi MC, Zaoutis LB (eds.) *The Philadelphia Guide: Inpatient Pediatrics.* LWW: Philadelphia 2005.

henselae infection frequently regresses before cervical adenopathy becomes manifest. The infectious/antigenic material triggers lymphocytic proliferation within the node, producing lymphadenopathy (nodal enlargement). Suppuration occurs if neutrophils are recruited by pyogenic bacteria (e.g., *Staphylococcus aureus*, *Streptococcus pyogenes*). Clinically, the node then resembles a skin abscess with warmth, tenderness, swelling, overlying skin erythema, and sometimes fluctuance. Subacute/chronic infection (e.g., *B. henselae*, fungi, and mycobacteria) may cause granulomatous changes within the lymph node.

Epidemiology

The incidence of cervical lymphadenitis is difficult to estimate because most cases result from reactive lymphadenitis from a viral URI.

Etiology

Common infectious causes of cervical adenitis are summarized in Table 6-1. Common noninfectious causes include malignancy (lymphoma, leukemia, thyroid cancer, neuroblastoma), collagen vascular disease (juvenile idiopathic arthritis, systemic lupus erythematosus), sarcoidosis, Kawasaki's disease, medications (e.g., phenytoin, carbamazepine), and postvaccination. PFAPA is a rare disease of unclear etiology characterized by the following symptoms: **p**eriodic **f**ever, **a**phthous stomatitis, **p**haryngitis, and cervical **a**denitis.

TABLE 6-1
Common Infectious Etiologies of Cervical Lymphadenitis

Bacteria	Viruses	Miscellaneous
Staphylococcus aureus	Rhinovirus	Toxoplasmosis
Streptococcus pyogenes	Influenza	Histoplasmosis
Bartonella henselae (cat-scratch disease)	Herpes simplex virus	Coccidiomycosis
Group B *Streptococcus*	Enterovirus	
Mycoplasma pneumoniae	Adenovirus	
Mycobacterium tuberculosis	Cytomegalovirus	
Nontuberculous mycobacteria	Epstein–Barr virus	
	Human immunodeficiency virus (HIV)	
Treponema pallidum (syphilis)		
Francisella tularensis		
Actinomyces		
Eikenella corrodens		

ACUTE MANAGEMENT AND WORKUP

The acute management and workup are focused on classifying patients into one of three subsets. The first includes patients who may require airway stabilization, support, and immediate therapeutic intervention. A second subset may require laboratory studies, diagnostic imaging, subspecialty consultation, and possible inpatient workup and care. For the third subset (the majority of patients), therapy should be targeted at the underlying etiology but not the reactive lymphadenitis itself.

The First 15 Minutes

In the toxic-appearing child, your initial assessment should determine whether airway, breathing, and circulation are adequate. If indicated, a definitive airway should be established. This may easily be determined by observation of distress, the presence of stridor, listening to the patient speak, and watching the chest rise.

The First Few Hours

In stable patients, a thorough history and physical examination, with particular attention to the HEENT exam, usually determines the extent of workup and action plan. Ill-appearing children may require monitoring, laboratory testing, imaging, subspecialty consultation, hydration, and pain management. Stable patients with self-limited or mild cervical lymphadenitis may be discharged home with appropriate follow-up.

History

Good history taking is of paramount importance in establishing an accurate diagnosis. Key features include the duration of symptoms, the laterality of findings (unilateral versus bilateral), and associated symptoms (e.g., fever, ear pain, rash, etc.). You should ask families about the history of ill contacts, recent trauma, risk factors for tuberculosis, exposure to animals, travel, medications, immunization status, and dental/sinus pain. Children with acute cervical lymphadenitis typically present with URI symptoms such as fever, cough, sore throat, runny nose, and malaise. Subacute unilateral lymphadenitis following a bite or scratch from a young kitten suggests cat scratch disease. Exposure to fleas, ticks, and farm animals points to less common etiologies such as tularemia, bubonic plague, or brucellosis. Finally, chronic symptoms such as fatigue and weight loss may indicate malignancy.

Physical Examination

Specific details of the lymph node exam should include their number, size (measured with a ruler), tenderness, shape, texture, and mobility as well as overlying skin changes. Infected nodes are difficult to differentiate clinically from subcutaneous skin infection; infected deep nodes are usually nonpalpable. The HEENT exam may reveal infections such as pharyngitis, dental caries, or tinea capitis. Figure 6-1 shows the typical locations of cystic and solid neck masses, including lymph nodes. Acute bilateral lymphadenopathy with small, rubbery, mobile nodes generally occurs in the setting of a viral URI; lymphadenitis from group A streptococcal pharyngitis is usually bilateral but more tender. Acute unilateral lymphadenitis is frequently the result of bacterial infection: the child may be febrile and the node is usually warm, tender, and swollen. Subacute/chronic lymphadenitis is generally indolent and less painful. Mycobacterial infection is a risk factor for sinus tract formation. Reactive or "shotty" nodes are small, discrete, mobile, and minimally tender. Malignant nodes are firm, painless, and fixed to underlying structures.

> ### CLINICAL PEARL
>
> *A complete exam of the lymphatic system should include the liver, spleen, and noncervical lymph nodes. These details will allow the clinician to classify the cervical lymphadenitis as acute versus subacute/chronic and generate a short list of likely diagnoses.*

Labs and Tests to Consider

Clinical history and physical examination should supersede all laboratory testing. In the setting of worsening or persistent lymphadenitis, useful tests might include a throat culture (or rapid strep), complete blood count (CBC) with differential, blood culture, erythrocyte sedimentation rate (ESR), C-reactive protein (CRP), and serologies. These nonspecific tests may suggest inflammation, bone marrow suppression/infiltration, or a specific etiology. Gram's stain and wound culture should be ordered for all drainage procedures.

Key Diagnostic Labs and Tests

There are no specific tests to order in the setting of cervical lymphadenitis. CBC with differential, ESR, and CRP may collectively suggest a bacterial or viral etiology but are best utilized for neonates or as baseline markers to monitor the patient's condition or response to treatment. If initial treatment fails after 6 to 8 weeks, the clinician should consider ordering serology/polymerase chain reaction (PCR) testing for cytomegalovirus (CMV), Epstein–Barr virus (EBV), human herpesvirus 6 (HHV6), *Histoplasma*, *Coccidiomycosis*, *Toxoplasma*, *Francisella tularensis*, *B. henselae*, and *Brucella* as well as a rapid plasma reagin test (RPR) for syphilis. The serologies have variable sensitivities and specificities. Patients with suspected mycobacterial lymphadenitis should undergo tuberculin skin testing. Excisional or tissue biopsy may reveal malignancy as well as a specific infectious etiology. A portion of the biopsy sample may be used for molecular studies.

Imaging

Radiologic imaging of the neck is required if a deep neck infection is suspected. A dental Panorex radiograph may reveal dental infection. Mediastinal widening on chest radiography implies extension of infection into the mediastinum. Lateral soft-tissue radiographs of the neck allow for imaging of the retropharyngeal and paratracheal spaces. If the depth of suppuration is unclear, neck ultrasound or contrast-enhanced computed tomography (CT) may better define the inflammatory boundaries. Ultrasonography is useful for superficial infections but has limited utility for deep neck infections. Bedside ultrasound is a useful adjunct to facilitate drainage procedures in experienced hands. Contrast-enhanced CT offers moderately good delineation of the extent of infection but involves a greater amount of ionizing radiation than plain radiography. Magnetic resonance imaging (MRI) offers excellent soft tissue resolution but has the disadvantages of expense, time consumption, or relative unavailability.

Treatment

Self-limited bilateral cervical lymphadenitis associated with a viral URI requires no treatment. Well-appearing patients with mild unilateral lymphadenopathy may be followed with serial exams over time. If febrile, these children should benefit from antibiotic treatment and may require needle aspiration. Cephalosporins, such as cephalexin, have been the mainstay of therapy for presumed cervical lymphadenitis due to *S. aureus*. Given the increasing prevalence of community-acquired methicillin-resistant *S. aureus* (CA-MRSA), clindamycin may be a better first-line agent in regions with a high incidence. Other options include trimethoprim–sulfamethoxazole, but this will not cover group A strep. Children with acute suppurative lymphadenitis may require needle aspiration or incision and drainage for either symptomatic relief or diagnostic testing. Large fluctuant nodes require incision and drainage. An otolaryngologist should be involved in all cases in which deep neck infection is suspected. As always, the treatment course should be directed at the underlying cause (e.g., chemotherapy for malignancy).

Admission Criteria and Level of Care Criteria

Most patients can be safely managed as outpatients with a few notable exceptions. Neonates less than 2-3 months of age should be admitted for parenteral antibiotic therapy for sepsis. Admission should be considered for patients with moderate to severe dehydration or pain, failed outpatient therapy, or an inability to tolerate oral fluids. Any child with potential airway compromise or mediastinal involvement should be admitted to an intensive care unit (ICU) with appropriate subspecialty management.

The case patient was able to drink well in the ER and was therefore felt to be safe for discharge on oral clindamycin for 10 days. His parents were instructed to follow up with his pediatrician in 2 days. At that point, his cervical mass was about the same size but was less tender and he was no longer febrile. After 7 days of antibiotics, the mass had essentially resolved, and he finished his 10-day course of clindamycin without any further issues.

EXTENDED IN-HOSPITAL MANAGEMENT

In-hospital management generally includes antibiotic therapy and the observation of changes in node size and neck swelling. The majority of patients can be discharged home after a few days. Prolonged stays are the result of a delay in reaching the right diagnosis, resistance to antimicrobial therapy, deep infections that require surgical involvement, or malignancy that requires extensive workup and care.

DISPOSITION
Discharge Goals

Patients may be discharged home after the inflamed node is no longer enlarging. Other considerations include adequate pain control, cessation of fever, improving lab markers (CBC, CRP, ESR), and institution of appropriate therapy (e.g., antituberculous medications for scrofula).

Outpatient Care

After hospital discharge, patients should follow up with their pediatricians within 2 to 3 days of treatment directed at the underlying cause. The recurrence of fever and increasing neck swelling are the hallmark features of failed outpatient therapy. For diagnosed mycobacterial infection, all family members and significant contacts should receive a skin test with purified protein derivative (PPD).

 WHAT YOU NEED TO REMEMBER

- Viral URI, the most common cause of cervical lymphadenitis, requires no ancillary testing or treatment.
- Acute unilateral cervical lymphadenitis is generally due to bacterial infection.
- The patient's history and physical examination should guide any laboratory testing or imaging.

SUGGESTED READINGS

Courtney MJ, Miteff A, Mahadevan M. Management of pediatric lateral neck infections: does the adage "never let the sun go down on undrained pus· · ·" hold true? *Int Pediatr Otorhinolarygol* 2007;71:95–100.

Cummings CW, Haughey BH, Thomas JR, et al. *Cummings Otolaryngology: Head and Neck Surgery.* St. Louis: Mosby, 2007.

Douglas SA, Jennings S, Owen VM, et al. Is ultrasound useful in evaluating paediatric inflammatory neck masses? *Clin Otolaryngol* 2005;30(6):526–529.

Elden LM, Grundfast KM, Vezina G. Accuracy and usefulness of radiographic assessment of cervical neck infections in children. *J Otolaryngol* 2001;30(2):82–89.

Luu TM, Chevalier I, Gauthier M, et al. Acute adenitis in children: clinical course and factors predictive of surgical drainage. *J Paediatr Child Health* 2005;41:273–277.

Moore SW, Schneider JW, Schaaf HS. Diagnostic aspects of cervical lymphadenopathy in children in the developing world: a study of 1877 surgical specimens. *Pediatr Surg Int* 2003;19(4):240–244.

Shaikh U. Lymphadenitis. *Emedicine* 2008 (serial online).

Swanson DS. Etiology and clinical manifestations of cervical lymphadenitis in children. *UpToDate* 2007 (serial online).

Swanson DS. Diagnostic approach to and initial treatment of cervical lymphadenitis in children. *UpToDate* 2007 (serial online).

Congenital Heart Disease

PATRICIO A. FRIAS

THE PATIENT ENCOUNTER

A 2-day-old infant is noted to be mildly tachypneic during predischarge evaluation in the newborn nursery. The infant was born at 38 weeks' gestation following an uncomplicated pregnancy, although with limited prenatal care. Apgar scores were 8 at 1 minute (off for color and tone), and 9 at 5 minutes (off for color). Since birth, the child has reportedly been nursing well, although recently with mild tachypnea.

OVERVIEW

Definition

Congenital heart disease (CHD) is defined as a cardiac structural abnormality that is present at birth. These defects can range from small, clinically insignificant holes to minor valve abnormalities to hypoplasia of a cardiac chamber. CHD can generally be divided into cyanotic and acyanotic lesions. This chapter focuses on the recognition and management of the cyanotic infant. It should be noted that current advances in fetal imaging have resulted in an increased incidence of prenatal diagnosis, allowing for detailed planning about the timing and location of delivery. However, because of a lack of prenatal care, difficult imaging, and/or misdiagnosis, many infants with cyanotic heart disease remain undiscovered before birth.

Pathophysiology

In the early hours and days of life, there are numerous changes in the transition from fetal to neonatal circulation. In utero, the ductus arteriosus and foramen ovale serve as a means for oxygenated maternal blood to bypass the fetal lungs and make its way to the systemic circulation. Shortly after birth, as pulmonary vascular resistance begins to drop, shunting across the ductus arteriosus and foramen ovale normally reverse, and these openings ultimately close in the majority of infants. In the cyanotic newborn, however, these in utero connections may serve as lifesaving shunts, allowing the following: (i) the mixing of systemic and pulmonary blood, (ii) the maintenance of systemic blood flow, or (ii) the maintenance of pulmonary blood flow. When the ductus arteriosus closes in infants with "ductal-dependent" lesions, such infants

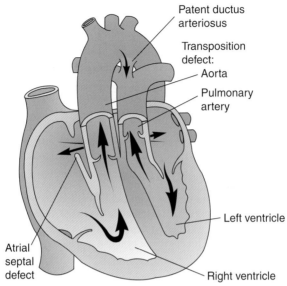

Patent ductus arteriosus

Transposition defect:
Aorta

Pulmonary artery

Left ventricle

Atrial septal defect

Right ventricle

FIGURE 7-1: Transposition of the great arteries. From Pillitteri, A. *Maternal and Child Nursing,* 4th ed. Philadelphia: Lippincott Williams & Wilkins, 2003, with permission.

can rapidly become critically ill. Likewise, if the foramen ovale is insufficient in lesions such as the complete transposition of the great arteries (D-TGA), there may be inadequate mixing of systemic and pulmonary blood.

Cyanosis in and of itself is not necessarily harmful to the newborn infant but rather a sign of potential illness that must be investigated. The appearance of cyanosis may be difficult to note in darker-skinned and/or anemic infants. Approximately 5 g/dL of reduced hemoglobin in cutaneous veins will lead to the appearance of cyanosis. Because there is normally 2 g/dL of reduced hemoglobin in venules, it takes only an additional 3 g/dL to give the outward appearance of cyanosis.

The most common cyanotic congenital cardiac malformations can be remembered as the 5 Ts of cyanotic CHD plus hypoplastic left heart syndrome (HLHS, 1% of all CHD): (i) D-transposition of the great arteries (D-TGA, 5% to 7% of all CHD), (ii) tetralogy of Fallot (TOF, 5% to 10% of all CHD), (iii) tricuspid atresia (1% to 3% of all CHD), (iv) total anomalous pulmonary venous return (TAPVR, 1% of all CHD), and (v) persistent truncus arteriosus (<1% of all CHD). Other forms of cyanotic CHD include pulmonary atresia with and without ventricular septal defect, Ebstein's anomaly, heterotaxy syndromes, and single-ventricle lesions; these are not addressed in this chapter. The basic pathology of the six lesions to be discussed is as follows:

1. **D-Transposition of the Great Arteries:** The aorta arises from the right ventricle (RV), recirculating desaturated blood to the systemic circulation, while the pulmonary artery arises from the left ventricle (LV) and recirculates oxygenated blood to the lungs. Survival is dependent on adequate mixing at the ductal, atrial, and/or ventricular levels (Fig. 7-1).

2. **Tetralogy of Fallot:** This includes large membranous (subpulmonary extension) ventricular septal defect (VSD), aortic override, RV outflow tract (RVOT) obstruction, and RV hypertrophy (RVH). Clinical presentation ranges from the acyanotic infant with minimal RVOT obstruction and clinical evidence of congestive heart failure to the cyanotic infant with severe RVOT obstruction and hypoplastic branch pulmonary arteries (Fig. 7-2).

3. **Tricuspid Atresia:** This is characterized by an atretic tricuspid valve with hypoplastic RV and varying degrees of RVOT obstruction. Systemic venous blood must cross an atrial septal defect (ASD, obligate) to the left heart with pulmonary circulation dependent on a patent ductus arteriosus (PDA) and VSD. The degree of cyanosis is dependent on the degree

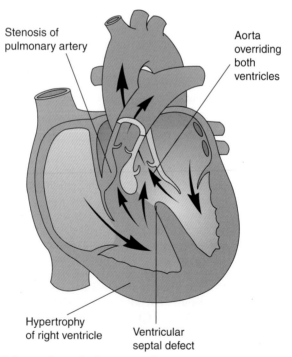

FIGURE 7-2: Tetralogy of Fallot. From Pillitteri, A. *Maternal and Child Nursing*, 4th ed. Philadelphia: Lippincott Williams & Wilkins, 2003, with permission.

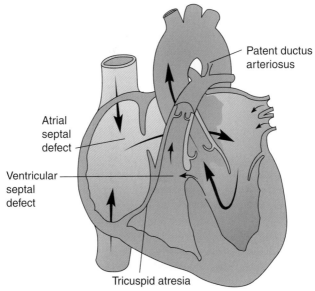

Patent ductus arteriosus

Atrial septal defect

Ventricular septal defect

Tricuspid atresia

FIGURE 7-3: Tricuspid atresia. From Pillitteri, A. *Maternal and Child Nursing,* 4th ed. Philadelphia: Lippincott Williams & Wilkins, 2003, with permission.

of obstruction at the VSD and/or the RVOT. It may have associated transposition of the great arteries (Fig. 7-3).

4. **Total Anomalous Pulmonary Venous Return:** This is characterized by pulmonary venous blood return via venous confluence to systemic venous circulation. Drainage can be supracardiac (the most common is vertical vein to innominate vein), cardiac (typically coronary sinus), infracardiac (below the diaphragm, often obstructed) or mixed. There is obligate right-to-left shunting across an ASD (Fig. 7-4).

5. **Truncus Arteriosus:** This is characterized by failure of the common trunk to septate, resulting in a common cardiac origin for systemic, coronary, and pulmonary blood flow. Subtypes are based on the location of the pulmonary artery origin. Obligate VSD is present and varying degrees of truncal valve abnormalities (stenosis and/or insufficiency) and aortic arch anomalies (interrupted aortic arch and/or right aortic arch) may be seen (Fig. 7-5).

6. **Hypoplastic Left Heart Syndrome:** As the name suggests, HLHS is characterized by varying degrees of left heart hypoplasia leading to inadequate delivery of blood to the systemic circulation. With ductal closure, these infants rapidly become critically ill.

Epidemiology

CHD is the most common congenital malformation in newborns and the number one cause of mortality from birth defects in the first year of life. The

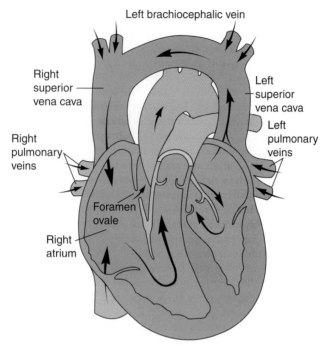

FIGURE 7-4: Total anomalous pulmonary venous return. From Pillitteri, A. *Maternal and Child Nursing*, 4th ed. Philadelphia: Lippincott Williams & Wilkins, 2003, with permission.

incidence of CHD is approximately 1%, with an estimated 35,000 children born annually with a cardiac defect. The American Heart Association estimates that about a million Americans are living with a congenital heart defect.

Etiology

The majority of congenital cardiac malformations occur as isolated defects, although some are related to chromosomal anomalies, maternal infection, maternal drug use, and/or familial causes.

ACUTE MANAGEMENT AND WORKUP

The acute management and workup should serve to stabilize the cyanotic infant and determine the underlying etiology for this clinical appearance. Once cardiac disease is confirmed, long-term planning and surgical disposition can be addressed.

The First 15 Minutes

The initial assessment of a cyanotic infant should include attention to the airway, breathing, and circulation (the ABCs) of basic cardiopulmonary

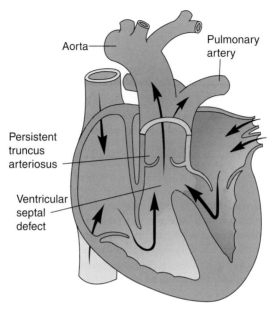

FIGURE 7-5: Truncus arteriosus. From Pillitteri, A. *Maternal and Child Nursing*, 4th ed. Philadelphia: Lippincott Williams & Wilkins, 2003, with permission.

resuscitation. Is this cyanosis related to airway positioning? Is the infant breathing? Are there clinical signs of poor circulation and/or decreased perfusion? Any acute issues identified during this initial evaluation should be treated accordingly. In general, the cyanotic newborn found in the setting described at the beginning of this chapter is comfortable and in no distress. Following the initial assessment, confirmation of systemic oxygen saturations should be performed pre- and postductally. Infants with significant pulmonary hypertension will demonstrate a lower saturation in the lower extremities owing to right-to-left shunting at the ductal level. This may also be seen in left-heart obstructive lesions with associated increase in pulmonary vascular resistance. The hyperoxia challenge may also be performed (see "Labs and Tests to Consider") in order to aid in the differentiation between cardiac and noncardiac causes of cyanosis.

The First Few Hours

Oxygen can be administered, yet keep in mind that children with single-ventricle lesions do not need saturations in the 90s. In fact, excessive use of oxygen in these children can lead to increased pulmonary blood flow at the expense of systemic circulation. This, in turn, can lead to congestive heart failure, metabolic acidosis, and end-organ damage (including but not limited to renal failure and necrotizing enterocolitis).

> ### CLINICAL PEARL
>
> *If there is clinical suspicion of a ductal-dependent lesion, initiate prostaglandin E_1 (PGE₁) via stable venous access (0.05 to 0.1 µg/kg/min starting dose). Be aware that common side effects of PGE₁ include apnea and fever.*

History

Maternal medical history (infection, meds, chronic disease, CHD, diabetes), birth history, and family history are all important in assessing the infant with cyanosis. Maternal infections such as rubella have been associated with various forms of congenital heart disease. In addition, maternal chronic disease can be associated with structural cardiac defects either primarily (i.e., diabetes has been associated with an increased incidence of congenital heart disease) or secondary to required medication use (lithium, antiepileptics). Difficulties at birth—such as maternal fever, heavy maternal sedation, or perinatal asphyxia—may point to noncardiac causes of cyanosis and shock.

Physical Examination

The physical examination of any infant should include inspection, palpation, and auscultation. Inspection of the infant will provide details such as the presence or absence of cyanosis, retractions, flaring, pallor, and lethargy and will also uncover associated congenital malformations that might be related to the underlying congenital heart disease. Palpation of the chest wall will reveal findings such as an increased RV impulse in the infant with TAPVR and pulmonary overcirculation or a prominent LV impulse in the infant with tricuspid atresia. Palpation of the extremities and pulses will provide insight into the systemic perfusion. Abdominal palpation might reveal hepatomegaly in the infant with tricuspid atresia and an obstructed interatrial communication or in the infant with HLHS and pulmonary overcirculation. Cardiac auscultation should focus not only on the presence or absence of murmurs but also on the other heart sounds (rub, click, gallop, single first and/or second heart sound). Auscultation of the lungs will typically prove normal in the infant with cyanotic congenital heart disease, although in those with excessive pulmonary blood flow, the exam may mimic that of an infant with primary pulmonary disease. See Table 7-1 for physical exam findings that might be seen in children with the cyanotic CHD described earlier.

Labs and Tests to Consider

Although the diagnosis of CHD is generally made by a combination of physical examination and imaging modalities, specific lab tests and imaging are also important to consider in the acute management of these

TABLE 7-1

Initial Findings in the Evaluation of Infants with Cyanotic CHD

	Physical Exam	Chest X-Ray	ECG	Echocardiogram
Transposition of the great arteries (D-TGA)	Cyanosis (may be profound), single S_2, often no murmur, comfortable tachypnea.	Cardiomegaly with normal to increased pulmonary vascularity; "egg" shaped appearance of cardiac silhouette.	Typically normal; may see RVH and RAD.	Assess ductal patency, presence and size of interatrial communication and VSD (if present), ventricular outflow obstruction, and coronary artery anatomy.
Tetralogy of Fallot (TOF)	Degree of cyanosis and quality of murmur dependent on degree of pulmonary obstruction.	Pulmonary vascularity generally decreased in cyanotic TOF; absent pulmonary trunk; right aortic arch may be present.	RVH, RAD, and possible RAE.	Assess degree of RV outflow tract obstruction; large membranous VSD with aortic override; evaluate coronary artery anatomy; arch sidedness (25% have right aortic arch).

(continued)

TABLE 7-1

Initial Findings in the Evaluation of Infants with Cyanotic CHD (Continued)

	Physical Exam	Chest X-Ray	ECG	Echocardiogram
Tricuspid Atresia	Dependent on degree of obstruction to pulmonary flow. Cyanosis (may be profound); harsh systolic murmur typical (left-to-right flow across VSD), single S_1, possibly single S_2, occasional S_3 (if ↑ PBF), hepatomegaly.	Decreased pulmonary vascularity, absent pulmonary trunk typical, heart size typically normal early.	RAE, LVH, leftward and superior QRS axis (unlike most other cyanotic lesions).	Assess presence and size of VSD, RVOT obstruction, and interatrial communication. 30% have associated TGA.
Total anomalous pulmonary venous return (TAPVR)	No obstruction—may show minimal cyanosis and asymptomatic at birth; early	↑ pulmonary blood flow, "figure of 8" appearance (snowman) in	RAE, RAD and RVH.	Delineate drainage of all pulmonary veins and determine whether or not obstruction is present.

	Physical Examination	Chest X-ray	ECG	Echocardiography/Catheterization
	months—tachypnea, cyanosis, RV heave, split S_2, S_3 and S_4 audible, 2/6 systolic flow murmur in pulmonary area. With obstruction – may be critically ill.	TAPVR to innominate vein; with obstruction, abnormal pulmonary vascular markings/pulmonary edema, Kerley-B lines.		
Truncus Arteriosus	Single S_2, systolic and diastolic murmurs possible; ejection click may be audible.	Cardiomegaly, increased pulmonary vascularity, right aortic arch.	BVH possible.	Determine origins of pulmonary arteries, degree/presence of truncal valve abnormalities, associated aortic arch anomalies.
Hypoplastic left heart syndrome (HLHS)	Tachypnea, dyspnea, poor pulses/perfusion, cyanosis, single S_2, no to soft murmur.	Cardiomegaly with pulmonary venous congestion after first few days	RVH/RV prominence.	Determine adequacy of intra-atrial communication for mixing; assess mitral valve, LV, and aorta for possible two-ventricle repair.

RAE, right atrial enlargement; RVH, right ventricular hypertrophy; PBF, pulmonary blood flow; LVH, left ventricular hypertrophy; RVOT, right ventricular outflow tract; BVH, biventricular hypertrophy; RAD, right axis deviation.

infants. These include the measurement of arterial blood gas, the hyperoxia test, the measurement of serum lactate, renal and hepatic profiles, chest x-ray (CXR), 12-lead electrocardiogram (ECG), and two-dimensional echocardiogram.

Key Diagnostic Labs and Tests

Arterial blood gas is helpful not only in the assessment of acid-base status but can also be used to differentiate pulmonary from cardiac causes of cyanosis. The hyperoxia test is carried out by exposing the cyanotic infant to 100% FiO_2 (via endotracheal tube or oxyhood) and measuring the partial pressure of oxygen (PaO_2). In general, the PaO_2 will not rise above 100 mm Hg in the setting of cyanotic CHD. As with everything in medicine, there are exceptions to this rule; patients with TAPVR may increase to >100 mm Hg and infants with severe pulmonary disease may not go above 100 mm Hg. A surrogate of systemic perfusion and acid–base status is the serum lactate, which has been shown to correlate with severity of clinical presentation and ultimate outcome. B-type natriuretic peptide (BNP) is synthesized and secreted by the ventricular myocardium in response to increases in volume or pressure and has a high positive predictive value for heart failure when elevated.

Infants presenting with cyanotic CHD may present in shock, with limited end-organ perfusion. Renal and hepatic profiles should be measured as a baseline assessment of such damage. Hypocalcemia is not uncommon in infants with CHD and should be treated accordingly.

Imaging

The CXR is a key part of the evaluation of the cyanotic infant. Its use is important not only to rule out pulmonary disease but also to assess the cardiac silhouette, arch sidedness, and pulmonary vascularity. The 12-lead ECG is an important adjunct in the evaluation of a child with suspected heart disease. In addition to providing a picture of the cardiac rhythm and conduction, the ECG provides clues to the anatomic diagnosis and severity of condition. The gold standard in the diagnosis of congenital CHD in the current era is a comprehensive two-dimensional echocardiogram with color-flow mapping and Doppler interrogation. Although echocardiography is discussed last in this sequence, the reality is that a quick look with an echocardiogram can give preliminary data regarding the presence or absence of critical CHD and the need for PGE_1. This by no means eliminates the need to evaluate the entire clinical picture yet takes into account the advances in technology that can often prove critical in making rapid decisions regarding need for transfer and/or emergent cardiac intervention, such as balloon atrial septostomy. See Table 7-1 for specific CXR, ECG, and echocardiographic findings of the previously mentioned forms of cyanotic CHD.

Treatment

As mentioned earlier, the initial stabilization of the infant with cyanotic congenital heart disease should focus on the ABC's of basic cardiopulmonary resuscitation. During this process, thought and attention should be given to whether or not this could be a duct-dependent lesion and cardiac consultation should be initiated. If concern exists for a duct-dependent lesion, the infant should be started on PGE_1, as noted earlier. Specific therapy depends on the cardiac diagnosis, although initial care should focus on stabilizing the infant, as mentioned earlier.

Admission Criteria and Level-of-Care Criteria

In general, all infants with cyanotic congenital heart disease should be admitted for detailed evaluation and management. These infants are usually already in house, many being diagnosed in the newborn nursery or neonatal intensive care unit (ICU) setting, although some present to the office of a primary care provider or ER once the ductus arteriosus closes or as a result of excessive pulmonary blood flow once pulmonary vascular resistance drops.

EXTENDED IN-HOSPITAL MANAGEMENT

Surgical repair depends on the lesion. For most cases of cyanotic CHD, neonatal repair is required and preferable in the current era. Although lesions such as D-TGA, TOF, truncus arteriosus, and TAPVR are generally amenable to anatomic/corrective repair, single-ventricle lesions such as tricuspid atresia and HLHS are treated with surgical palliation in multiple stages. In addition, surgical correction in some lesions (TOF, truncus arteriosus) will almost certainly require subsequent additional operations. Brief summaries of the typical cardiac repairs for the previously mentioned lesions are as follows:

1. **D-Transposition of the Great Arteries:** Repair consists of arterial switch with ASD and VSD closure as needed and reimplantation of coronary arteries (first few days of life).
2. **Tetralogy of Fallot:** Complete repair—consisting of VSD closure and augmentation of pulmonary outflow (with or without transannular patch)—is required, typically after 4 months of age.
3. **Tricuspid Atresia:** Repair consists of staged palliation, depending on the degree of pulmonary obstruction. If there is adequate pulmonary blood flow (PBF), the first stage will be a cavopulmonary anastomosis (SVC to pulmonary arteries, Glenn) at approximately 4 months of age (variable). If limited PBF and severe cyanosis are present, the first stage might be a systemic-to-pulmonary shunt, followed by a Glenn procedure at 4 to 6 months of age (variable). The final stage is typically total cavopulmonary anastomosis (Fontan) at 2 years of age (variable).

4. **Total Anomalous Pulmonary Venous Return:** Surgical repair depends on the type of anomalous drainage (i.e., direct anastomosis of common pulmonary vein, unroofing of coronary sinus, ASD closure such that pulmonary venous blood channels to the left atrium). If obstruction is present, repair must occur early, given the risks of pulmonary hypertension related to obstruction.

5. **Truncus Arteriosus:** Most centers repair in the early newborn period with VSD closure and anastomosis from the right ventricle (RV) to the pulmonary artery (PA), depending on the subtype.

6. **Hypoplastic Left Heart Syndrome:** Repair consists of a staged approach with systemic-to-pulmonary connection and arch reconstruction in the newborn period, followed by a Glenn/hemi-Fontan procedure at approximately 4 months of age and fenestrated Fontan at approximately 2 years of age. Some larger centers are now looking at a hybrid approach to the initial stage in order to avoid cardiopulmonary bypass in the early newborn period. Some centers offer neonatal heart transplantation, and some still offer compassionate care for this lesion.

DISPOSITION

Discharge Goals

The discharge goals and long-term disposition of children with cyanotic CHD are dependent on the diagnosis, whether or not a full anatomic correction was feasible, or if the infant underwent staged palliation. For the immediate term, however, all infants must show adequate weight gain on their particular feeding regimen (oral or tube). Depending on the surgical approach, the infant's oxygen saturation goal will be different and must be managed accordingly.

Outpatient Care

The course and frequency of outpatient follow-up is also dependent on the initial diagnosis and the operative approach. In the child with complete "repair," lifetime follow-up will still be required, as some will need revision of homograft conduits that were placed in infancy and will not grow; others will need placement of pulmonary valves perhaps many years later; and all will be at risk of reentrant arrhythmias in the setting of surgical scars in the atria and/or the ventricles. Infants who embark on surgical palliation for tricuspid atresia, HLHS, or TOF not amenable to infant repair must be watched closely in the early stages, as the initial palliation is often a systemic-to-pulmonary shunt on which all or most of the infant's pulmonary circulation is dependent. Community-acquired illnesses are generally less well tolerated by these infants than by their peers and in many cases might warrant inpatient observation to ensure adequate oxygenation and hydration. Prophylaxis against respiratory syncytial virus (RSV) is recommended for all infants with cyanotic congenital heart disease.

WHAT YOU NEED TO REMEMBER

- Congenital heart disease is the most common congenital malformation in newborns.
- Cyanosis with a prominent murmur should prompt cardiac evaluation.
- The absence of a murmur does not rule out critical congenital heart disease.
- Infants with critical heart lesions might look quite well and have ductal patency.
- Cautious oxygen use in infants with mixing lesions (i.e., single ventricle) is recommended, as they will have compromised systemic circulation in the setting of excessive pulmonary blood flow.

SUGGESTED READINGS

Allen HD et al. *Moss and Adams' Heart Disease in Infants, Children, and Adolescents: Including the Fetus and Young Adult*, 6th ed. Philadelphia: Lippincott Williams and Wilkins, 2001.

Chang A. *Pediatric Cardiac Intensive Care*. Philadelphia: Lippincott Williams & Wilkins, 1998.

Driscoll DJ. Left-to-right shunt lesions. *Pediatr Clin North Am* 1999;46:355–368.

Gessner I, Victoria B. *Pediatric Cardiology: A Problem-based approach*. Philadelphia: Saunders, 1993.

Grifka RG. Cyanotic congenital heart disease with increased pulmonary blood flow. *Pediatr Clin North Am* 1999;46:405–425.

Park M. *Pediatric Cardiology for Practitioners*, 5th ed. Philadelphia: Elsevier, 2007.

Welke KF, Komanapalli C, Shen I, et al. Advances in congenital heart surgery. *Curr Opin Pediatr* 2005;17(5):574–578.

Croup

DEBORAH J. ANDRESEN

THE PATIENT ENCOUNTER

An 18-month-old girl was brought to the emergency department at midnight one night in September with an acute onset of a seal-like, barking cough, a moderate degree of difficulty breathing, and inspiratory stridor. Throughout the day her parents had noted a low-grade fever and runny nose, but her breathing was fine when they put her to bed. On examination, her respiratory rate was 48 and oxygen saturation 97% in room air. She appeared to be in mild to moderate distress, and inspiratory stridor could be heard from across the room. Subcostal retractions were noted and air entry was diminished in both lung fields; however, the lung exam was obscured by the loud inspiratory noises.

OVERVIEW

Definition

Croup, also referred to as *laryngotracheitis*, is a virally induced childhood illness in which swelling and inflammation occur in the larynx and subglottic regions of the trachea. It generally presents as a viral prodrome with 1 to 2 days of upper respiratory infection (URI) symptoms and low-grade fever followed by the acute onset of a harsh, seal-like, barking cough and frequently inspiratory stridor. Croup has the potential to cause a significant degree of respiratory distress in young children because their airways are still very narrow.

Pathophysiology

Croup is caused by viral agents that trigger inflammation and edema of the larynx and the subglottic region of the trachea. This region within the cricoid cartilage is the narrowest area of a toddler's already narrow airway. Swelling of the vocal cords causes the barking cough and hoarse voice, and narrowing of the airway causes increased resistance to airflow, which leads to respiratory distress, as the child has to exert more energy to obtain sufficient oxygen.

Epidemiology

Croup generally occurs between the ages of 6 months and 5 years. Reportedly, 5% of all children experience an episode of croup in their second year of life. Rates of hospitalization are between 1.5% and 5.0% of cases; of those hospitalized, <1% require intubation. Interestingly, males are affected by croup 1.5 times more often than females. Croup peaks in autumn, when parainfluenza viruses types 1 and 2 are most prevalent; there is a trough in midsummer.

Etiology

The most common causes of croup are parainfluenza viruses types 1, 2, and 3. Together they cause 75% of cases. Overall, parainfluenza 1 is the most common etiology. Influenza A, respiratory syncytial virus (RSV), adenovirus, and rhinovirus are other triggers of croup. Influenza has been associated with more severe cases of croup.

ACUTE MANAGEMENT AND WORKUP

Although the majority of patients with croup can be managed as outpatients, it is important to recognize that it can lead to severe respiratory compromise.

The First 15 Minutes

Generally, everyone knows when a patient with croup has arrived to a medical facility because of the characteristic cough. The severity of the illness must be rapidly assessed and other more serious problems, such as bacterial tracheitis and epiglottitis, must be considered. If the patient has stridor at rest, significant retractions on exam, saturations below 93%, altered mentation, or cyanosis, the patient's airway status must be addressed immediately. Nebulized racemic epinephrine is given to alleviate airway obstruction in patients who have a moderate to severe degree of distress. Corticosteroids, which take a minimum of 2 hours to begin to take effect, are generally indicated as well.

The First Few Hours

As always, a thorough history and physical are important. Patients that require nebulized racemic epinephrine must be observed for 3 to 4 hours after the treatment, as the effect of this medication is short-lived and the patient's stridor can recur when its effects wear off.

History

Children with croup generally have a 1- to 2-day history of URI symptoms with associated low-grade fevers. The fevers can be higher if influenza is the causative agent. As the night progresses, the patient develops the classic barking cough, followed by varying degrees of inspiratory stridor and respiratory distress. The illness generally lasts for 3 to 7 days. Croup is believed to be more common in children who have allergies, and there is a familial tendency. It is important to ask about the possibility of foreign-body aspiration and about past medical history (prematurity, intubations, reactive airway disease [RAD]). It is frequently noted that the patient has been exposed to family members with respiratory illnesses.

Physical Examination

It is helpful to keep the patient as calm as possible during the exam because increased anxiety will lead to increased respiratory distress. It is important to note if inspiratory stridor at rest is present, as this will help to guide decision making. The chest wall should be examined for the presence of retractions. Air entry should be assessed. It may be diminished, but wheezes and crackles should not be present unless the patient also has bronchiolitis, asthma, or pneumonia. Oxygenation should be checked via pulse oximetry. The patient's skin color and level of consciousness should also be considered. Patients often have a hoarse voice and an inflamed oropharynx. The typical patient with croup, however, does not look seriously ill. If the patient appears toxic, then other illnesses must be strongly considered.

> ## CLINICAL PEARL
>
> *Croup should not cause hypoxia until the degree of upper airway obstruction is severe, because the alveoli are not affected.*

Labs and Tests to Consider

In the patient with a straightforward case of mild croup, no labs are indicated. In atypical cases in which diagnoses such as bacterial tracheitis and epiglottitis are being considered, appropriate labs include a blood culture and complete blood count (CBC) with differential. These tests are also indicated in patients who appear toxic. Most patients with croup will have a normal CBC and C-reactive protein. Viral testing for influenza, RSV, and parainfluenza may be considered but generally do not affect management.

Imaging

Imaging is not indicated for a patient with a typical case of croup. If antero-posterior (AP) and lateral images of the neck are obtained, the AP image frequently shows the "steeple sign," which is evidence of airway edema and narrowing in the subglottic region that extends approximately 5 to 10 mm below the vocal cords. The steeple sign is not always present with croup.

If a foreign body is suspected based on history or physical exam, x-rays of the chest and neck should be obtained. If other diagnoses such as epiglottitis, bacterial tracheitis, or retropharyngeal abscess are being considered, neck films can aid in the diagnosis; however, airway management must take precedence. On x-ray, epiglottitis reveals a swollen epiglottis, bacterial tracheitis reveals a ragged tracheal column, and a retropharyngeal abscess reveals a widening of the prevertebral tissues. On occasion, airway fluoroscopy can be helpful in atypical cases.

Treatment

The mainstay of treatment in croup is airway management. The majority of patients with mild croup can be treated as outpatients. Using corticosteroids for croup has been controversial, but there is now enough evidence to support its use even in milder cases. Steroids have been proven to decrease symptoms, the need for racemic epinephrine treatments, the number of admissions, and the length of stay in the emergency department. The most commonly administered steroid is a single dose of dexamethasone at 0.6 mg/kg. IM and PO forms have been proven to be equally efficacious. The IM form, therefore, should be reserved for cases in which the patient is vomiting or cannot take an oral medication. Other smaller studies have suggested that dexamethasone 0.15 mg/kg may be equally efficacious for mild croup. The steroids act by decreasing the edema of the airway, and they have not been shown to have any adverse effects when given as a single dose. In more severe cases, some pediatricians give a second dose of dexamethasone the following day, or they may give 2 to 3 days of prednisone.

Nebulized racemic epinephrine causes constriction of the arterioles via stimulation of the alpha receptors. In turn, this leads to decreased capillary hydrostatic pressure, increased fluid resorption around the airway, and decreased edema. It is indicated for the patient who has stridor at rest or moderate respiratory distress. Since it is fast-acting, racemic epinephrine can bring almost immediate relief. Additionally, it has been proven to decrease the need for intubations and tracheotomies in patients with severe croup. Generally, it should not be given more frequently than every 2 hours because of cardiac side effects. Patients who require racemic epinephrine must then be observed for at least 3 to 4 hours because respiratory distress may recur as its effects wear off.

For centuries, cool mist and humidity have been recommended for croup; however, a number of more recent studies do not support their use. Mist tents should not be used, as they can cause several problems: Patients can become hypothermic, they often become more agitated when separated from their parents, they are harder to assess, and the tents can accumulate mold.

Antibiotics, antitussives, and decongestants are not indicated.

Heliox is being examined as a mode of therapy for severe croup as a means to avoid intubation. It is usually administered in an intensive care setting. Helium has one-third the viscosity of air and can decrease resistance to airflow through the narrowed airway. It is mixed with oxygen. Heliox is currently being investigated further, and results have been somewhat promising.

The case patient was treated with nebulized racemic epinephrine and oral Decadron. Fifteen minutes after receiving the racemic epinephrine, she no longer had stridor at rest. She was observed in the emergency department for 4 more hours and then discharged home.

Admission Criteria and Level-of-Care Criteria

Criteria for admission include stridor at rest that returns after treatment with racemic epinephrine and steroids. Patients with significant retractions, altered mental status, or cyanosis warrant further observation as well. The corticosteroid will generally take a minimum of 2 hours to take effect, so this factor can be taken into account when disposition decisions are made. Admission to the ICU is necessary for severe cases that do not respond to racemic epinephrine, as these patients may require intubation to secure the airway.

EXTENDED IN-HOSPITAL MANAGEMENT

The most common cause for ongoing stridor is a prolonged viral illness. Anatomic abnormalities such as polyps, hemangiomas, and vocal cord paralysis must be considered in patients with persistent stridor. These abnormalities can be readily visualized by an ear/nose/throat (ENT) specialist via laryngoscopy. Patients with a history of past intubations can develop subglottic stenosis, leading to narrowing of the airway. Laryngomalacia is a common diagnosis in infancy. Parents will describe a history of loud breathing since birth. These patients generally grow out of this as the cartilage around the airway becomes more firm; however, croup can affect these patients more severely. It is common for patients with underlying gastroesophageal reflux to have baseline airway edema secondary to exposure to gastric acid; it is, therefore, important to address this problem with acid suppressants. The possibility of a foreign-body aspiration should always be considered in cases of persistent stridor.

Obstruction to the airway below the level of the thoracic inlet causes biphasic stridor as opposed to the inspiratory stridor seen with croup. If biphasic stridor is present, an upper gastrointestinal (UGI) series should be considered in order to identify a vascular ring or sling or compression on the airway from another source.

If the patient begins to appear toxic or his or her respiratory status deteriorates, bacterial tracheitis should be considered, as bacterial superinfection can occur secondary to a straightforward case of croup. Typical pathogens include *Staphylococcus aureus*, *Streptococcus pyogenes*, *Streptococcus pneumoniae*, and *Moraxella catarrhalis*. These patients require broad-spectrum antibiotics after a blood culture is obtained, and they frequently require intubation.

DISPOSITION

Discharge Goals

The typical patient with croup generally requires only an overnight stay. Patients are ready for discharge when they no longer have stridor at rest, they have adequate oral intake, and they have not required nebulized racemic epinephrine for at least 4 to 6 hours.

Outpatient Care

It is important to educate parents on signs of respiratory distress associated with croup and to teach them when they need to seek medical help. More often than not, croup is a short-lived viral illness and symptoms subside completely within 3 to 7 days. During an outpatient visit for mild croup, a single dose of dexamethasone is generally indicated. A single dose of dexamethasone has been found to be superior to a single dose of prednisone because of its longer half-life. Frequently, providers will recommend carrying the child out into the cool night air, but this recommendation is based on anecdotal reports, not on strong evidence.

 WHAT YOU NEED TO REMEMBER

- Croup is generally mild and self-limiting; however, airway management takes precedence and must be addressed immediately in moderate to severe cases.
- In atypical cases, other diagnoses should be considered.
- Corticosteroids have been proven to be an effective therapy.

SUGGESTED READINGS

Bjornson CL, Johnson DW. Croup treatment update. *Pediatr Emerg Care* 2005; 21(12):873–870.

Cherry JD. Clinical practice: croup. *N Engl J Med* 2008;358(4):384–391.

Kaditis AG, Wald ER. Viral croup: current diagnosis and treatment. *Pediatr Infect Dis J* 1998;17(9):827–834.

Moore M, Little P. Humidified air inhalation for treating croup. *Cochrane Database Syst Rev* 2006;(3):CD002870.

Russell K, Wiebe N. Glucocorticoids for croup. *Cochrane Database Syst Rev.* 2004; (1):CD001955.

Wright RB, Rowe BH. Current pharmacologic options in the treatment of croup. *Exp Opin Pharmacol* 2005;6(2):255–261.

Cystic Fibrosis

JONATHAN POPLER

THE PATIENT ENCOUNTER

A 2-year-old girl presents with 1 week of cough, congestion, and fever. On examination, she appears to have moderately increased work of breathing, with a respiratory rate of 60 breaths per minute and an oxygen saturation of 92%. Her pediatrician notes that the patient appears thin and has clubbing of her fingernails. Auscultation reveals crackles throughout all lung fields.

OVERVIEW

Definition

Cystic fibrosis (CF) is an autosomal recessive disease caused by mutation of a single gene on the long arm of chromosome 7. The affected gene encodes the polypeptide cystic fibrosis transmembrane regulator (CFTR). More than 1,000 mutations of the CF gene have been identified, with the most common mutation, ΔF508, being a deletion of three base pairs. The CFTR polypeptide functions as a chloride-conducting channel within epithelial membranes (1). Altered or deficient function of the CFTR channel leads to abnormal conduction of water and salt, which in turn leads to derangement of CFTR-containing organs: airways, biliary tree, intestines, vas deferens, sweat ducts, and pancreatic ducts (2).

Pathophysiology

The derangement in the movement of water and salt across cell membranes leads to abnormally thick and viscous secretions. The greatest effect is seen in the airways, where thick, tenacious secretions impair mucociliary clearance, allowing for chronic colonization with bacteria and other organisms. Common bacterial pathogens include *Pseudomonas aeruginosa*, *Staphylococcus aureus*, *Haemophilus influenzae*, and *Stenotrophomonas maltophilia*. Airway colonization with these pathogens leads to prolonged neutrophilic invasion and chronic inflammation of the airway. The organ system most affected in CF is the lung; however, other organ systems are commonly involved.

Virtually all CF patients have exocrine pancreatic insufficiency. Pancreatic secretions are greatly decreased and pancreatic enzymes are not secreted, which in turn leads to autodigestion of the pancreas by its own enzymes. As a result, CF patients suffer from malabsorption and malnutrition. The biliary tract is also affected by CF; almost 30% of CF patients have abnormal liver function tests (3). CF patients are at increased risk for fatty infiltration of the liver, gallstones, and biliary cirrhosis.

Most men with CF (98%) are infertile and have abnormalities of the seminal vesicles and vas deferentia. Women have normal reproductive function, although there are alterations in the viscosity of cervical mucus.

Epidemiology

CF is one of the most common genetic disorders in whites, with an estimated incidence of 1 in 3,000. There are close to 30,000 patients with CF in the United States and approximately 60,000 patients worldwide. CF is less common in Asian, African American, and Hispanic patients.

Etiology

The most common mutation in CF is a three-base-pair deletion at position 508 of the CFTR protein, which codes for phenylalanine. There are >1,000 CF mutations identified, with the majority resulting in amino acid substitutions or nonsense mutations (2). Neonatal screening for CF is currently available in 37 states.

ACUTE MANAGEMENT AND WORKUP

Many CF patients presenting with an acute pulmonary exacerbation will have previously been diagnosed, and the pathogens colonizing their airways will likely already have been cultured on previous clinical visits. However, in areas where neonatal screening is not available, a pulmonary exacerbation may mark the first time that a CF patient seeks medical attention (as with our patient encounter).

The First 15 Minutes

You must first assess the patient's level of respiratory distress. The presence of tachypnea, retractions, significant hypoxia, and markedly increased work of breathing, including accessory respiratory muscle use, are worrisome and may signify impending respiratory failure.

The First Few Hours

Most CF patients with a pulmonary exacerbation require hospitalization. CF patients should routinely be admitted to a children's hospital and, if possible, to a CF care center accredited by the Cystic Fibrosis Foundation. The typical care of a CF patient will include intravenous and inhaled antibiotics, airway clearance therapy, and enzyme supplementation.

History

The diagnosis of CF should be suspected in any patient with chronic respiratory symptoms, including chronic cough, wheezing, or poor exercise capacity. Meconium ileus, caused by thick, inspissated meconium, is a common presentation in the neonatal period. As pancreatic insufficiency increases, failure to thrive is a common presentation in infancy and childhood. CF should be suspected in patients with weight loss, failure to gain weight, or oily stools.

Although CF patients often have chronic respiratory symptoms, including productive cough and exercise intolerance, CF patients with a pulmonary exacerbation will often present with increased cough and sputum, increased work of breathing, or hemoptysis. A thorough and careful history will often aid in the management of the CF patient. The history should focus on the patient's acute symptoms as well as on chronic outpatient management. For example, it is helpful to assess the length of time the patient has been feeling short of breath or has had increased difficulty in breathing. However, it is also helpful to find out what pathogens have been cultured from the patient in the past, as this will guide empiric antibiotic therapy.

Physical Examination

CF patients will often have physical examination findings consistent with endobronchitis, including tachypnea, grunting, and nasal flaring. On auscultation, rales, rhonchi, and wheezing may be heard. In addition to physical exam findings indicative of acute illness, CF patients often have findings of chronic disease. These include nasal polyps, clubbing of the digits, cachexia, hepatosplenomegaly, increased anteroposterior diameter of the chest, scoliosis, and kyphosis.

Labs and Tests to Consider

Although the diagnosis of a CF exacerbation is often apparent, laboratory testing and imaging can help with both the initial management and chronic care.

Key Diagnostic Labs and Tests

In patients with suspected CF who have not received neonatal screening, a sweat chloride test is commonly performed; this test often shows high concentrations of chloride and sodium within sweat. A concentration in sweat >60 mmol/L is considered diagnostic of CF (3). CF genotyping to diagnose the most common CF mutations should be considered when the diagnosis is uncertain.

Initial testing of a CF patient with an acute pulmonary exacerbation should include a complete blood count, C-reactive protein, erythrocyte sedimentation rate, and a complete metabolic profile. Sputum should be obtained for culture. For patients unable to produce a sputum sample, sputum collection may be aided by administration of nebulized hypertonic saline. For younger patients, a throat swab can be sent for culture on the assumption that pathogens obtained on throat culture will correlate with the pathogens colonizing the airway. Fiberoptic bronchoscopy is another method used to obtain sputum for culture in patients unable to provide an adequate sputum sample. Pulmonary function testing is often helpful in both acute and chronic settings. The progressive airway and parenchymal lung damage of CF patients causes airflow obstruction, which can be well characterized by pulmonary function testing. The forced expiratory volume in 1 second (FEV_1) of CF patients is often decreased. As the disease progresses, the FEV_1 continues to decrease; as pulmonary fibrosis and scarring progress, associated air trapping will cause an increased ratio of residual volume to total lung capacity (RV/TLC). CF patients often know their baseline FEV_1 and forced vital capacity (FVC); an acute drop in these values can help characterize the severity of the exacerbation.

Imaging

Chest radiography is an important part of evaluating both acute pulmonary exacerbations and chronic progression of disease. Findings on chest radiography include hyperinflation, peribronchial thickening, air trapping, and consolidation. The Brasfield scoring system exists to help standardize the severity of CF as it appears on chest radiography. CF is best imaged by using high-resolution computed tomography (HRCT). On HRCT, CF often evokes the appearance of bronchiectasis, consolidation, bronchial wall thickening, the tree-in-bud sign, mucous plugging, and thickening of interlobular septa.

Treatment

On an inpatient basis, the typical care of a CF patient with a pulmonary exacerbation includes antibiotic therapy tailored to the pathogens colonizing the airways, airway clearance therapy, and enzyme supplementation. Typical pathogens include *P. aeruginosa*, *S. aureus*, *H. influenzae*, and *S. maltophilia*. CF patients are often initially colonized with *S. aureus* and *H. influenzae*, thus requiring antibiotic treatment to cover both bacteria. As CF patients grow older, most become colonized with *P. aeruginosa* and may suffer from a more rapid decline in pulmonary function and a corresponding increase in the number and severity of hospitalizations. Pulmonary exacerbations of patients known to be colonized with *P. aeruginosa* must include appropriate pseudomonal coverage, such as aminoglycosides and fluoroquinolones. Patients colonized with *Burkholderia cepacia* have more severe disease and worse clinical outcomes.

The case patient was admitted for further evaluation and management. A sweat test was positive for CF at 80 mmol/L, and a chest x-ray revealed right-upper- and left-lower-lobe opacities consistent with pneumonia. She was treated with intravenous antibiotics and aggressive airway clearance and was started on pancreatic enzymes. Sputum cultures did not reveal evidence of colonization with *Pseudomonas* or *Cepacia*.

Admission Criteria and Level-of-Care Criteria

Most CF patients presenting with an acute exacerbation will require hospitalization. They often do not need to be admitted to the intensive care unit unless they have progressed to end-stage disease. Their hospital stay can be anywhere from 1 to 4 weeks, depending on their rate of improvement and clinical symptoms.

EXTENDED IN-HOSPITAL MANAGEMENT

The inpatient treatment of a CF patient will consist of directed antibiotic therapy, airway clearance, and nutritional supplementation. Intravenous antibiotic therapy will be tailored to known pathogens that colonize the patient's airways. The patient will also receive intensive airway clearance treatment. The clearance of mucus and inflammatory debris from the airways will help improve the patient's lung function. To this end, patients will often receive nebulized hypertonic saline, which will induce the expectoration of mucus. Inhaled dornase alfa is also used as a twice-daily nebulized medication. Dornase alfa is thought to decrease the viscosity of purulent sputum and thus help to relieve mucous plugging. In addition, patients will receive mechanical airway clearance treatment, such as manual chest physiotherapy, autogenic drainage with forced expirations, and high-frequency oscillating vest therapy.

CLINICAL PEARL

An important part of both acute and chronic management of CF patients is nutrition maintenance.

Patients with CF have severe malabsorption, requiring supplementation of the fat-soluble vitamins (vitamins A, D, E, and K). CF patients must also supplement their meals and snacks with pancreatic enzymes because the exocrine function of the pancreas is destroyed.

DISPOSITION

Discharge Goals

CF patients will often spend 2 to 3 weeks in the hospital during a pulmonary exacerbation. There are several discharge criteria. These include resolution of respiratory symptoms, such as decreased cough and normal respiratory rate. The patient must be afebrile. The FEV_1 should return to baseline values or at least demonstrate clear improvement. Other discharge criteria include good caloric intake and nutrition. CF patients often lose weight during a pulmonary exacerbation and should show weight gain and improved nutritional status before discharge.

Outpatient Care

The outpatient care of CF patients is often challenging. They may require monthly or semimonthly clinical visits. CF patients often require prophylactic antibiotics even when they are asymptomatic. This may include coverage for *S. aureus*, *H. influenzae*, and *S. maltophilia*. Patients who are colonized with *P. aeruginosa* will be treated with several-month-long courses of inhaled aminoglycides each year in an effort to decrease colonization of the airways. Patients will also continue their airway clearance maneuvers at home, to include both autogenic and manual drainage. Macrolide antibiotics, as well as ibuprofen, are being increasingly used for their anti-inflammatory properties. CF patients are also advised to carefully maintain their weight and nutritional status by continuing vitamin and pancreatic enzyme supplementation. They may often add nutritional supplements to their meals in an effort to increase caloric intake. Patients who continue to have trouble maintaining an appropriate weight will be offered a gastrostomy tube to aid with nutritional supplementation.

CF is a progressive disease. Median life expectancy is currently 33 years (2). As FEV_1 decreases and the number and severity of exacerbations increases, many patients will require more frequent hospital admissions. When CF patients reach end-stage disease, often signified by an $FEV_1 < 30\%$, many will be offered lung transplantation.

WHAT YOU NEED TO REMEMBER

- Meconium ileus should always prompt an investigation for CF.
- The diagnosis of CF should be suspected in any pediatric patient with chronic respiratory symptoms and/or failure to thrive.
- Common pathogens colonizing the airways of CF patients include *P. aeruginosa*, *S. aureus*, *H. influenzae*, and *S. maltophilia*.
- Aggressive antibiotic therapy, airway clearance, and nutritional supplementation are the mainstays of CF treatment.

REFERENCES

1. Cystic Fibrosis Foundation. *Cystic Fibrosis Foundation Patient Registry Annual Report 2000.* Bethesda, MD: Cystic Fibrosis Foundation, 2001.
2. Kerby GS, Accurso FJ, Deterding RR, et al. Respiratory tract and mediastinum. In Hay WW, Levin MJ, Sondheimer JM, Deterding RR, eds. *Current Diagnosis and Treatment in Pediatrics,* 18th ed. New York: Lange Medical Books/McGraw-Hill, 2007.
3. Ratjen F, Doring, G. Cystic fibrosis. *Lancet* 2003;361:681.

Delivery Room

SARAH D. KEENE AND DAVID A. MUNSON

THE PATIENT ENCOUNTER

The pediatric staff is called to the vaginal delivery of an infant in his 35th week of gestation. The mother had rupture of membranes the previous day. She noted a fever on the morning of admission. Her pregnancy was uneventful with the exception of gestational diabetes mellitus. The obstetrics staff reports that the infant has begun to experience heart rate decelerations following contractions. They have also noted meconium staining of the amniotic fluid.

After delivery, the infant is noted to be limp, blue, and lacking notable respiratory effort. He is intubated and suctioned to remove meconium from the airway. At 30 seconds of life, he is again assessed and remains limp, blue, and apneic. Intubation and meconium aspiration is repeated. At 1 minute of life, his heart rate is approximately 50 beats per minute (bpm). The infant is dried and stimulated, and positive-pressure ventilation is initiated with an available bag-mask. The heart rate increases to >100 bpm over the next 20 to 25 seconds, and the infant begins to breathe spontaneously. His skin color remains blue on his chest, face, and extremities. A pulse oximeter is placed in his hand and the value is 82%. This is improved with 100% oxygen delivery. He is therefore placed on oxygen via nasal cannula and transferred to the neonatal intensive care unit for extended management.

OVERVIEW

Definition

At delivery, an infant must successfully transition from the intrauterine environment to the external one. The term *perinatal depression* refers to the state of an infant who is not vigorous at birth and needs help with this transition. Perinatal depression can result from almost any factor affecting the pregnancy, be it a remote occurrence or something related to the birth process itself. It can be mild and reversible or severe, resulting in asphyxia, lack of oxygen, and permanent neurologic sequelae. Delivery room management centers on providing supportive care at the time of transition and assessing and treating those infants that need assistance.

Pathophysiology

Birth is a complicated and challenging process that requires an infant to transition rapidly from having fluid-filled lungs and experiencing placental gas exchange to breathing air and experiencing pulmonary gas exchange. A newborn must possess sufficient respiratory drive to breathe as well as the muscle power to take in air, recruit functional residual capacity, mobilize lung fluid into the interstitium, and expel fluid from the large airways. Alveolar recruitment is accompanied by relaxation of pulmonary arterioles mediated by mechanical changes and chemical and paracrine signals, including the generation of thromboxane and nitric oxide. The resulting circulatory changes include transitioning from a high-resistance pulmonary vascular system with minimal blood flow to separated circulatory systems with the entire body's blood flow passing through the lungs. The heart must compensate for this change as well as the rapid increase in blood pressure that results from the removal of the placenta from the circulation. The infant must also be able to maintain his temperature in the extrauterine environment and rapidly convert over the next hours from placental nutrition to oral.

Epidemiology

The complex interactions required after birth make it a high-risk time. Infants are more likely to die in the neonatal period (0 to 28 days) than at any other time in childhood. General estimates are that 10% of infants will require some assistance to transition into the extrauterine environment and 1% will require significant help, such as chest compressions or epinephrine treatments. The neonatal death rate is low in the United States (<5 per 1,000) and the developed world; such deaths stem mainly from prematurity and congenital anomalies.

Etiology

Any factor that compromises the health of the mother or fetus or affects placental–fetal blood exchange can result in a depressed or ill infant that needs active resuscitation. Maternal factors including maternal illness (e.g., diabetes, hypertension), anesthesia or medication use, and intrauterine infections (e.g., chorioamnionitis) can affect oxygenation, blood flow, and the overall health of the fetus. The aspiration of meconium or blood or simply a slower than usual clearance of fluid from the lungs, usually referred to as *delayed transition*, can cause respiratory distress. Placental anomalies, placental abruption, and umbilical cord complications can all result in a chronically or acutely compromised infant. Congenital malformations and infections along with prematurity can also result in an infant who needs assistance in the delivery room.

Respiratory Distress Syndrome

Neonatal respiratory distress syndrome (RDS), once more commonly referred to as *hyaline membrane disease*, is a disorder common to premature infants, but it can also present in late preterm (weeks 34 to 37) and full-term infants. RDS occurs in most infants born before 28 weeks' gestation, although the incidence is lower if glucocorticoid therapy is given to the mother prior to delivery. Even with several effective treatments, RDS can lead to morbidity and mortality. RDS results from insufficient amounts of surfactant, a mixture of lipids and proteins that lines the alveoli. Surfactant aids respiration by decreasing alveolar surface tension, thereby lessening the work required for lung expansion. In premature infants, the combination of surfactant deficiency and a highly compliant chest makes lung inflation difficult to maintain. Chest radiographs often demonstrate underinflation of the lungs and a characteristic ground-glass appearance. Treatment includes maintaining lung volumes, either through continuous positive airway pressure (CPAP) delivered nasally or mechanical ventilation, and surfactant replacement.

Infection

Infection is a common cause of respiratory distress in infants, whether it occurs as a result of pneumonia or systemic infection, known as *sepsis*. Bacteria or other pathogens may enter through the maternal bloodstream, pass into the uterus after the rupture of membranes during labor, or infect the baby from the maternal genitourinary tract during delivery. Risk factors for infection (Table 10-1) heighten concern and, with symptomatology, should prompt treatment. A blood culture may reveal the causative bacteria, but many cultures are negative even in infants who clinically appear to have fulminant sepsis. A chest radiograph may demonstrate hazy lung fields or areas of opacification in cases of pneumonia, but true focal disease is unusual.

The two most common organisms in neonatal sepsis are group B *Streptococcus* (GBS) and *Escherichia coli*. Other enteric organisms—*Enterococcus* spp., *Enterobacter* spp., *Klebsiella* spp., and *Listeria monocytogenes*—are also

TABLE 10-1
Risk Factors for Perinatal Infection

Maternal fever

Maternal chorioamnionitis

Maternal GBS, especially a urinary tract infection or affected sibling

Other maternal infection at delivery

Prolonged rupture of membranes (>18 hours)

Prematurity

Premature rupture of membranes

Male gender

GBS, group B *Streptococcus*.

causes of neonatal infection. The neonatal immune system is, in fact, so underdeveloped that almost any organism can be pathogenic.

GBS causes pneumonia and sepsis and has historically been the leading infectious cause of neonatal morbidity and mortality in the United States. The Centers for Disease Control and Prevention (CDC) currently recommend universal maternal screening for rectovaginal colonization with GBS during the 35th to 37th week of pregnancy and the use of intrapartum antibiotic prophylaxis for GBS carriers. This has resulted in a reduction by more than half of the cases of GBS; the incidence is currently approximately 0.33 cases per 1,000 live births (CDC 2005 data). *E. coli* and other gram-negatives have become more prevalent as a result of this change.

Meconium

The passage of meconium into the amniotic fluid is a sign of fetal distress that occurs following some degree of hypoxemia during labor, which causes increased bowel contractility. Meconium is present in 10% to 20% of deliveries and is estimated to cause respiratory distress in 2% of infants. This can be anywhere on the spectrum from mild tachypnea to fulminant respiratory failure and can include pulmonary hypertension and death. Chest x-ray characteristically shows patchy lung disease with areas of collapse, or atelectasis, and areas of hyperinflation.

Respiratory distress associated with meconium occurs through two pathways. First, the presence of meconium may simply be a marker of in utero distress rather than a true cause of the respiratory insufficiency. Second, the meconium itself can cause an obstructive and inflammatory process after entering the airways. Pulmonary hypertension is one of the feared consequences of meconium aspiration syndrome (MAS) and is associated with significant morbidity and mortality. Severe pulmonary hypertension is treated with oxygenation, ventilation, pulmonary vasodilatory agents (e.g., nitric oxide), and surfactant replacement therapy.

Maternal Factors

Specific maternal factors may also cause distress in the child. As stated earlier, evidence of acute maternal fever or infection can be indicative of a heightened risk for fetal infection. Maternal gestational diabetes mellitus results in delayed lung maturity and surfactant production, so a full-term infant may present with surfactant deficiency. Infants of diabetic mothers are also often large for gestational age, placing them at risk for difficult and complicated deliveries. Magnesium is used in the treatment of preeclampsia and eclampsia but has a side effect of muscle relaxation, which can present as poor respiratory effort or apnea. Anesthetic given to the mother for delivery can also pass across the placenta and cause respiratory distress or apnea. Maternal use of narcotics or sedatives, whether prescribed or illicit, can also affect the newborn.

Infant-Specific Factors

Congenital anomalies in the newborn infant may also present immediately after delivery because of the physiologic changes required in the first few minutes of life. Many airway, lung, and cardiac anomalies are asymptomatic in utero and may go undiagnosed, especially if prenatal care has been limited. A small jaw (micrognathia), choanal atresia, vocal cord abnormalities, airway stenosis, and tracheoesophageal fistula may all present in the immediate postpartum period with respiratory distress. More distal airway malformations and lung abnormalities may also become apparent with the first few breaths. Isolated congenital heart disease often causes cyanosis, with tachypnea secondary to hypoxia. Central nervous system disease often presents with impaired respiratory drive, whether it is related to asphyxia during labor and delivery or to congenital malformation or disease in the newborn infant.

ACUTE MANAGEMENT AND WORKUP

The goal of the acute management period is to assess whether infants need immediate intervention or continued care and monitoring outside of standard well-infant care.

The First 15 Minutes

The Neonatal Resuscitation Program (NRP) and the American Association of Pediatrics (AAP) recommend that every hospital with a delivery program have staff whose sole responsibility is care of the newborn infant, with the skills required for resuscitation if necessary. The key to preparation is having the necessary equipment available and anticipating difficulty in high-risk situations. Essential equipment is listed in Table 10-2.

Assessment and treatment should begin immediately after birth. With the exception of the nonvigorous infant who was exposed to meconium, neonatal resuscitation universally begins with drying, suctioning, and stimulation. This initial step is given 30 seconds, during which time initial estimates of respiratory effort and heart rate should be made. For most newborns, these maneuvers will be adequate to facilitate ventilation and ensure temperature control.

The Apgar scoring system (Table 10-3), which includes five components of the exam that are indicators of the neonate's condition, is commonly used in the initial assessment. The functions of the Apgar scoring system are to identify infants who need intervention (usually a total Apgar score <7) and to assess the response to treatment. Scoring is done starting at 1 minute, although assessment and treatment should begin immediately. Scoring is repeated at 5 minutes and then after every 5 minutes until an infant no longer requires intervention. The Apgar score also provides a fairly universal method of communicating initial delivery and resuscitation information

TABLE 10-2
Essential Equipment for Delivery Room Resuscitation

Requirement	Equipment
Temperature control	Radiant warmer Towels for drying
Airway clearance	Bulb syringe, suction source and catheters, meconium aspirator
Assistance with respiration	Stethoscope Apparatus for bag-mask ventilation, oral airway, equipment for intubation (laryngoscope numbers 0 and 1, endotracheal tubes [sizes 2.5–4.0])
Obtaining intravenous access	Sterile gloves, masks, gowns Umbilical catheter equipment
Medications for emergent resuscitation	Epinephrine (ET/IV), naloxone (ET/IV), atropine (ET/IV), sodium bicarbonate, calcium gluconate Volume expanders (normal saline), 10% dextrose solution

TABLE 10-3
Apgar Scoring System

	Score		
Sign	**0**	**1**	**2**
Heart rate	Absent	<100	>100
Respirations	Absent	Irregular	Regular or crying
Color	Blue or white	Pink body, blue extremities	Fully pink
Muscle tone	Limp	Some flexion	Active motion
Reflex irritability[a]	No response	Grimace	Cough, sneeze, or cry

[a]Generally refers to response to suctioning or stimulation

about a baby to other caregivers. The 5-minute Apgar score is sometimes referred to as the "prognostic Apgar," and indeed a 5-minute Apgar score <3 is associated with poor neurologic outcomes, although this is by no means universal.

CLINICAL PEARL

After initial assessment and along with stimulation and suctioning, the AAP guidelines for infant resuscitation (available at www.aap.org/nrp/nrpmain.html) prioritize establishment of successful ventilation. This is the single most important factor in the resuscitation of a depressed neonate and will often be adequate for recovery of heart rate, followed by oxygenation and tone.

If the infant is not breathing spontaneously after stimulation and suctioning during the first 30 seconds of life, assisted ventilation should be provided using a bag-mask apparatus. The infant's head and mask position should be adjusted until adequate air entry is established. Some infants will require intubation for successful ventilation.

Cardiac maneuvers (e.g., chest compressions, medications) may be initiated once ventilation has been established and provided for 30 seconds. Chest compressions should be commenced for a heart rate <60 bpm and stopped after it is has risen to >60 bpm. Continued care will be required until the infant has reached a normal heart rate and is breathing spontaneously. Infants who require this level of care at delivery will often need continued support or, at a minimum, observation in an intensive care unit.

The First Few Hours

The infant in our case scenario is observed and continues to require 100% oxygen to keep his saturation level >95%. He develops nasal flaring and intercostal retractions. An arterial blood gas (ABG) reading is performed and reveals decreased arteriolar oxygen concentration, with a PaO_2 of 45 mm Hg. He is intubated to maintain gas exchange and oxygenation. Blood is obtained for culture, and fluids containing dextrose as well as antibiotics (ampicillin and gentamicin) are administered. A chest radiograph reveals hazy lung fields with poor expansion and a ground-glass appearance, so the infant is treated with endotracheal surfactant.

History

A detailed maternal and pregnancy history is essential to care for the infant appropriately. Maternal age and past medical history, legal and illegal drug use, and laboratory work, including blood type and infectious disease screening labs, should be obtained. Information about vertically transmissible diseases (hepatitis, HIV, syphilis) should be obtained early. The results of GBS cultures are also important in treating the infant. The pregnancy course—including complications such as premature labor, gestational diabetes, and pregnancy-induced hypertension—may also have an impact on the newborn.

Physical Examination

The general physical exam of a newborn infant should include an evaluation for congenital anomalies as well as evidence of acute distress. The essential initial components are those contained in the Apgar scoring system: heart rate, respiratory effort, color, and passive tone. The infant should then have a brief head-to-toe physical exam to evaluate for any congenital anomalies that could be life-threatening. The general appearance of the infant's face is important because many syndromes, including the trisomies, present with recognizable patterns of abnormality. Positioning of the eyes and ears, as well as cataracts, can all be indicators of disease. The mouth and palate should be assessed for clefts and other deficits that may impair feeding. The infant's head shape should be assessed both as an indicator of blood loss into the scalp from birth (a cephalohematoma or subgaleal bleeding) and to look for normal anterior and posterior fontanelles and cranial sutures.

The remainder of the body should be examined systematically. You should observe the infant's breathing to look for nasal flaring, abdominal desynchrony, and retractions that indicate respiratory distress. Auscultation should be done for symmetric air entry and stridor. The newborn cardiac exam focuses on murmurs and other abnormal heart sounds as well as on peripheral pulses and perfusion. A normal finding in a newborn infant is a single second heart sound (S_2), which will begin to split over the next hours to days. You should assess the abdomen for distention, which can indicate an obstructive process or abdominal mass. The anus should be assessed for patency and the gender should be confirmed with a careful examination of the genitalia. A basic neurologic exam for alertness, response to stimuli, and spontaneous movement of all extremities should also be performed as part of the initial assessment.

Labs and Tests to Consider

The evaluation of a sick infant is complicated by the lack of specific findings on the physical exam, although markers in the history can be useful. Laboratory evaluation should be multifaceted along several pathways until a diagnosis can be made.

Key Diagnostic Tests and Labs

Handheld machines for monitoring blood glucose and blood gases allow for the rapid reporting of results. Blood glucose is often abnormal in ill infants and will require treatment. A blood gas monitor provides the pH as well as information on oxygenation (PaO_2) and ventilation (PCO_2). This reading allows assessment of ventilator strategy and treatment for significant acidosis if present. Onsite blood gas readings also frequently report ionized calcium as well as hemoglobin and hematocrit values. These are useful when anemia or acute blood loss is suspected.

Other laboratory studies are useful in the first few minutes to hours. A complete blood count (CBC) will evaluate for anemia and screen for infection (low or high white blood cell count) and thrombocytopenia. A C-reactive protein may aid in the diagnosis of infection, although this may be mildly elevated after delivery. If infection is suspected, a blood culture and lumbar puncture should be obtained.

Imaging

In acute delivery room management, portable x-ray may occasionally be required to evaluate an infant who is not responding to therapies. A chest x-ray may show a pneumothorax, which requires a chest tube, or anomalies, such as a congenital diaphragmatic hernia or cystic lung lesion, which require specialized care. Other necessary imaging can usually be performed after transfer to the intensive care unit (ICU). Chest and abdominal x-rays can provide specific information on the cause of lung disease and abdominal distention or emesis. They are also necessary to verify proper positioning of endotracheal tubes, nasogastric tubes, chest tubes, and umbilical lines if placement was required in the delivery room. In infants in whom an acute neurologic complication is suspected, ultrasound or computed tomography of the head is indicated.

Treatment

After initial delivery room care, as guided by the NRP algorithm, the majority of infants will require only standard care in the newborn nursery. The essential components are monitoring of cardiac and respiratory status, feeding behaviors, hydration status, blood sugar maintenance, and temperature control. An infant with difficulty in any of these areas may require care in the ICU.

Focal treatment is possible for some illnesses. An infant of a diabetic mother may require glucose infusion until he is able to maintain blood sugars in a normal range. Infants with suspected or diagnosed infections will be treated with antibiotics or with antiviral or antifungal drugs. An infant with respiratory distress may require oxygen supplementation by nasal cannula, CPAP for lung distention, or mechanical ventilation.

Admission Criteria and Level of Care Criteria

Levels of newborn care vary according to the specific hospital and may include the well-newborn nursery, special care nursery, and various levels of neonatal intensive care.

EXTENDED IN-HOSPITAL MANAGEMENT

Extended in-hospital management is beyond the scope of this chapter.

DISPOSITION

Several hours later, the nurse reports that the patient is breathing more comfortably. He remains intubated for 2 days and is then extubated and requires a nasal cannula for 2 more days. Blood cultures done the day of admission grow GBS, but a lumbar puncture reveals no evidence of meningitis. The baby receives a full 10-day course of antibiotics. Following extubation, he begins to take breast milk by mouth, and by the time of discharge is eating well.

Discharge Goals

Discharge goals are similar for all newborns regardless of gestational age and problems at delivery. They must have completed the transition to extrauterine life. Temperature control, stable respirations and gas exchange, and the ability to take in adequate nutrition are key, whether these markers occurs at a few minutes of life or several months later.

Outpatient Care

Frequent outpatient visits are required for all newborn infants. Infants with uncomplicated deliveries will often be discharged by 2 days of life. Follow-up is needed to assess weight gain and often to track jaundice. Infants who were born prematurely, have congenital anomalies, or had significant illness at birth are at higher risk for later illness and readmission. In newborns who require active resuscitation, considerably more follow-up care may be required. Infants with perinatal depression who have asphyxia require neurodevelopmental follow-up and may require lifelong care.

 WHAT YOU NEED TO REMEMBER

- The maternal and pregnancy history will provide key information about which infants are at high risk for needing assistance in the delivery room.
- Every delivery team should include at least one member whose primary responsibility is the infant and who is trained in resuscitation.
- Effective ventilation is the single most important step in the resuscitation of the compromised newborn.
- There are multiple causes of perinatal depression, but they are all managed initially by following the NRP resuscitation protocol.

SUGGESTED READINGS

Baltimore RS. Consequences of prophylaxis for group b streptococcal infections of the neonate. *Semin Perinatol* 2007;31(1):33–38.

Contributors and Reviewers for the Neonatal Resuscitation Guidelines. International Guidelines for Neonatal Resuscitation: an excerpt from the guidelines 2000 for cardiopulmonary resuscitation and emergency cardiovascular care: International Consensus on Science. *Pediatrics* 2000;106:e29.

NRP Web site for current recommendations: http://www.aap.org/nrp/pdf/nrp-summary.pdf

Vain NE, Szyld EG, Prudent LM, et al. Oropharyngeal and nasopharyngeal suctioning of meconium-stained neonates before delivery of their shoulders: multicentre, randomised controlled trial. *Lancet* 2004;364:597–602.

Diabetic Ketoacidosis

MELINDA PENN AND ADDA GRIMBERG

THE PATIENT ENCOUNTER

An 8-year-old boy presents to his pediatrician's office with a 2-day history of abdominal pain and vomiting. He reports 2 weeks of increased thirst, frequent urination, and nocturia. On examination, he is found to have had a 10-pound weight loss since his well-child exam 2 months prior. He appears ill and is tachycardic and tachypneic, with a sighing-like respiratory pattern and a fruity smell to his breath. His mucous membranes are dry and his extremities cool, but he is alert, oriented, and cooperative. He is found to have a "critical high" reading on a finger-stick glucose monitor and positive glucose and ketones in his urine.

OVERVIEW

Definition

Diabetic ketoacidosis (DKA) is defined by hyperglycemia (blood glucose >200 mg/dL), a venous pH <7.3, and a bicarbonate reading <15 mmol/L. DKA can be further classified as mild (pH 7.2 to 7.3), moderate (pH 7.1 to 7.19), or severe (pH <7.1).

Pathophysiology

Diabetic ketoacidosis is caused by insulin deficiency. It can occur in patients with type 1 diabetes mellitus (DM), either at the time of disease onset (after progressive beta cell destruction) or later, after omission of exogenous insulin. The imbalance between insulin and its counterregulatory hormones (glucagon, catecholamines, cortisol, and growth hormone) leads to increased gluconeogenesis and glycogenolysis, resulting in hyperglycemia, hyperosmolarity, an osmotic diuresis, progressive electrolyte loss, and dehydration. Increased lipolysis produces free fatty acids and ketones (betahydroxybutyrate and acetoacetate), leading to a metabolic acidosis (1).

Epidemiology

Approximately 25% of patients in the United States with new-onset type I DM will present with DKA. It occurs more frequently in younger children, children of lower socioeconomic status, and children without diabetic family members. In patients with known diabetes, the risk of DKA is 1% to 10% per year (2).

Etiology

Ketoacidosis can occur in patients with new-onset type I DM as a result of progressive beta-cell destruction and resulting insulin deficiency. It is also seen in patients with known type I DM when insulin is omitted or at times of stress or illness, resulting in increased stress-hormone response and a relative insulin deficiency.

ACUTE MANAGEMENT AND WORKUP

The appropriate setting in which to treat a child with DKA must be determined based on the severity of the illness and whether the diagnosis of diabetes was previously known. Any patient with a history of polyuria and polydipsia should be evaluated for diabetes; if found to have glucosuria or hyperglycemia, further evaluation for DKA should be pursued. In patients with known type I DM, hyperglycemia and ketosis can often be managed on an outpatient basis with close supervision. However, patients with vomiting, persistent ketosis, severe dehydration, respiratory symptoms, altered mental status, or a history of noncompliance should be evaluated emergently.

The First 15 Minutes

The major cause of morbidity and mortality in DKA is cerebral edema, but patients are also at risk for severe dehydration, electrolyte imbalance, and the associated complications. Patients should first be evaluated for evidence of severe obtundation, as this can compromise the airway and be evidence of cerebral edema. The degree of dehydration should also be assessed, with close attention to signs of cardiovascular failure (e.g., tachycardia, poor pulses, and cool extremities). All patients should be placed on cardiac monitors, and intravenous access should be obtained for fluid resuscitation and frequent laboratory sampling. Severe cases may require arterial lines.

The First Few Hours

The severity of DKA at presentation determines the early management. Care should be taken to correct fluid and electrolyte imbalances without placing the patient at greater risk for cerebral edema, and close attention should be paid to the patient's neurologic status.

History

Children with DKA typically present with symptoms of diabetes (polyuria, polydipsia, polyphagia, and weight loss). Vomiting and abdominal pain are often seen, especially when acidosis is present. Dehydration, abnormal breathing (known as *Kussmaul respirations*), and mental status changes are also frequently noted. Evidence for infection or other inciting illness should be assessed. In children with known diabetes, the omission of insulin, insulin pump failure, the use of expired insulin, or failure to follow "sick day" rules should be evaluated.

Physical Examination

The degree of dehydration and level of consciousness are of greatest importance in evaluating a patient with DKA, but you should perform a full physical exam, paying close attention to signs of infection that can lead to DKA. An accurate weight should be obtained to use for fluid replacement calculations and to help determine the level of dehydration (by comparing with the weight prior to the onset of illness). The severity of dehydration may be difficult to assess because of the presence of hyperosmolarity, but evidence of dehydration includes dry mucous membranes, sunken eyes, cool extremities, decreased strength of pulses, prolonged capillary refill, tachycardia, and hypotension. A funduscopic exam to look for papilledema is also important to evaluate for potential cerebral edema. Deep, labored breathing (Kussmaul respirations) is present in severe acidosis and occurs as a compensatory mechanism to "blow off" excess carbon dioxide. A fruity odor to the patient's breath may be noted and is caused by the presence of acetone. Abdominal pain and tenderness can be a result of acidosis, but appendicitis and other causes of an acute abdomen can result in DKA in patients with diabetes and should not be overlooked. Mucocutaneous candidiasis is frequently seen in patients with new-onset or poorly controlled diabetes.

Labs and Tests to Consider

Initial labs help to determine the degree of acidosis, dehydration, electrolyte abnormalities, and hyperglycemia. Additional labs are sent in patients presenting with their first episode of ketoacidosis in order to confirm the diagnosis and differentiate between type 1 and type 2 diabetes.

Key Diagnostic Labs and Tests

Patients presenting with a history and physical exam concerning for DKA should initially have a venous blood gas, serum betahydroxybutyrate, serum or plasma glucose, and electrolyte panel, including sodium, potassium, bicarbonate, creatinine, blood urea nitrogen, calcium, magnesium, and phosphorus ordered to assess for the severity of acidosis, dehydration, and electrolyte abnormalities. Pseudohyponatremia is often seen as a result of hyperglycemia and osmotic dilution. The following formula is used to determine the true sodium level:

$$\text{Measured [Na]} + 1.6 \times [(\text{glucose in mg/dL} - 100)/100]$$

Children with DKA have a total body potassium deficit but may present with normal, increased, or decreased potassium levels owing to transcellular shifts. Intracellular phosphate levels are also decreased with DKA, and phosphate is likewise lost through the osmotic diuresis.

Patients with hyperkalemia should be placed on cardiac monitors and an electrocardiogram should be performed to assess for cardiac abnormalities that occur in the context of abnormalities in serum potassium, magnesium, or phosphorus.

A urinalysis should be ordered to evaluate for glucosuria, ketonuria, and evidence of urinary tract infection. A complete blood count (CBC) should also be obtained; it is not unusual to have leukocytosis in DKA without the presence of infection. However, if there is concern for underlying infection, appropriate cultures should be obtained (i.e., blood, urine, and throat).

A hemoglobin A1c test can help to evaluate prior control of diabetes and the degree of hyperglycemia that has preceded the episode of DKA. Patients with new-onset diabetes should have diabetes autoimmune antibodies (anti–glutamic acid decarboxylase [GAD]), anti-insulin and anti–islet cell antibodies (ICA) as well as insulin and C-peptide levels determined to help the clinician discriminate between type 1 and type 2 diabetes; patients with type I DM have low insulin and C-peptide levels whereas patients with type 2 DM typically have high insulin and C-peptide levels.

The case patient was sent to the ER, where initial lab results revealed a glucose level of 475 mg/dL, a sodium level of 128 mmol/L, a potassium level of 5.5 mmol/L, a CO_2 level of 5 mmol/L, and a venous pH of 7.03.

Imaging

Routine imaging is not required in patients with DKA unless the patient history or physical exam points to an identifiable concern. Patients with altered mental status may require computed tomography (CT) of the head to assess for cerebral edema. A CT of the abdomen and pelvis may be necessary to rule out appendicitis and other causes of acute abdomen.

Treatment

There are many different protocols for the management of DKA, but the goals of treatment are the same: to restore the intravascular volume, reverse the acidosis, and correct the electrolyte and fluid deficiencies. First the patient's fluid deficit should be determined; most patients with DKA are at least 10% dehydrated. Normal saline boluses must be used initially to establish cardiovascular stability, although full repletion of the fluid deficit will continue more slowly over the next 36 to 48 hours. Most patients will require 10 to 20 mL/kg of normal saline, but patients with severe dehydration may require more to reverse hypovolemic shock. After each bolus of 10 mL/kg, the patient's cardiovascular status should be reevaluated to avoid excess fluid administration, which can place a patient at higher risk for cerebral edema. Once the patient is hemodynamically stable, you should begin to replace the remainder of the fluid deficit. In addition to maintenance fluid requirements, half of the fluid deficit should be replaced over the first 16 hours with normal saline (a rate of 1.5 to 2.0 times maintenance will usually achieve this goal). While the patient is hyperglycemic, urinary losses may be excessive and may also require replacement with normal saline.

Blood glucose must be monitored hourly and should not decrease by more than 50 to 100 mg/dL/hr. If this rate of decline is exceeded or when blood glucose is <300 mg/dL, dextrose should be added to the intravenous fluids. A two-bag system consisting of one bag of normal saline and electrolytes and one bag of 10% dextrose with normal saline and the same electrolytes allows for titration of the dextrose infusion rate without varying the electrolyte or volume replacement (3).

Electrolytes should be monitored every 2 to 4 hours during treatment of DKA. Potassium levels are often initially elevated because of the acidosis, but patients in DKA experience overall potassium depletion and will become hypokalemic as the acidosis resolves. Therefore potassium should be added to replacement fluids as long as urine output is adequate and signs of hyperkalemia are not present. If potassium levels are normal, 40 mEq/L should be added to the replacement fluids, but up to 80 mEq/L may be needed as potassium decreases. Patients often also experience phosphate depletion. A portion of the potassium replacement should be given as potassium phosphate to replete phosphate levels.

CLINICAL PEARL

Insulin is the only treatment to reverse the metabolic acidosis of DKA.

An insulin infusion should be initiated once initial fluid resuscitation has begun. The insulin infusion rate should be 0.1 units/kg/hr and should not be decreased until the acidosis has resolved. The use of bicarbonate in DKA treatment is controversial and should be considered only in severe cases of acidosis.

An approach to the treatment of DKA is summarized in Table 11-1.

Admission Criteria and Level-of-Care Criteria

All patients with DKA require hospitalization. Management in the intensive care unit (ICU) is suggested if the pH is <7.1, blood glucose is

TABLE 11.1
A Protocol for the Management of DKA

	First Hour	First 16–48 Hours	After Resolution of Acidosis
Fluids	Normal saline (NS)	Two-bag system: NS with electrolytes and 10% dextrose/NS with electrolytes Urine output replacement: NS	Oral rehydration
Fluid rate	Boluses of 10–20 mL/kg	Fluid deficit + maintenance requirements (using a two-bag system) + ongoing losses (NS)	
Electrolytes		K >6 mEq/L: hold K replacement until urine output confirmed K = 5.5–6 mEq/L: 20 mEq Kcl K = 4–5.5 mEq/L: 40 mEq K (20 mEq Kcl + 20 mEq Kphos) K <4 mEq/L: 60 mEq K	
Insulin		0.1 unit/kg/hr	Subcutaneous insulin regimen
Labs	Urinalysis, venous blood gas, BMP, HbA1c	BMP q2–4h, Glucose q1hr	Glucose and ketonuria q2h until ketones clear; maintenance glucose monitoring when ketones have cleared
Monitoring	Neurologic status, cardiovascular status, strict ins/outs	Neurologic status hourly, strict ins/outs	

BMP, basic metabolic profile; HbA1c, hemoglobin A1c.

>1,000 mg/dL, or the patient is <5 years of age or exhibits an altered mental status.

EXTENDED IN-HOSPITAL MANAGEMENT

Patients should remain on the insulin infusion until the serum bicarbonate is >15 mmol/L and they are able to tolerate oral fluids. The transition to subcutaneous insulin should optimally occur around a mealtime. The subcutaneous insulin should be administered, the insulin infusion and intravenous fluids simultaneously discontinued 15 to 30 minutes later, and the meal should be eaten. The clearance of ketonuria may lag behind the resolution of the acidosis, but it should resolve with continued oral hydration and subcutaneous insulin. Electrolytes may not be completely normal, but they should be followed until they are approaching normalization.

In patients with new-onset type I DM, education regarding diabetes should begin once the DKA has resolved. In patients with known type I DM, the cause of the DKA should be addressed and education and interventions to prevent its recurrence should be performed.

In the emergency department, the case patient was given a total of 20 mL/kg of normal saline and then started on an insulin infusion and a two-bag system of intravenous fluids. He was transferred to the pediatric intensive care unit, where he remained overnight on a continuous insulin infusion. The following morning he was feeling much better; his glucose was 147 mg/dL and his CO_2 had improved to 17 mmol/L. At that point, he was changed to subcutaneous insulin injections. He was transferred out of the ICU and onto the endocrine service for continued management as well as for diabetes education.

DISPOSITION

Discharge Goals

Discharge can be considered when the patient is stable on a subcutaneous insulin regimen, is tolerating oral intake, and is adequately educated to safely manage his or her diabetes at home.

Outpatient Care

A comprehensive diabetes care team that can address nutritional, educational, and social issues related to diabetes should follow patients with type I DM. Studies have shown that access to 24-hour "help lines" can decrease the occurrence of DKA by offering advice and instructions for diabetes care during illness and before the onset of DKA.

WHAT YOU NEED TO REMEMBER

- DKA is the result of insulin deficiency.
- DKA can masquerade as (or coexist with) an acute abdomen.
- The major causes of morbidity and mortality in DKA are cerebral edema, dehydration, and electrolyte abnormalities.
- Characteristics that place patients with DKA at an increased risk for poor outcomes are pH <7.1, blood glucose >1,000 mg/dL, initial true hyponatremia, new-onset type I DM, age <5 years, and altered mental status.
- In patients with known type I DM, the cause of DKA must be determined and addressed.

REFERENCES

1. Wolfsdorf J, Glaser N, Sperling M. Diabetic ketoacidosis in infants, children and adolescents: a consensus statement from the American Diabetes Association. *Diabetes Care* 2006;29(5):1150–59.
2. Dunger DB, Sperling MA, Acerini CL, et al. ESPE/LWPES consensus statement on diabetic ketoacidosis in children and adolescents. *Arch Dis Child* 2004;89: 188–194.
3. Grimberg A, Cerri RW, Satin-Smith M, et al. The "two bag system" for variable intravenous dextrose and fluid administration: benefits in diabetic ketoacidosis management. *J Pediatr* 1999;134:376–378.

12

Febrile Neonate

GRACE E. LEE

THE PATIENT ENCOUNTER

A 3-week-old infant presents to the emergency department (ED) with a 1-day history of fever of 38.3°C (100.9°F) at home. She has otherwise been well, with no apparent signs of illness. She was born at 40 weeks' gestation by vaginal delivery. The mother had vaginal group B streptococcal (GBS) colonization and, therefore, received two doses of intrapartum penicillin. There were no complications after delivery. In the ED, the infant's temperature is 38.1°C (100.6°F) rectally, with otherwise normal vital signs. She is alert and well-appearing with a nonfocal examination.

OVERVIEW

Definition

By convention, fever in the neonate refers to infants 60 days or younger who present with a rectal temperature ≥38.0°C (100.4°F) of uncertain source after a thorough history and physical examination. Many studies regarding the management of febrile neonates have used slightly different age ranges (e.g., 0 to 56 days). The approaches described in this chapter do not apply to neonates in the immediate postpartum period (i.e., those in the well-baby nursery or intensive care unit).

Pathophysiology

Infants <2 months of age are especially vulnerable to serious bacterial infection (SBI), including meningitis, bacteremia, urinary tract infection (UTI), and bacterial enteritis. Infection may be community-acquired, intrauterine–transplacental, or perinatally acquired, either through maternal colonization with pathogenic bacteria (e.g., GBS, *Enterococcus* species, and enteric gram-negative bacteria), passage through an infected canal (e.g., herpes simplex virus [HSV], *Chlamydia trachomatis*) or through complications of maternal infections (e.g., chorioamnionitis). Neonates are particularly susceptible to bacterial infection because of several factors, including decreased opsonin activity, macrophage function, and neutrophil activity.

Epidemiology

Viral infections, the most common cause of fever in the neonate, exhibit seasonal variation. Respiratory viruses such as respiratory syncytial virus and influenza are more commonly seen during the fall to spring, whereas enteroviral infections are more prevalent in the summer and early fall. Bacterial infections are a less common but typically more serious cause of fever in the neonate. The prevalence of SBI varies by age, ranging from 8.8% to 13.7% for infants <1 month of age and 5.0% to 8.7% for infants between 1 and 2 months of age.

Etiology

The most common causes of neonatal SBI vary by site of infection. UTIs account for most neonatal SBIs, with enteric gram-negative bacteria (most commonly *Escherichia coli* and *Klebsiella* species), *Enterococcus*, and GBS being the most common etiologies. Bacteremia is the second most common neonatal SBI, with enteric gram-negative bacteria, *Staphylococcus aureus*, GBS, and *Streptococcus pneumoniae* being the most likely causes. Bacterial meningitis is often caused by enteric gram-negative bacteria, GBS, and *S. pneumoniae;* in neonates <1 month of age, *Listeria monocytogenes* also occurs. In the summer and early fall, enteroviruses frequently cause aseptic meningitis. Although rare, herpes simplex virus (HSV) infections are associated with substantial morbidity and mortality and should also be considered in cases of aseptic meningitis.

Historically, GBS has been associated with a high proportion of neonatal SBI. The use of intrapartum chemoprophylaxis in GBS-colonized mothers has led to a decline in incidence of GBS sepsis from 1.5 per 1,000 live births to 0.5 per 1,000 live births (1).

ACUTE MANAGEMENT AND WORKUP

The acute management and workup of the febrile neonate should identify which patients are at low risk and may be managed with observation or as outpatients, and which patients are at high risk and require hospitalization and empiric antibiotic therapy.

The First 15 Minutes

Clinical stability should be rapidly assessed with an initial review of the infant's vital signs and general appearance for the presence of lethargy, dehydration, respiratory distress, and shock. The critically ill neonate will require rapid identification and hemodynamic stabilization.

The First Few Hours

The evaluation of the febrile neonate requires a thorough history, physical examination, and laboratory assessment to identify potential sources of SBI, as well as to determine the overall risk of SBI and the need for further inpatient management and antibiotic therapy.

History

Your risk assessment for SBI in the febrile neonate should begin with the birth history, including the presence of intrapartum and postpartum complications. A history of prematurity (i.e., ≤37 weeks' gestation), a chronic or underlying condition (e.g., a duplicated renal collecting system), and an intrapartum history of maternal fever, GBS colonization, or antibiotic treatment is associated with a higher likelihood of neonatal SBI.

Risk factors for neonatal HSV infection should also be assessed. Most (85%) neonatal HSV transmission occurs in the peripartum period, while the remaining cases are acquired postnatally (10%) or in utero (5%) (2). The single greatest risk factor for perinatal HSV transmission is primary maternal genital HSV disease at delivery. Primary genital HSV poses a greater risk to the neonate, because compared with recurrent genital HSV, primary HSV is associated with higher viral loads, a longer duration of viral excretion, and the absence of transplacentally acquired protective antibodies. However, the presence of primary maternal infection is frequently difficult to identify because two thirds of women who acquire genital herpes during pregnancy are asymptomatic. Infants born by cesarean section within 4 hours of membrane rupture are at substantially lower risk of perinatal HSV acquisition, even during primary maternal infection.

CLINICAL PEARL

In many cases of neonatal HSV, the patient's mother is unaware that she is infected. Thus, a negative maternal history of HSV does not rule out the possibility of HSV in the neonate.

Symptoms associated with SBI may be nonspecific; reports of lethargy, poor feeding, and cyanosis may be the only presenting signs of sepsis. Other concerning symptoms include irritability, tachypnea, apnea, vomiting, and diarrhea. Decreased urine output (<4 wet diapers per 24 hours) and absent tears suggest dehydration.

Physical Examination

Clinical appearance alone does not accurately predict the presence of SBI. In one landmark study (3), 66% of neonates ultimately diagnosed with SBI appeared well at the initial evaluation. In contrast, SBI is present in up to one-third of ill- or toxic-appearing infants. Clinical features associated with ill appearance include lethargy, poor or absent eye contact, poor extremity perfusion, acrocyanosis or mottling, a slow capillary refill time (>2 seconds in a "warm" environment), hyperventilation, marked hypoventilation, and cyanosis.

Aside from the overall clinical appearance, an effort should be made to discover a focal source of infection, including evidence of otitis media, skin or soft-tissue infection, or bone or joint infection. If applicable, the umbilical stump and surrounding skin should be assessed for signs of omphalitis, such as erythema, purulent drainage, and duskiness. The mouth and skin should be assessed for vesicles, which suggest HSV, although up to one third of infants with HSV never develop vesicles during the course of their acute infection. Meningismus rarely occurs in this age group; however, the presence of a bulging fontanelle may indicate meningitis. Pulse quality (femoral, brachial) should be assessed; thready or nonpalpable pulses signify shock.

Labs and Tests to Consider

Febrile infants ≤60 days of age should, with rare exception, undergo a complete evaluation to identify potential bacterial causes. In select patients in the appropriate season, consider respiratory virus, enterovirus, and HHV-6 testing, recognizing that a positive viral assay does not exclude SBI but is associated with a decreased risk of SBI in some infants. For example, a prospective multicenter study (4) found that while the rate of SBI was lower in RSV-positive infants (7.0%) compared with RSV-negative infants (12.5%) 29 to 60 days of age, the rate of SBI among RSV-positive and RSV-negative infants ≤28 days of age did not differ.

Key Diagnostic Labs and Tests

The standard laboratory evaluation for bacterial infection includes a complete blood count with differential, blood culture, urinalysis, urine culture, and lumbar puncture with cell count as well as total protein, glucose, culture, and Gram's stain. Urine specimens should be obtained by transurethral bladder catheterization or, when necessary, suprapubic aspiration. Perineal bag specimens are more likely to be contaminated and are of little utility in this population. Two methods of urinalysis (UA), standard and enhanced, have been traditionally used for UTI screening. Standard UA uses centrifuged specimens that are then resuspended, with white blood cells (WBCs) and bacteria enumerated per high-power field. Enhanced UA, which counts WBC per cubic millimeter in unspun specimens and includes Gram's stain for bacteria, has been shown to be more sensitive in screening for UTI compared with standard UA (94% versus 83%) and is recommended for neonates (5). Stool cultures, Hemoccult testing, and a fecal WBC smear should be obtained if diarrhea is present. Laboratory parameters for result interpretation vary by institution. Interpretation of these test results is included in the "Admission Criteria and Level-of-Care Criteria" section.

Laboratory evaluation for HSV should be considered in infants ≤30 days of age with vesicles, seizures, hypotension, or unexplained coagulopathy. HSV should also be considered in infants with cerebrospinal fluid (CSF) pleocytosis without bacteria on Gram's stain, particularly during the winter months (i.e., when enteroviruses are unlikely). Appropriate evaluation for HSV includes CSF HSV polymerase chain reaction (PCR) testing, pro-thrombin and partial thromboplastin times or D-dimers (to detect coagulopa-thy), and a hepatic function panel (to detect liver involvement). A negative CSF HSV PCR test does not exclude systemic or cutaneous perinatally acquired HSV infection. Therefore, swabs of the conjunctiva, nasopharynx, rectum, and any skin lesions should be sent for HSV detection by PCR (most sensitive), culture, or direct fluorescent antibody (most rapid but least sensi-tive); most infants with perinatally acquired HSV will have HSV detected from one of these sites.

The case patient underwent a lumbar puncture, complete blood count, blood culture, urinalysis, and urine culture. Pertinent results included the following: WBCs 15,000/mm^3, CSF WBCs 8/mm^3, and negative urinalysis.

Imaging

A chest radiograph should be obtained in all infants with respiratory symp-toms, abnormal chest exam, or hypoxia. Focal infiltrates suggest pneumonia.

Treatment

The need for antibiotic therapy is determined by clinical assessment and screening lab results as described in the next section. If acyclovir is consid-ered for empiric HSV coverage, HSV testing is recommended prior to or shortly after initiation.

Admission Criteria and Level-of-Care Criteria

Clinical practice varies by institution. Several protocols have been developed for the evaluation of febrile neonates in the ED setting to facilitate decisions regarding the site of care and empiric therapy. Because no single protocol successfully identifies all infants 0 to 28 days of age with SBI, all febrile neonates in this age group should be hospitalized, and empiric antibiotic therapy initiated with ampicillin for GBS, *Listeria*, and *Enterococcus* coverage plus a third-generation cephalosporin or gentamicin for gram-negative bac-terial coverage. See Table 12-1 for a summary of commonly used protocols. The Philadelphia protocol applies to neonates 29 to 56 days of age and is presented in detail here.

Infants 29 to 56 days of age who are clinically well-appearing, meet low-risk laboratory criteria, have a normal chest radiograph (if obtained), and are available for reevaluation by a medical provider 24 hours after their screen-ing assessment may be managed at home without antibiotics. Infants 29 to 56 of age days not determined to be at low risk should be admitted for empiric intravenous antibiotic therapy and observation. Although ampicillin and gentamicin have been the traditional choice for infants 29 to 56 days of age without CSF pleocytosis, *Listeria* and *Enterococcus* species are uncommon

TABLE 12-1

Protocol Summaries for the Management of Febrile Infants

	Philadelphia Criteria (Baker, 1993)	Rochester Criteria (Jaskiewicz, 1994)	Boston Criteria (Baskin, 1992)
Age	29–56 days	≤60 days	28–89 days
History	Not specified	• Term infant • No perinatal antibiotics • No underlying disease • Not hospitalized longer than the mother	• No immunizations within preceding 48 hours • No antimicrobials within 48 hours • Not dehydrated
Physical	• Well-appearing	• Well-appearing	• Well-appearing
Low-risk laboratory parameters	• WBCs <15,000/mm^3 • Band–total neutrophil ratio <0.2 • UA <10 WBCs per hpf • Urine Gram's stain negative • CSF WBCs <8/mm^3 • CXR: no infiltrate[a] • Stool: no blood, few or no WBCs on smear[a]	• WBCs >5,000 and <15,000/mm^3 • Absolute bands <1,500/mm^3 • UA ≤10 WBCs per hpf • Stool smear ≤5 WBCs per hpf[a]	• WBCs <20,000/mm^3 • UA WBCs <10/hpf • CSF WBCs <10/mm^3 • CXR: no infiltrate[a]

(continued)

TABLE 12-1

Protocol Summaries for the Management of Febrile Infants (Continued)

	Philadelphia Criteria (Baker, 1993)	Rochester Criteria (Jaskiewicz, 1994)	Boston Criteria (Baskin, 1992)
High-risk	Hospitalize + empiric antibiotics	Same	Same
Low-risk	• Home • No antibiotics • Follow-up required	• Home • No antibiotics • Follow-up required	• Home • Empiric Ceftriaxone • Follow-up required
Screening performance	Sensitivity: 100%[b] Specificity: 42%	Sensitivity: 92% Specificity: 50%	Sensitivity: N/A Specificity: 94.6%

[a]If indicated

[b]Including modified criteria of band–total neutrophil ratio <0.2; see original study, Boher, 1993.

Adapted from Bachur RG, Harper MB. Predictive model for serious bacterial infections among infants younger than 3 months of age. *Pediatrics* 2001; 108(2).

TABLE 12-2

Suggested Empiric Antimicrobial Therapy for the Febrile Neonate

0–28 Days	Ampicillin^a + gentamicin or cefotaxime^b
29–56 Days	Cefotaxime alone OR ampicillin^a + gentamicin
0–56 Days	*Ill-appearing or high-level of suspicion for bacterial meningitis:* Vancomycin + cefotaxime
HSV: high-level suspicion	High-dose IV acyclovir: 60 mg/kg/day divided every 8 hours

^{a}High-dose ampicillin should be given if suspicion of meningitis.
^{b}High-dose cefotaxime is preferred to gentamicin for suspected meningitis due to improved CSF penetration.

causes of infection in the second month of life. In fact, one systematic review found that 527 febrile infants 1 to 2 months of age would require therapy with ampicillin to empirically treat one infection caused by either microbe (6). Either ampicillin plus gentamicin or a third-generation cephalosporin alone would be appropriate for this age group; if findings suggest a UTI, ampicillin should be included for empiric enterococcal coverage. In infants 56 days of age or younger with a high level of suspicion for bacterial meningitis (i.e., CSF pleocytosis with low glucose and bacteria present on Gram stain, the presence of seizures, or lethargy), consider broader coverage with vancomycin and a third-generation cephalosporin for empiric *S. pneumoniae* coverage. See Table 12-2 for a summary of recommendations for empiric antimicrobial therapy.

EXTENDED IN-HOSPITAL MANAGEMENT

In general, the duration of observation and initial antibiotic therapy should cover a treatment period of 24 to 48 hours. The probability of identifying SBI in febrile infants 28 to 90 days of age by blood, urine, or CSF cultures after 24 hours is 1.1% (7). In addition, 95% of blood cultures with critical pathogens (*S. pneumoniae*, enteric gram-negative bacteria, *Neisseria meningitidis*, *S. aureus*, and groups A and B streptococci) will become positive by 24 hours, and 98% will become positive by 48 hours (8). Neonates with SBI will require prolonged antibiotic therapy as determined by the pathogen and source of infection.

The case patient was admitted to the general pediatric service and treated with ampicillin and cefotaxime. After 48 hours, her blood, urine, and CSF cultures were all negative. At that point, she was afebrile and drinking well. Her antibiotics were discontinued and she was discharged home.

DISPOSITION

Discharge Goals

Consider discharge when the patient is well-appearing and eating well. Culture results should be negative prior to discharge, with a true minimum incubation period of 24 to 48 hours. Antimicrobial therapy should be complete or able to be continued at home with the appropriate home environment. The family and the primary care physician should be comfortable with the discharge plan and in agreement regarding follow-up.

Outpatient Care

Neonates 29 to 56 days of age identified as low-risk children by the Philadelphia protocol may be managed as outpatients if follow-up can be assured within 1 day of the initial evaluation. Otherwise, hospitalized patients should have follow-up with their primary care provider within 2 to 3 days of discharge. Additional follow-up may be necessary depending on the final diagnosis.

WHAT YOU NEED TO REMEMBER

- Neonatal SBI cannot be reliably diagnosed by clinical exam alone.
- The presence of viral infection does not exclude the possibility of concurrent SBI.
- All infants <1 month of age with fever should be empirically treated with intravenous antibiotics while cultures are pending.
- Some patients between 1 month and 2 months of age can be managed as outpatients.

REFERENCES

1. Gerdes JS. Diagnosis and management of bacterial infections in the neonate. *Pediatr Clin North Am* 2004;51:939–959.
2. Kimberlin DW. Neonatal herpes simplex infection. *Clin Microbiol Rev* 2004; 17:1–13.
3. Baker MD, Bell LM, Avner JR. Outpatient management without antibiotics of fever in selected infants. *N Engl J Med* 1993:329:1437–1441.
4. Levine DA, Platt SL, Dayan PS. Risk of serious bacterial infection in young febrile infants with respiratory syncytial virus infections. *Pediatrics* 2004;113:1728–1734.

5. Shaw KN, McGowan KL, Gorelick MH. Screening for urinary tract infection in infants in the emergency department: which test is best? *Pediatrics* 1998;101:E1.
6. Brown JC, Burns JL, Cumming P. Ampicillin use in infant fever. *Arch Pediatr Adolesc Med* 2002;156:27–32.
7. Kaplan RL, Harper MB, Baskin MN. Time to detection of positive cultures in 28–90 day old febrile infants. *Pediatrics* 2000;106:E74.
8. McGowan KL, Foster JA, Coffin SE. Outpatient pediatric blood cultures: time to positivity. *Pediatrics* 2000;106:251–255.

SUGGESTED READINGS

Baskin MN, O'Rourke EJ, Fleisher GR. Outpatient treatment of febrile infants 28–89 days of age with intramuscular administration of ceftriaxone. *J Pediatr* 1992; 120:22–27.

Jaskiewicz JA, McCarthy CA, Richardson AC. Febrile infants at low risk for serious bacterial infection – an appraisal of the Rochester criteria and implications for management. *Pediatrics* 1994;94:390–396.

Sadow KB, Derr R, Teach S. Bacterial infections in infants 60 days and younger. *Arch Pediatr Adolesc Med* 1999;153:611–614.

Febrile Neutropenia

JOSEPH A. HILINSKI

THE PATIENT ENCOUNTER

A 12-year-old boy with acute lymphoblastic leukemia (ALL) develops fever to 39°C (102.2°F) while at home. He complains of chills but has no specific focal complaints. He is brought to the pediatric emergency department by his parents immediately after the development of fever. His ALL is in remission at the delayed intensification phase after a successful 4-week induction. His recent chemotherapy regimen started 18 days ago and included cyclophosphamide, cytarabine (Ara-C), 6-mercaptopurine, and intrathecal methotrexate. On physical examination, he was febrile to 39.5°C (103.1°F) and moderately unwell-appearing with chills, but alert and appropriate. His physical exam was remarkable for oral mucositis.

OVERVIEW

Definition

Malignancy and related chemotherapeutic drugs are the most common cause of immune compromise in children. Chemotherapy-induced granulocytopenia is the most common risk factor that predisposes children being treated for cancer to infectious complications. The term *febrile neutropenia* is often used to refer to patients who present with fever in the context of chemotherapy-induced granulocytopenia. Febrile neutropenia is defined as a single oral temperature ≥38.3°C (101°F) or a temperature of ≥38.0°C (100.4°F) for ≥1 hour occurring in a patient with an absolute neutrophil count (ANC) <500/mm³ or a count of <1,000/mm³ with an expected decrease to <500/mm³.

Pathophysiology

Multiple factors in children being treated for malignancy act together to predispose them to infection, often with unusual sites or infecting organisms. Cancer itself often causes immune deficiency by impairing normal bone marrow function or production. The use of cytotoxic chemotherapeutic agents leads to further immune suppression and subsequent serious infections.

Other factors are also important to consider in children being treated for malignancy. Damage to mucosal surfaces (e.g., chemotherapy-induced mucositis of the gastrointestinal tract mucosa) creates portals of entry for normally harmless bacterial flora. The bacteria may translocate across the impaired oral or gut barrier, causing transient or sustained bacteremia. The severity of mucosal disruption is a significant factor in the likelihood of developing invasive infection. Receipt of high-dose cytarabine (Ara-C) is a risk factor for severe infection with the *viridans* group streptococci. Indwelling catheters—including short-term devices such as peripheral intravenous catheters and long-term devices such as implantable central venous lines—pose a substantial risk for invasive infections. Ventriculoperitoneal shunts or devices may also serve as a source of potential infection in those patients requiring them for the management of brain tumors. Other factors, such as prolonged parenteral nutrition, may predispose to invasive fungal infections. Patients requiring transfusions of either red blood cells or platelets may be at risk for fever from transfusion reactions or from transfusion-related bacteremias.

Epidemiology

Episodes of febrile neutropenia in children being treated for cancer occur commonly. Approximately one third of children with a sustained neutropenia (neutrophils $<500/mm^3$ for a week or more) will develop an episode of fever. Sustained neutropenia >2 weeks is almost certain to result in development of fever. Up to one-half of neutropenic patients with fever have an established or occult infection, with up to one-fifth of those with severe neutropenia (neutrophils <100 /mm^3) having bacteremia. Despite these high rates of likely infection, a specific microbiologic cause is found in only one-third of cases.

Etiology

The bacteria that cause invasive infections during periods of febrile neutropenia have undergone several substantial shifts over time. During the 1950s, *Staphylococcus aureus* predominated as the major pathogen. During the 1960s and 1970s, gram-negative pathogens predominated; in particular *Pseudomonas aeruginosa*. During this period, a high mortality of up to 80% was frequently associated with bacteremic episodes during febrile neutropenia. More recently, from the late 1980s to the present day, gram-positive pathogens have again predominated, although associated mortality rates are lower, ranging from 1% to 5%. At present, the most common bacterial pathogens related to therapies for cancer are the coagulase-negative staphylococci, followed by enterococci and *S. aureus*. When gram-positive infections are suspected, methicillin-resistant *S. aureus* (MRSA) must also be considered, along with several other pathogens that are not routinely isolated from normal hosts, such as *Corynebacterium jeikeium*, the *viridans* group streptococci, *Bacillus* species, and *Stomatococcus mucilaginosus*, some of which are resistant to commonly used classes of antibiotics. Despite the overall significance of gram-positive bacteria, very recent trends have indicated another resurgence of gram-negative bacteria, including *Escherichia coli*, *Enterobacter* species, *Klebsiella* species, and *P. aeruginosa*. These may increasingly be associated with inducible or extended-spectrum beta-lactamases, making the choice of empiric antibiotic coverage more challenging.

Fungal infections have increasingly assumed more importance in the management of patients undergoing therapy for malignancy. This may be due to several factors, including the prolonged survival of children with cancer because of advances in chemotherapy and medical technology; more invasive interventions such as long-term indwelling venous catheters; parenteral nutrition; and longer periods of severe neutropenia related to dose-dependent chemotherapeutic agents. Although fungal infections may present as a primary site of infection, they are more commonly associated with secondary infections in the setting of prolonged neutropenia while the patient is being treated with broad-spectrum antibacterial agents. *Candida* species account for the highest rates of invasive fungal infections. Approximately one-half of invasive infections are now due to *Candida albicans*, with the remaining infections accounted for by *C. parapsilosis*, *C. glabrata*, *C. tropicalis*, *C. krusei*, and *C. lusitaniae*. These shifts are important, as some nonalbicans species may be resistant to azoles or amphotericin. *Aspergillus* species account for the second most common cause of invasive fungal infections, with *A. fumigatus* being the most prominent. These infections typically occur in the most severely suppressed patients with prolonged neutropenia. Other invasive fungal infections, such as the Zygomycetes (*Mucor, Rhizopus, Rhizomucor*), *Fusarium*, *Trichosporon*, and other environmental molds are occasionally seen. *Pneumocystis jiroveci* (formerly *P. carinii*) rarely causes interstitial pneumonia in children undergoing treatment for cancer.

Viruses may occasionally cause severe infections in children undergoing treatment for cancer. Most commonly, herpes simplex viruses may be associated with significant mucositis. Varicella zoster virus may manifest as severe primary varicella (chickenpox) or as reactivated shingles. Other common agents, such as respiratory pathogens, enteroviruses, Epstein–Barr virus, and cytomegalovirus should also be considered in the differential.

ACUTE MANAGEMENT AND WORKUP

Appropriate and timely acute management and workup are critical in preventing morbidity and mortality in children who present with chemotherapy-induced febrile neutropenia. These children should be triaged rapidly in the emergency department for immediate evaluation and therapy.

CLINICAL PEARL

Delays in antibiotic administration may lead to worsening of existing illness or death. A parental report of fever should always be accepted, even if fever is not present at the time of arrival.

The First 15 Minutes

Many centers have pathways for the evaluation of children with chemotherapy-induced neutropenia in the emergency department. Such protocols allow for rapid and consistent assessment and treatment, including drawing specimens for required laboratory studies such as blood cultures, blood counts, and serum chemistries as soon as possible after arrival. On first evaluation of the child, an assessment of the severity of illness should occur to guide you as to whether to continue with the rest of the history and physical findings or to intervene immediately, by providing intravenous fluids, inotropic support, blood products, or respiratory support. Once the child has been deemed to be stable or stabilized, a thorough but directed history and physical examination should be performed. Antibiotics should be ordered as soon as possible based on local protocol guidelines (if available) and modified by specific findings in the history and physical.

The First Few Hours

Once the patient has been initially evaluated, with an appropriate workup obtained and antibiotics administered, it is advisable to re-evaluate the patient to confirm prior historical and physical exam points as well as to obtain more detailed information regarding the presenting symptoms and exposures and to perform a thorough physical exam.

History

A history of underlying malignancy; the stage of chemotherapy; and the specific chemotherapy regimen, including the last doses received; are important in stratifying the risk of many infections. Knowledge of prophylactic antimicrobials and a recent history of infections may guide the workup and therapy. If the patient has indwelling hardware, such as central venous lines, determine when the device was placed and whether there have been episodes of device infection. Determine whether symptoms of common infections are present, making sure to inquire about findings in the upper and lower respiratory tracts, gastrointestinal system, skin and nails, bones and joints, and neurologic system. In this particular patient population, a specific history should be sought regarding the symptoms of mucositis, dental pain or swelling, abnormal findings related to intravenous lines or devices (redness, drainage, pain, swelling), abdominal findings (pain, diarrhea), symptoms of rectal or anal cavity pain or tenderness (often associated with abscesses), and symptoms of pain or swelling associated with fingernails or toenails. Although often muted because of the effects of neutropenia, a history of chills, rigors, vomiting, or myalgias may be associated with bacteremia.

Physical Examination

A thorough physical examination with close monitoring of vital signs may be critical to pinpoint the source of an infection. A complete examination should be performed, with specific emphasis on certain areas, including the oral cavity (to evaluate for mucositis and dental infections); findings related to indwelling hardware devices, such as intravenous lines or prior surgical incisions; abdominal tenderness (which may prompt consideration of typhlitis [inflammation of the cecum], which is a potentially serious infection in this population); the rectal area and anal cavity (avoid digital rectal exams in neutropenic patients, especially in patients with mucositis); prior bone marrow aspiration sites; and the evaluation of fingernails and toenails for possible sites of cellulitis or abscess. **During periods of neutropenia, many classic findings of inflammation, such as redness, warmth, tenderness, and swelling, may initially be absent in these children, even though specific focal or systemic pyogenic infections are present.**

Labs and Tests to Consider

At a minimum, all children presenting with febrile neutropenia require blood cultures, complete blood counts, and serum chemistries. **If a patient has a multilumen central venous catheter, obtain cultures through each lumen.** Further diagnostic workup can be guided by individual symptoms or findings.

Key Diagnostic Labs and Tests

Appropriately drawn blood cultures prior to the receipt of antibiotics are essential, as rates of identified bacteremia vary but range between 10% and 40% for pediatric episodes of febrile neutropenia. Pathogen recovery is important to guide therapy, especially in the case of unusual or resistant pathogens that may not be covered by an empiric regimen.

Initial serum chemistries to evaluate renal function and hepatic transaminases may be important guides in antibiotic dosing and selection. Patients with renal insufficiency will need to receive renally dosed medications and consideration for reducing additional nephrotoxic agents if possible, and those with evidence of elevated hepatic transaminases may require modification to or a change in some antimicrobial regimens.

Additional laboratory studies should be obtained as appropriate based on the age of the patient and the presenting symptoms. For those with signs of upper or lower respiratory tract infection, viral diagnostic studies, such as rapid antigen testing, polymerase chain reaction (PCR) testing, or viral cultures, may be diagnostic. Sputum Gram stain and culture is indicated for children with suspected pneumonia able to produce adequate samples. Urinalysis and urine culture should be obtained from those with compatible symptoms and from very young children. If findings of skin abscess are present, cultures of involved sites should be obtained. If diarrhea is present, consider stool cultures as well as a rapid test for pathogens such as rotavirus. Herpes simplex cultures of the mouth should be obtained for mucositis that is unusually severe, prolonged, or presents with compatible, visible ulcers.

Given the significant mortality associated with untreated invasive infections in the neutropenic host and the need for specific diagnosis to guide therapy, it may often be necessary to obtain diagnostic specimens through more invasive means, including such measures as tissue biopsy, bronchoalveolar lavage (BAL), and lumbar puncture.

A complete blood count (CBC) on the case patient revealed the following findings: white blood cells, 1,000/mm^3 with 5% segmented neutrophils and 95% lymphocytes; a hemoglobin level of 7 g/dL; and platelets 30,000/mm^3. Electrolytes were obtained and were within normal limits, and blood cultures were obtained prior to the administration of antibiotics.

Imaging

Chest radiography should be obtained for all patients with pulmonary symptoms or findings. Additionally, a high-resolution computed tomography (CT) scan of the chest is indicated if invasive fungal infection is suspected clinically, and this may be considered for patients with a prolonged (>4- to 7-day) history of neutropenic fever. Typical radiographic findings may not be present at the initial evaluation of these patients, given their lack of neutrophils.

For patients with candidemia, a routine diagnostic workup should also include examination by an ophthalmologist, to detect dissemination of infection to the retina, as well as ultrasound or CT imaging of the liver, spleen, kidneys, and bladder (to evaluate for microabscesses and renal fungal balls). An echocardiogram should be performed in patients with signs of endocarditis and in those with persistent candidemia. For patients with bacteremia or candidemia and compatible neurologic symptoms, imaging of the brain should be performed, with contrast-enhanced magnetic resonance imaging (MRI) being generally preferred to CT.

Treatment

Several acceptable regimens for the inpatient management of febrile neutropenia in children exist. Most institutions will have site-specific guidelines for preferred agents. All regimens should include drugs active against *P. aeruginosa*. Regimens available include single-drug therapy (monotherapy), combination therapy (generally a monotherapy agent in combination with an aminoglycoside), and combination regimens, including vancomycin. Although many centers use combination therapy with an aminoglycoside, outcomes may not be improved compared with monotherapy agents, and these drugs may be associated with significant renal toxicity. In general, the empiric addition of vancomycin to the initial regimen has not been shown to reduce mortality; therefore, this agent should not be routinely used unless certain risk factors are present. Risk factors include institutions with high rates of infection with resistant gram-positive organisms (*viridans* group streptococci, *C. jeikeium*, *Bacillus* species); clinically suspected

TABLE 13-1
Recommended Monotherapy Agents for the Empiric Treatment of Febrile Neutropenia

Drug	Dose	Maximum Daily Dose
Ceftazidime	Infants >1 month and children: 150 mg/kg/day divided every 8 hours	6 g
Cefepime	Infants >2 months and children: 150 mg/kg/day divided every 8 hours	6 g
Meropenem	Infants >3 months and children: 60 mg/kg/day divided every 8 hours	6 g
Imipenem–cilastatin	Infants >3 months and children: 60–100 mg/kg/day divided every 6 hours (imipenem component)	4 g
Piperacillin–tazobactam	Infants >6 months and children: 300–400 mg/kg/day divided every 6–8 hours (piperacillin component)	16 g

catheter infections (bacteremia or localized cellulitis/abscess) or gram-positive infections; known colonization with resistant pathogens, such as MRSA; known positive blood or tissue cultures for gram-positive organisms prior to final identification and susceptibility testing; hypotension; signs of severe illness; and, at some centers, the receipt of high-dose Ara-C, given its association with streptococcal infections related to the severe *viridans* group. Table 13-1 lists the most commonly recommended monotherapy agents for febrile neutropenia. Two recent meta-analyses have called into question the efficacy of cefepime for this and other indications, with some centers no longer considering cefepime for monotherapy.

Admission Criteria and Level of Care Criteria

Inpatient hospitalization with the administration of intravenous antibiotics remains the standard of care for pediatric patients with febrile neutropenia. Most such patients can be admitted to a general pediatric or oncology ward. Patients with signs of shock, respiratory distress, altered mental status, severe abdominal pain, or other signs at presentation that suggest the potential for rapid decompensation should be admitted to the intensive care unit.

EXTENDED IN-HOSPITAL MANAGEMENT

It is important to reevaluate the patient on a daily basis after admission, reviewing symptoms and repeating the physical examination to determine if focal findings have developed. In general, broad-spectrum therapy should be continued while the patient is neutropenic and febrile; however, if a defined focus of infection is found by examination or cultures, adjust therapy to cover the causative pathogens. For central line–related infections, removal of the catheter is essential for some pathogens (especially *Candida* species and *S. aureus*).

The duration of therapy can be individualized for those with documented infections. Most patients with febrile neutropenia become afebrile within 2 to 7 days. If no infection is present, antibiotics can be discontinued 48 hours after achieving an ANC $\geq$500/mm^3 (and rising) for most patients who are afebrile by 3 to 5 days. In those who remain neutropenic but defervesce by days 3 to 5 and who were initially at low risk and clinically well-appearing, antibiotics may be stopped after 5 to 7 total days if no infection is found. Antibiotics will have to be continued longer for those who are initially at high risk (ANC <100/mm^3, mucositis, severe illness), even with an early resolution of fever.

For those who remain persistently febrile, the duration of antibiotics will be guided by the resolution of neutropenia. For those who remain persistently neutropenic, reassessment should occur and antibiotics adjusted as necessary. Most experts continue for at least 2 weeks, at which point consideration could be given to stopping if the patient is clinically well. **For patients who remain persistently febrile and neutropenic after 4 to 7 days of broad-spectrum therapy, add an antifungal agent to cover occult fungal infection.** Recommended agents include liposomal amphotericin B, caspofungin, or voriconazole.

The case patient was treated with intravenous cefepime. After 48 hours, he had defervesced and his absolute neutrophil count had risen to 650. His cultures remained negative and he was discharged home.

DISPOSITION

Discharge Goals

Discharge may be considered when fever and signs or symptoms of infection have resolved and the patient has completed the previously determined antibiotic course.

Outpatient Care

Patients require follow-up with their hematologist or oncologist within 3 days of discharge. At that time, a history of any subsequent symptoms or fever, physical exam findings, and complete blood counts should be reviewed. Further management, such as prolonged antibiotic courses, laboratory studies, and imaging, should be done as clinically appropriate for specific conditions.

WHAT YOU NEED TO REMEMBER

- Immediate evaluation and antibiotic administration are critical in reducing mortality from infectious causes of febrile neutropenia.
- Many classic findings of inflammation may initially be absent, even though focal or systemic pyogenic infections are present during neutropenic episodes.

SUGGESTED READINGS

Bal AM, Gould IM. Empirical antimicrobial treatment for chemotherapy-induced febrile neutropenia. *Int J Antimicrob Agents* 2007;29:501–509.

Hartel C, Deuster M, Lehrnbecher T, et al. Current approaches for risk stratification of infectious complications in pediatric oncology. *Pediatr Blood Cancer* 2007;49: 767–773.

Hughes WT, Armstrong D, Bodey GP, et al. 2002 Guidelines for the use of antimicrobial agents in neutropenic patients with cancer. *Clin Infect Dis* 2002;34:730–751.

Koh AY, Pizzo PA. Fever and granulocytopenia. In Long SS, Pickering LK, Prober CG, eds. *Principles and Practice of Pediatric Infectious Diseases,* 3rd ed. Philadelphia: Elsevier, 2008.

Paul M, Yahav D, Fraser A, et al. Empirical antibiotic monotherapy for febrile neutropenia: systematic review and meta-analysis of randomized controlled trials. *J Antimicrob Chemother* 2006;57:176–189.

Viscoli C, Varnier O, Machetti M. Infectious in patients with febrile neutropenia: epidemiology, microbiology, and risk stratification. *Clin Infect Dis* 2005;40: S240–S245.

Fever of Unknown Origin

GRACE E. LEE

THE PATIENT ENCOUNTER

A 14-month-old boy is brought to the emergency room for evaluation of daily fevers of 38.3°C (101°F) or higher for almost 3 weeks. His mother reports that he has been less active and increasingly fussy, with decreased oral intake. He presents with mild, intermittent abdominal pain, but his review of systems is otherwise unremarkable. He was evaluated by his pediatrician and noted to have a 2-pound weight loss since his well-child visit at 12 months of age; screening labs were notable for elevated inflammatory markers and an elevated liver enzymes. His temperature in triage today is 39.2°C (102.5°F). On examination, he is ill appearing, with bilateral cervical lymphadenopathy and mild hepatosplenomegaly.

OVERVIEW

Definition

Fever of unknown origin (FUO) in children has had variable definitions in the medical literature; however, the most commonly used definition is that of daily fever ≥38.3°C (101°F) for a minimum of 14 days without apparent cause after physical examination and screening laboratory tests. This definition excludes periodic fever syndromes, which are characterized by recurrent fever and predictable symptoms lasting days to weeks, with intervening symptom-free periods.

Pathophysiology

The pathophysiology of FUO is widely variable and is dependent on the underlying etiology.

Epidemiology

The epidemiology of FUO has not been well described and is likely to vary by geographic region depending on the relative incidence and prevalence of the myriad underlying etiologies.

Etiology

The most common cause of FUO in children is infection, ranging from 28% to 52% of cases in published pediatric case series, depending on the definition of FUO that is used. However, autoimmune disorders (7.5% to 20%) and malignancy (3% to 8%) are also notable causes. FUO resolves without identification of a specific cause in 20% to 40% of cases. See Table 14-1 for a summary of diagnostic considerations for FUO in children.

ACUTE MANAGEMENT AND WORKUP

The acute management and workup of the child with FUO should exclude life-threatening etiologies of FUO and identify the well-appearing and/or chronically ill child whose investigation can take place on an outpatient basis. It should also include identifying the ill-appearing child who requires further management in the inpatient setting.

The First 15 Minutes

Clinical stability should be rapidly assessed. Is the patient comfortable (well), agitated (sick), or lethargic (toxic)? Reviewing the patient's vital signs and mental status will aid in the assessment of hemodynamic stability. The critically ill patient will require rapid identification and hemodynamic stabilization with or without simultaneous evaluation of the FUO etiology.

The First Few Hours

The investigation of FUO requires a thoughtful history and physical examination. Clues from the initial evaluation should direct the need for specific laboratory, imaging, and diagnostic studies, eliminating the need for a costly, low-yield "shotgun" approach.

History

The initial task should be the categorization of fever. It should be determined if fever was truly present, as confirmed by a temperature ≥38.3°C (101°F) and ideally documented by a health-care provider. Characterization of the pattern of fever may be helpful in distinguishing among *recurrent fever* (characterized by a series of self-limited febrile periods, most commonly due to recurrent upper respiratory infections or additional unrelated infections, such as urinary tract or gastrointestinal), *periodic fever* (recurrent fever and predictable symptoms lasting days to weeks, with intervening symptom-free periods of variable duration), and true FUO. Pattern recognition may also give clues to the etiology. The classic "quotidian" fever of systemic juvenile idiopathic arthritis (JIA) consists of twice-daily spiking fever, with interval subnormal temperatures. Malaria may also present with a characteristic cyclic fever, ranging from every other day to every third day, depending on the species, although it may be persistent in the early period of infection.

A thorough history of potential infectious exposures is key. An extensive travel history should be sought, as malaria, tuberculosis, histoplasmosis, and coccidioidomycosis may present years after travel

TABLE 14-1
Causes of Fever of Unknown Origin

Infectious

Common

Infectious mononucleosis[a] (Epstein–Barr virus, cytomegalovirus), systemic viral illness, upper or lower respiratory tract infection, osteomyelitis,[b] bartonellosis, urinary tract infection

Less common

Tuberculosis, CNS infection, endocarditis, enteric infection,[c] enterovirus, rickettsial diseases, ehrlichioses, endemic mycoses

Unusual

Intra-abdominal abscess, dental infection, atypical mycobacterium, Q-fever, brucellosis, tularemia, rat-bite fever, malaria, congenital syphilis, leptospirosis, toxoplasmosis, chronic meningococcemia, HIV, *Toxocara* spp.

Autoimmune

Vasculitis: Kawasaki disease, polyarteritis nodosa, granulomatous vasculitis, hypersensitivity vasculitis

Rheumatologic disorders: Systemic juvenile idiopathic arthritis (JIA), systemic lupus erythematosus, acute rheumatic fever

Inflammatory bowel disease

Hematologic–oncologic

Hemophagocytic syndromes

Leukemia/lymphoma

Solid tumors: Neuroblastoma, Wilms tumor, hepatoblastoma

Other

Drug fever[d]	Munchausen by proxy
Sarcoidosis	Anticholinergic toxicity
Central fever[e]	Thyrotoxicosis
Primary immunodeficiency	

[a]Children <6 years are less likely to present with classic signs of infectious mononucleosis.

[b]Notable sites of osteomyelitis presenting as FUO include vertebral and pelvic osteomyelitis.

[c]*Yersinia enterocolitica, Salmonella typhi* and nontyphoid *Salmonella* may cause prolonged fever with delayed or brief gastrointestinal symptoms.

[d]Most commonly implicated are sulfa drugs, beta-lactam agents, and antiepileptic drugs.

[e]Suspected in patients with central nervous system injury or anomalies.

or residence in an endemic area. Exposure to domestic and wild animals increases the risk of numerous zoonotic infections. Tularemia may be suspected in a patient with recent exposure to rabbits or other rodents; exposure to domestic or wild animals may increase the risk of leptospirosis or brucellosis. Bartonellosis should be considered in the patient with exposure to cats or, more commonly, kittens. A history of travel or residence (such as camping) in wooded or tick-infested areas may increase the risk of rickettsial infections as well as Lyme disease. Rat-bite fever may be considered in the patient who reports ingestion of food or liquids contaminated by rodents or who has a history of a rodent bite or scratch. Diet is an important source of infectious exposure because consumption of unpasteurized dairy products may increase the risk of brucellosis and Q-fever, and a history of pica increases the risk of infection with *Toxocara* spp.

A medication history should be elicited, including both recently initiated and established medications. Although drug fever is more likely to be related to medications initiated in the 1 to 2 weeks prior to fever onset, it may also be an idiosyncratic reaction manifesting itself several months after drug initiation. A history of anticholinergic medication use (present in some cold, allergy, and antiemetic medications) may lead to hyperthermia due to anticholinergic toxicity.

Last, the genetic background of the patient should be considered. Familial dysautonomia (Riley–Day syndrome) is more common in persons of Jewish heritage, while sarcoidosis is more common in the African-American population. Various periodic fever syndromes have particular association with ethnicity, including familial Mediterranean syndrome (non-Ashkenazi Jews, Armenians, Arabs, and Turks), hyperimmunoglobulinemia D syndrome (Dutch, French), and tumor necrosis factor receptor–associated periodic syndrome (Irish, Scottish).

Physical Examination

A review of the patient's vital signs may reveal certain clues about the underlying etiology. Bradycardia in the setting of fever may indicate the presence of heart block, as may be seen with acute rheumatic fever, infective endocarditis, Lyme disease, or viral myocarditis. Relative bradycardia (a low-normal pulse rate in the setting of fever) is suggestive of typhoid fever, brucellosis, leptospirosis, or drug fever.

An ophthalmic exam may reveal bulbar conjunctivitis, as seen with Kawasaki disease or leptospirosis, or it may point to uveitis, as seen with JIA or sarcoidosis. The sinuses should be examined for signs of sinusitis, including tenderness, erythema, and swelling. (Note that transillumination is unreliable in children <10 years of age.) Hyperemia of the pharynx can be seen with infectious mononucleosis, Kawasaki disease, leptospirosis, or oropharyngeal tularemia.

The heart should be examined for the presence of murmurs, as this increases suspicion for infective endocarditis, acute rheumatic fever, and Kawasaki disease. A pericardial friction rub may be appreciated in the presence of pericardial effusion, seen in systemic JIA, systemic lupus erythematosus, and Kawasaki disease. Lung exam may reveal evidence of consolidation, adventitial sounds, or a pleural friction rub, which may suggest tuberculosis, endemic mycoses, or rheumatologic processes.

Many disease processes may manifest themselves with organomegaly, including malignancy, systemic JIA, typhoid fever, malaria, bartonellosis, and hepatic or splenic abscess. An abdominal mass, particularly in a child <2 years of age, is a common presenting sign of neuroblastoma and Wilms' tumor. Abdominal and/or perirectal tenderness may be suggestive of an intra-abdominal, retroperitoneal, or pelvic abscess.

A detailed musculoskeletal examination for tenderness of the muscles or bones, range of motion, and swelling as well as an examination of gait should be performed. In the preverbal child, this portion of the examination is crucial, as this may be the only means of identifying the presence of a deep myositis, osteomyelitis, or inflammatory/infectious arthritis.

Certain disease processes produce distinctive skin findings. An evanescent macular salmon-colored rash may appear during fever spikes with systemic JIA. Subcutaneous nodules and erythema marginatum may be present with acute rheumatic fever, while splinter hemorrhages, Janeway lesions, and Osler nodes are classically described in infective endocarditis. The presence of petechiae may indicate thrombocytopenia, as seen with bony infiltrative processes such as leukemia, while petechiae and purpura in the ill-appearing child may be ominous signs of bacteremia and sepsis.

Labs and Tests to Consider

In the patient with neurologic and/or meningeal signs, a lumbar puncture with cell count, protein, glucose, bacterial and mycobacterial cultures, and Gram and acid-fast stains should be performed. Additional cerebrospinal fluid (CSF) may be saved for other tests. A bone marrow aspirate may be indicated in the patient with suspected malignancy or infectious infiltrative process (e.g., mycobacterial, fungal). If gastrointestinal symptoms are present, stool cultures for enteric pathogens should be ordered. Enterovirus often presents as nonspecific febrile illness and may be detected by polymerase chain reaction (PCR) tests or by cell cultures from stool, urine, CSF, and/or blood. Patients suspected of having malaria or babesiosis should have a blood smear analysis.

Serologic testing may be helpful if the clinical presentation is suggestive of specific etiologies, such as tularemia, brucellosis, rickettsial disease, and leptospirosis. If cytomegalovirus is suspected, paired acute and convalescent serologies may indicate primary infection. Immunoserologies such as antineutrophil cytoplasmic antibodies (ANCA) and antinuclear antibody (ANA) profile may be helpful if specific rheumatologic processes are being considered. Note that systemic JIA is rarely associated with a positive ANA finding.

Key Diagnostic Labs and Tests

The following screening tests should be performed: complete blood cell count with differential, inflammatory markers (erythrocyte sedimentation rate [ESR] and C-reactive protein), hepatic enzyme levels, urinalysis and urine culture, blood culture, tuberculin skin test, and chest radiograph. An ESR ≥100 mm/hr increases the likelihood of processes such as Kawasaki disease, malignancy, or rheumatologic disorders. Multiple blood cultures may be required to detect bacteremia associated with infective endocarditis; for fastidious organisms (e.g., those associated with culture-negative infective endocarditis, as well as zoonotic organisms such as *Francisella* and *Brucella* spp.), a prolonged incubation time may be required. Because of the high frequency of Epstein–Barr virus (EBV) infection presenting as FUO in children, EBV serologies should be strongly considered, especially if hepatic enzymes are abnormal. Bartonellosis is another frequent infectious cause of FUO; its presence should be assessed by serology in children with exposure to cats.

Imaging

CLINICAL PEARL

The literature does not support the use of nonselective imaging for patients with FUO in the absence of diagnostic evidence from the history and physical examination.

The initial evaluation and screening workup should direct the use of imaging modalities. In the patient with gait changes, localized pain, or a decreased range of motion, osteomyelitis and other bony infiltrative processes should be considered, leading to a nuclear bone scan (if unable to localize), or magnetic resonance imaging (MRI). Abdominal ultrasonography and/or abdominal computed tomography (CT) are useful studies if intra-abdominal processes are suspected. A chest CT may be helpful in patients with persistent respiratory symptoms or abnormalities on chest radiography. Head CT or brain MRI may reveal the presence of abscess, leptomeningeal enhancement, or other infectious lesions in the patient with neurologic signs or altered mental status. In children >1 year of age with evidence of sinusitis, a CT of the sinuses may assist in making the diagnosis. Note that sinusitis is rare in infants, and the presence of sinus abnormalities on CT in the absence of clinical evidence is not diagnostic. An echocardiogram should be obtained in patients suspected of having infective endocarditis.

Treatment

The use of empiric therapy should be considered only for those patients whose health is significantly compromised. The use of empiric antibiotics is inappropriate unless a specific bacterial cause is considered likely. Fever may be managed by the use of antipyretics as necessary for the patient's comfort. If drug fever is suspected, cessation of the drug exposure for 48 hours or 3 to 5 half-lives should result in fever resolution, although hypersensitivity reactions, such as serum sickness or erythema multiforme, may take longer to resolve.

Admission Criteria and Level-of-Care Criteria

FUO in itself is not an indication for hospitalization, although in the well-appearing child, hospitalization may be warranted for coordination of a diagnostic workup. The critically ill child with FUO may warrant intensive care management for close monitoring and emergent intervention.

Because of his ill appearance and dehydration, the case patient was admitted to the hospital for intravenous fluids and further management. After receiving two 20-mL/kg boluses of normal saline and acetaminophen, he was much more active and his exam was less concerning. He was started on maintenance intravenous fluids and multiple lab tests were ordered to look for possible infectious etiologies of his fever. These included daily blood cultures, EBV and CMV serologies, cat-scratch titers, serum adenovirus and enterovirus PCR, routine stool culture, stool for adenovirus, and a respiratory viral direct flourescent antibody panel. On the third day of hospitalization, his EBV serologies, consistent with acute infection, came back. At that point, he continued to have daily fevers but was otherwise active and well appearing; he was therefore discharged.

EXTENDED IN-HOSPITAL MANAGEMENT

The duration of inpatient management is wholly dependent upon the etiology of FUO and the patient's clinical course.

DISPOSITION

Discharge Goals

At a minimum, consider discharge in the well-appearing patient with stable vital signs who is able to maintain adequate hydration through oral intake. Defervescence is not necessarily required if serious and/or treatable conditions have been excluded, close follow-up can be established, and the patient's caregivers are comfortable with discharge.

Outpatient Care

Outpatient follow-up should be determined by the final diagnosis. Patients with self-limited or undetermined etiology but resolved symptoms should have follow-up within 2 to 3 days of discharge. Patients with persistent or recurring fever should have close follow-up, as reevaluation for additional diagnostic clues and further workup may be indicated.

WHAT YOU NEED TO REMEMBER

- Most FUOs are uncommon manifestations of common diseases.
- Avoid a shotgun approach to evaluation! A careful history and physical examination will produce a higher-yield investigation.
- Some 20% to 40% of all FUOs will self-resolve without diagnosis.

SUGGESTED READINGS

Jacobs RF, Schutze GE. *Bartonella henselae* as a cause of prolonged fever and fever of unknown origin in children. *Clin Infect Dis* 1998;26:80–84.

Long SS. Distinguishing among prolonged, recurrent, and periodic fever syndromes: approach of a pediatric infectious disease specialist. *Pediatr Clin North Am* 2005;52:811–835

Long SS, Edwards KM. Prolonged, recurrent, and periodic fever syndromes. In Long SS, Pickering LK, Prober CG, eds. *Principles and Practice of Infectious Diseases*, 3rd ed. New York: Churchill Livingstone, 2008:126–135.

Powell KP. Fever without a focus. In: Kliegman RM, Behrman RE, Jenson HB, Stanton BF, eds. *Nelson textbook of pediatrics*, 18th ed. Philadelphia: Saunders Elsevier, 2007.

Steele RW, Jones SM, Lowe BA, Glasier CM. Usefulness of scanning procedures for diagnosis of fever of unknown origin in children. *J Pediatr* 1991;199:526–530.

Gastroenteritis

TRACY ANN MERRILL

THE PATIENT ENCOUNTER

A 4-year-old male presented to the emergency room with a 2-day history of vomiting followed by a 1-day history of watery, non-bloody, nonmucoid diarrhea. His mother had spoken to the pediatrician by phone the day prior and started him on small amounts of clear fluids frequently. Though the child's vomiting had improved, he had suffered eight watery stools the day of presentation. He was tachycardic at 134 beats per minute, his temperature was 37.9°C (100.2°F), and his respiratory rate and blood pressure were normal. He was pale, with dry, cracked lips, but was alert and cooperative. His capillary refill was 2 seconds, and he had mild, diffuse abdominal tenderness without localizing signs.

OVERVIEW

Definition

Gastroenteritis refers to the acute onset of diarrhea with or without nausea, vomiting, fever, or abdominal cramps. Diarrhea can be further defined as the increased frequency and decreased consistency of stool, often with increased stool weight owing to excess water. Excess water comes from increased intestinal secretion, decreased absorption, or both. This chapter focuses on acute diarrheal illnesses in children lasting ≤14 days. Diarrhea that persists beyond 14 days is classified as chronic or protracted diarrhea and warrants a separate evaluative approach.

Pathophysiology

Infectious gastroenteritis develops when the gastrointestinal tract is colonized or invaded by viruses, bacteria, or parasites or when a preformed toxin is ingested. This occurs mainly through the ingestion of contaminated water or food or directly from another person through fecal–oral contact. The small and large intestines may be affected separately or together, depending on the pathogen. Diarrhea can further be classified as noninflammatory or inflammatory.

Noninflammatory diarrhea occurs by three mechanisms: (i) the adherence of bacteria or parasites to the intestinal mucosa, (ii) the production of bacterial enterotoxin, and (iii) the viral destruction of the villis' surface cells. Pathogens adhere to the mucosa via plasmid-encoded adhesion proteins, including fimbriae or pili. Adherence causes thinning of the lumenal enterocyte membrane with subsequent destruction of the microvillis' brush border. Enterotoxins, such as cholera toxin, are polypeptides that are made by some bacteria. They cause intestinal secretion of fluid and electrolytes by binding to the gut cell membrane and inserting part of their structure into the cell, usually without causing direct tissue damage. Viruses tend to attach to and damage surface cells, leading to blunting of the villi without infecting the crypt cells. The surface epithelium of the villi is then repopulated by secretory cells. Coupled with the loss of absorptive cells, the net secretion of water and electrolytes occurs. Incompletely absorbed nutrients contribute to an increased osmotic load, further contributing to diarrheal losses. Fecal leukocytes are not present in these cases.

Inflammatory diarrhea is usually caused by bacteria that invade the intestinal mucosa directly or that produce cytotoxins. These bacteria usually contain a virulence plasmid that allows them to enter the cells by endocytosis. Once inside the cell, they replicate and cause cell lysis, after which they continue to spread to other cells. Some bacteria, such as *Salmonella*, can spread directly between neighboring cells by transcytosis. Cytotoxins are polypeptides, such as Shiga toxin, that cause direct tissue damage and necrosis of epithelial cells. Fecal leukocytes are present in the stool of these patients.

Epidemiology

Worldwide, it is estimated that 3 to 5 billion cases of acute gastroenteritis occur each year in children <5 years of age. Up to 35 million of these cases occur in the United States, which translates to an approximate incidence of 1.3 to 2.3 cases of gastroenteritis per child annually, which is surpassed in frequency only by the common cold. Approximately 13 out of every 1,000 of these cases results in a hospitalization, accounting for 9% of all pediatric hospitalizations under the age of 5 years. Gastroenteritis is the second most common cause of death globally in children <5 years old and is estimated to cause about 1.8 million deaths per year.

Etiology

In developed countries like the United States, viruses account for 87% of gastroenteritis cases, with rotavirus being most common, followed by adenovirus, calicivirus, Norwalk virus in older children, and astrovirus. In developing countries, bacterial pathogens are more frequent; however, rotavirus is still highly prevalent and a cause of significant morbidity and mortality. The following paragraphs summarize the most frequently encountered pathogens.

Rotavirus is transmitted person to person through the fecal oral route and can also survive on fomites. Rotavirus often results in epidemic spread because most infected patients shed the virus for several days before developing symptoms. The incubation period is 2 to 4 days, illness can last from

3 to 8 days, and stool excretion can persist for up to 21 days. The illness begins with fever and vomiting, followed by 1 to 4 days of profuse, watery diarrhea. Diagnosis is by enzyme immunoassay (EIA) or latex agglutination assay for group A rotavirus antigen in stool. Treatment is supportive. Two oral rotavirus vaccines, RotaTeq (Merck) and Rotarix (GlaxoSmithKline), are now available for use in young infants.

Campylobacter is a comma-shaped gram-negative bacillus that causes bloody diarrhea, abdominal cramps, malaise, and fever. It usually causes a mild 1- to 2-day illness, but the relapse rate can reach 20%. It can mimic appendicitis, intussusception, and inflammatory bowel disease in prolonged cases. Treatment is recommended to decrease illness duration and stool excretion and to prevent relapse. Treat affected patients with erythromycin or azithromycin for 5 to 7 days.

Clostridium difficile, a gram-positive spore-forming bacillus, is found in soil. It causes bloody mucoid diarrhea with significant abdominal pain and fever. Some infected patients develop a severe pseudomembranous colitis. *C. difficile* commonly affects patients who have recently been on antibiotics and whose mucosal barrier is altered, allowing the pathogen to proliferate. Asymptomatic carriage is common in newborns and young infants. Diagnosis is by stool enzyme immunoassay for *C. difficile* toxin. Treatment is with oral or IV metronidazole or oral vancomycin for 10 days.

Cryptosporidium is an oocyst-forming protozoan. Transmission occurs by direct contact with infected animals, as at petting zoos; through person-to-person contact, as at daycare centers; and through the ingestion of contaminated municipal drinking water or public swimming pool water (because the organism is resistant to chlorine). It causes nonbloody watery diarrhea with or without cramps, vomiting, anorexia, weight loss, and fever, but it can also be asymptomatic. Incubation is 2 to 14 days and disease is usually self-limited, lasting from 1 to 20 days. Diagnosis is by microscopic examination of stool for oocytes, antigen detection by EIA, or antibody-based fluorescein stain. Treatment (with nitazoxanide) is necessary only in patients with protracted illness or a compromised immune system.

Escherichia coli is a gram-negative bacillus transmitted by food and water that is contaminated with the stool of infected people or animals such as cattle, deer, and sheep. Frequent sources of infection include the consumption of undercooked ground beef, unwashed produce, and unpasteurized milk or apple cider, as well as visits to petting zoos. There are five main strains of *E. coli*, but only one of them is common in the United States: Shiga toxin–producing *E. coli*, or STEC. The most virulent strain is STEC 0157:H7. Serious complications include hemolytic uremic syndrome (HUS) in children and thrombotic thrombocytopenic purpura (TTP) in adults. The other four *E. coli* strains include enteropathogenic *E. coli* (EPEC), enteroinvasive *E. coli* (EIEC), enteroaggregative *E. coli* (EAEC), and enterotoxigenic *E. coli* (ETEC; a major cause of traveler's diarrhea).

Diagnosis is by stool culture or Shiga toxin immunologic assay. There is no benefit to treatment of STEC, but traveler's diarrhea can be treated with 3 days of Bactrim, azithromycin, or ciprofloxacin. Children need two negative stool cultures before returning to day care.

Giardia, a flagellate protozoan, is transmitted person to person or via contaminated food or water. The infection is localized to the small intestine and biliary tract. It causes an intermittent, watery, foul-smelling diarrhea with flatulence, anorexia, and abdominal distention and cramps. Chronically infected patients may develop weight loss and anemia. Reservoirs for *Giardia* include humans, dogs, cats, and beavers. Incubation is 1 to 4 weeks and infectious cysts can be excreted in stool for several months. Diagnosis is by examination of fecal smear or duodenal contents (obtained by the "string test"), by immunofluorescent antibody testing, or by direct fluorescent antibody (DFA) testing of stool. Treatment options for symptomatic patients include 7 days of metronidazole, 3 days of nitazoxanide, or a single dose of mebendazole.

Salmonella, a gram-negative bacillus, can be transmitted by direct contact with infected livestock, pets, and reptiles (frogs, salamanders, turtles, lizards, snakes) or by the ingestion of contaminated poultry, beef, raw eggs, dairy products, or water. Incubation is only 12 to 36 hours. Acute infection causes diarrhea with abdominal cramps and fever, which can progress to colitis or bacteremia. Diagnosis is by stool culture. Antibiotic therapy prolongs excretion; therefore treatment is appropriate only in infants <3 months of age or in hosts who are immunocompromised. Ampicillin, amoxicillin, or Bactrim may be used but resistant cases may require ceftriaxone, cefotaxime, or fluoroquinolones.

Shigella, a gram-negative bacillus, is transmitted via the fecal–oral route from person to person, through contact with primates, through housefly-contamination of food, or from the ingestion of contaminated water. Incubation is 2 to 4 days and the site of infection is the large intestine. *Shigella sonnei* causes 88% of cases and produces watery diarrhea. *Shigella flexneri*, *boydii*, and *dysenteriae* account for remaining cases and produce bloody mucoid diarrhea, fever, abdominal pain, and tenesmus. Diagnosis is by stool culture. Most cases are self-limited and last 2 to 3 days; therefore therapy is warranted only in severe cases of dysentery or if the patient is immunocompromised. Treatment is with 5 days of either ampicillin (resistance in the United States approaches 77%), Bactrim, ceftriaxone, fluoroquinolones, or azithromycin.

ACUTE MANAGEMENT AND WORKUP

Acute gastroenteritis can lead to varying levels of dehydration, electrolyte imbalance, and acidosis, so acute management requires rapid risk assessment of the severity of the patient's condition and support of vascular volume as needed, followed by stabilization and attempts to halt disease progression.

The First 15 Minutes

Upon the initial survey, it is important to assess the ABCs (airway, breathing, and circulation). Severely dehydrated patients may be acidotic, hypokalemic, or hypoglycemic and may present with altered mental status, tachycardia, or tachypnea; or they may be in hypovolemic shock. Quick assessment of vital signs and a clinical estimate of the severity of dehydration are crucial to determining whether aggressive volume resuscitation is required (see "Physical Examination," below). For severe dehydration, obtain IV or IO access and begin a rapid fluid bolus of normal saline or lactated Ringer's solution, 20 mL/kg, before moving on to your secondary survey.

The First Few Hours

A thorough history and physical exam will help you develop a differential for the etiology of the illness as well as to decide what laboratory or imaging evaluation may be useful. Treatment can then be tailored to the individual patient's clinical status and adjustments made as the patient responds to therapy. Ultimately, a disposition will be made to discharge the patient home or admit him or her for further care.

History

A thorough history must include a history of present illness, a review of systems, past medical history, family history, social history, and exposure history. The history of present illness details when the symptoms started, the order in which the symptoms appeared, the number of episodes of vomiting and diarrhea, when the most recent episodes occurred, the physical quality of the vomitus and diarrhea (such as bilious, bloody, watery, mucoid), and any remedies tried so far. A review of systems should discern whether or not fever, weight loss, abdominal pain, rectal discomfort, dysuria, oliguria, headache, dizziness, weakness, or syncope is present. The past medical history should assess the patient's vaccination status and prior gastrointestinal or autoimmune disease. The family history may reveal other noninfectious causes of diarrhea to include in the differential diagnosis, such as inflammatory bowel disease (Crohn's disease or ulcerative colitis), irritable bowel syndrome, lactose intolerance, polyposis, a gastrointestinal neoplasm, or malabsorption syndromes such as celiac disease. The social history should include day care attendance or habitation in a shelter or treatment center where large numbers of people live in close proximity. Exposures should include sick contacts, recent antibiotic use, recent travel, freshwater or well-water ingestion, pets (especially reptilian), visits to petting zoos, or public pool use.

Physical Examination

The most critical aspect of the physical exam is to identify the degree of dehydration. *Mild dehydration* (<5% fluid deficit) is characterized by normal vital signs, slightly dry mucous membranes, brisk capillary refill, and normal to slightly decreased urine output. Patients with *moderate dehydration* (5% to 10% fluid deficit) are tachycardic but have normal blood pressures. They may be listless and may have mildly sunken eyes, a capillary refill of ≥2 seconds, and dry mucous membranes. Patients who are *severely dehydrated* (>10% fluid deficit) may be lethargic or unresponsive. They will be tachycardic and might be hypotensive. They are likely to have poor skin turgor with cool extremities and a capillary refill >2 seconds.

Another important exam finding is tachypnea, which suggests the presence of metabolic acidosis. Assess the fontanelle in infants, which might be depressed in dehydrated patients. Evaluate the abdomen for peritoneal signs, such as rebound and guarding, and, if present, consider other diagnoses, such as intussusception or appendicitis. Hypokalemia causes electrocardiographic (ECG) changes, including flattened T waves and the appearance of U waves, and it may lead to dangerous dysrhythmias, such as torsades.

Labs and Tests to Consider

Patients can lose a large amount of sodium, potassium, chloride, and bicarbonate in diarrheal stools, warranting electrolyte testing in some cases. Patients also tend to become hypoglycemic if they have had poor intake or vomiting. If diarrhea is bloody, testing the patient's hemoglobin level is reasonable, and if a family history of inflammatory bowel disease (IBD) is present, inflammatory markers, including the erythrocyte sedimentation rate (ESR) and C-reactive protein (CRP), may be helpful. If HUS is suspected, renal function tests and a platelet level are essential. Assessment of renal function is also important in severe dehydration to look for acute renal insufficiency or failure. Optional stool studies are case-specific, depending on the suspected etiology, and include stool culture, *Giardia*, Rotazyme, ova and parasites, *Cryptosporidium*, *C. difficile*, *V. cholerae*, and Hemoccult for blood.

Key Diagnostic Labs and Tests

A serum electrolyte panel should be done in patients who are moderately dehydrated and for whom there is no straightforward diagnosis from the history and physical, in those who are severely dehydrated, and in any patient who receives IV fluids. The most common abnormalities found are decreased bicarbonate levels, hypoglycemia, hypokalemia, and hypernatremia.

Imaging

Abdominal radiographs are indicated in cases of suspected ileus (e.g., vomiting and hypoactive or absent bowel sounds), obstruction, or in processes other than gastroenteritis, such as intussusception. Any child with hypoactive or absent bowel sounds, high-pitched tinkling bowel sounds, or peritoneal signs on exam should have plain films done to evaluate the bowel gas pattern. The appearance of air–fluid levels on an upright film or a paucity of distal bowel gas suggests obstruction. The presence of free air underneath the diaphragm indicates bowel perforation.

Treatment

If a child is not dehydrated, oral fluid replacement should be maintained for each diarrheal stool passed, with a goal of 10 mL/kg per stool. Otherwise the patient may continue to consume a diet appropriate for age. Infants may continue to breast-feed or receive formula and older children may continue to drink milk. Although lactase enzyme release will be reduced in an injured intestinal brush border, most patients can tolerate foods containing lactose without worsening symptoms or signs of malabsorption.

In mildly to moderately dehydrated children, oral rehydration therapy is as effective as IV fluid rehydration. The goal for fluid replacement in mild dehydration is 50 mL/kg plus replacement of ongoing losses to be administered over a 4-hour period. The goal in moderate dehydration is 100 mL/kg plus replacement of ongoing losses over a 4-hour period. Oral rehydration solutions should contain appropriate amounts of electrolytes and glucose. The World Health Organization promotes the use of an oral rehydration solution containing a high concentration of sodium (75 mmol/L). Rehydration using this type of solution has had a profound effect on morbidity and mortality in developing countries with high rates of diarrheal disease. There are also a variety of commercially made products in the United States, including Pedialyte and Infalyte, whose sodium concentrations are lower (45 to 50 mmol/L) but that can be effectively used to rehydrate infants and children. Sports drinks are commonly used in older children but caution is advised because of their even lower sodium content of approximately 20 mmol/L and usually higher glucose content. Inappropriate beverages to use include juice and soda products whose sodium concentrations are extremely low.

Early refeeding as soon as the patient is rehydrated can decrease the duration of diarrhea by approximately 0.5 days. Fatty foods and foods containing high quantities of simple sugars should be avoided, as they may exacerbate the diarrhea.

IV fluid therapy is required for patients who are severely dehydrated, have altered mental status, have an intestinal ileus, present in hypovolemic shock, or are moderately dehydrated and have failed attempts at oral rehydration due to persistent vomiting. Normal saline or lactated Ringer's solution should be administered at 20 mL/kg over an hour and more rapidly in cases of poor perfusion. Additional fluids may be necessary in cases of hypernatremia, in clinically relevant bicarbonate loss (<16 mmol/L), in ongoing losses, or with an unimproved clinical picture. Dextrose water in the form of D10W or D25W should be administered if the serum glucose level is <60 mg/dL, and potassium replacement should be considered if potassium is ≤3.0 mmol/L.

Recent studies have shown that nasogastric (NG) fluid administration is as effective as IV infusion and is an option for moderately dehydrated patients. However, NG tubes should not be used in patients with persistent emesis, an altered mental status, or an ileus, and placement must be confirmed prior to fluid administration. Isotonic glucose–electrolyte solutions should be used at the same rate as IV fluids.

> ## CLINICAL PEARL
>
> *Antidiarrheal medications are not recommended in children owing to the chance of adverse side effects. They tend to increase organism carriage in the stool and can increase the risk for ileus and intestinal perforation.*

Probiotics are live microorganisms that are used to replenish normal intestinal flora. They are often used concomitantly with antibiotics to reduce the overgrowth of pathogenic bacteria. Recent studies have shown that they can also help reduce the duration of diarrhea in cases of acute viral gastroenteritis, especially that due to rotavirus. The three most common forms are *Lactobacillus*, *Saccharomyces*, and *Bifidobacterium*. They have been used in all ages without significant adverse effects, but further studies are required before routine use can be recommended.

Admission Criteria and Level-of-Care Criteria

Children requiring more than 50 mL/kg of IV or NG fluids over 3 hours or who have intestinal ileus should be admitted. Admission should also be considered for children who have electrolyte abnormalities, such as hypoglycemia, hypokalemia, or hypernatremia. The use of bicarbonate levels to assess the severity of dehydration and the need for admission has been controversial. A bicarbonate level ≤16 mmol/L is considered clinically significant and a level ≤13 mmol/L identifies most children who will not be able to tolerate oral rehydration therapy at home. Most children can be managed on the inpatient general pediatric service, but patients with an altered mental status, severe metabolic acidosis, and those who are in hypovolemic shock should be considered for ICU admission.

EXTENDED IN-HOSPITAL MANAGEMENT

Once stabilized and admitted to the hospital, patients should receive maintenance IV fluids. Antiemetics such as ondansetron (ages ≥6 months) or promethazine (ages ≥2 years) reduce the frequency and duration of vomiting. Frequent blood glucose checks may be needed in hypoglycemic patients and electrolyte panels may be needed every 12 to 24 hours, depending on the initial abnormalities. Patients with intestinal ileus may benefit from NG decompression and bowel rest until resolved. All patients should be placed on contact precautions to prevent nosocomial spread.

DISPOSITION

Discharge Goals

Patients must have normalized electrolytes, have decreased pain and emesis, be afebrile, and be able to tolerate oral intake before being discharged from the hospital.

Outpatient Care

Once rehydrated, patients can resume a normal diet at home and can continue to replace fluid losses for any ongoing diarrhea. Specific antimicrobials may be required depending on the responsible pathogen, and probiotics and/or antiemetics can be administered at home as needed. All hospitalized patients should be rechecked by their pediatrician 2 days after hospital discharge. Patients should not return to school or day care until the diarrhea has resolved and, in some cases, until one to three stool cultures on different days are negative. Patients should not use recreational water areas such as pools, rivers, lakes, or oceans for 2 weeks after the cessation of diarrhea.

The patient in the case study was admitted for moderate dehydration and hypoglycemia. His glucose level was 47 mg/dL and his bicarbonate level was 10 mmol/L. He received IV fluids overnight and was discharged home after 24 hours. His final diagnosis was rotavirus.

 WHAT YOU NEED TO REMEMBER

- Send stool studies in cases in which nonviral causes are suspected, especially if the patient has bloody or mucoid diarrhea or significant fevers.
- Electrolyte abnormalities cannot be predicted clinically, so all patients receiving IV fluids, especially <1 year of age, should have a serum electrolyte panel.
- Never use antimotility agents in children.

SUGGESTED READINGS

American Academy of Pediatrics. Summaries of infectious diseases. In Pickering LK, Baker CJ, Long SS, McMillan JA, eds. *Red Book: 2006 Report of the Committee on Infectious Diseases*, 27th ed. Elk Grove Village, IL: American Academy of Pediatrics; 2006:201–734.

Faust H, Jakobsen PS, Rabouhans ML. *Oral Rehydration Salts: Production of the New ORS*. World Health Organization online publication. 2006:2–5. Available at http://www.who.int/child-adolescent-health

Nager AL, Wang VJ. Comparison of nasogastric and intravenous methods of rehydration in pediatric patients with acute dehydration. *Pediatrics* 2002;109:566–572.

United Health Foundation. Gastroenteritis in children. Dalby-Payne J, Elliott E, eds. *BMJ: Clinical Evidence Handbook*. Tavistock Square, London, UK: BMJ Publishing Group, 2007:83–84.

Wathen JE, MacKenzie T, Bothner JP. Usefulness of the serum electrolyte panel in the management of pediatric dehydration treated with intravenously administered fluids. *Pediatrics* 2004;114:1227–1234.

Gastroesophageal Reflux Disease

DAVID E. HALL

THE PATIENT ENCOUNTER

A 4-month-old female infant is brought to the clinic for a routine checkup. During the visit, her mother tells you that she is concerned about the baby's frequent spitting up, which began at about 1 month of age. After a meal, she sometimes vomits her formula. She does this in an effortless way and does not seem distressed. The emesis is the color of milk and is not projectile. The baby is fed a formula based on cow's milk. She is otherwise healthy and developmentally normal. The infant's weight and height are 75th and 50th percentile, respectively. The physical examination, including head circumference and fontanelle, is normal.

OVERVIEW

Definition

Gastroesophageal reflux (GER) is the normal physiologic passage of gastric contents into the esophagus. Regurgitation, which refers to the passage of gastric contents into the oropharynx or mouth, may also be normal. Vomiting is expulsion of gastric contents out of the mouth. Gastroesophageal reflux disease (GERD) occurs when GER persists and produces symptoms or complications such as pain, irritability (usually due to esophagitis), poor weight gain, wheezing or other respiratory symptoms, dysphagia (difficulty swallowing), odynophagia (pain with swallowing), or abnormal posturing during feedings. GERD-related symptoms can also include esophageal bleeding, apnea, or an acute life-threatening event (ALTE).

Sandifer syndrome, an abnormal posturing associated with reflux, is sometimes incorrectly diagnosed as a seizure. The infant may suddenly and briefly rotate the head and neck to one side, arch the back, extend the legs, and flex the elbows. Unlike a child having a seizure, the patient remains alert during the episodes, there is no postepisode sleepiness, and there is usually a history of these movements being related to meals or other symptoms consistent with reflux.

Pathophysiology

GERD occurs when the lower esophageal sphincter relaxes transiently and often inappropriately. Intraesophageal pressure is typically lower than intragastric pressure, so gastric contents may normally reflux into the esophagus.

In children with GERD, once the sphincter relaxes and gastric contents reflux into the esophagus, the intraesophageal muscle tone relaxes further and esophageal peristalsis fails to occur. In addition, decreased intrathoracic pressure, which can occur during respiratory distress, increases reflux. Transient increases in abdominal pressure can also do so. Other factors include delays in the duration of gastric emptying, increases in gastric volume, the position of the crural diaphragm in relation to the esophagus, the effect of gravity and position on gastric contents, and abnormalities in esophageal motility. The esophagus of infants has a small capacity, so reflux is more likely to cause vomiting in infants than in adults. In addition, the angle between the esophagus and stomach is larger in infants than in older children and adults, which contributes to the increased prevalence of reflux in this age group.

GERD can present in many ways; symptoms vary depending on the age of the child. In neonates and young infants, failure to thrive or poor weight gain can occur owing to excess vomiting of feedings, causing caloric deprivation. The esophagus is poorly protected against the digestive enzymes and the low pH of gastric contents. Patients with GERD can develop esophagitis and pain. Infants may also present with irritability, excessive crying, or arching of the back. If feeding is associated with pain, children may eat less and demonstrate poor weight gain even without vomiting. Older children and adults may complain of heartburn, upper abdominal pain, or chest pain. Less commonly, esophageal bleeding can develop and lead to iron deficiency anemia.

In some infants, GERD is associated with apnea or ALTEs, although this association is somewhat controversial and may be overdiagnosed. GERD is also associated with recurrent wheezing caused by the frequent aspiration of small amounts of liquid or food into the lungs, causing inflammation, or by stimulation of chemoreceptors in the airway or esophagus. In neurologically impaired patients, particularly those who lack coordinated oropharyngeal function, reflux can lead to aspiration and pneumonia. Neurologically normal patients are less likely to develop pneumonia from reflux because they are better able to protect their airways. Some studies have demonstrated that reflux can cause hoarseness or laryngitis, presumably from direct irritation of the vocal cords by acidic gastric contents. Some studies suggest that recurrent sinusitis and otitis media are associated with reflux.

Epidemiology

GER, or normal physiologic reflux, is extremely common in infants. One study reported that half of babies 3 months of age regurgitated at least once a day. Regurgitation peaked at 4 months, and more than 60% of parents reported this symptom. However, by 12 months of age, only 5% of patients were reported to have regurgitation; after age 18 months, it was even less common. In children 3 to 17 years of age, the prevalence of symptoms of GERD has been reported to range from 1.4% to 8.2%.

Etiology

GER falls within the spectrum of normal variation in infants and is probably due to neurologic and physical immaturity. There appears to be a genetic component to GERD in many patients. It is exacerbated by caffeine, tobacco (including passive smoking), alcohol, and possibly spicy foods. GERD is especially common in children with cerebral palsy and other forms of neurologic impairment. Patients with congenital esophageal abnormalities, such as those with tracheoesophageal fistulas, have a high prevalence of GERD. Children with cystic fibrosis are at long-term risk for GERD because they have abnormal esophageal motility, dysfunction of the lower esophageal sphincter, and a poor saliva-buffering capacity.

ACUTE MANAGEMENT AND WORKUP

GER is not an emergency; however, GERD may require acute management if the condition is causing a new problem, such as an ALTE or pneumonia.

The First 15 Minutes

Determine whether the patient is at risk for aspiration. This may occur if the patient is neurologically impaired. If the patient is in respiratory distress, order that the child take nothing by mouth until the situation can be clarified. Make sure that the patient does not have any signs of a bowel obstruction, which is a medical emergency in an infant. Bilious (green, "pea soup" colored) vomiting is a clue to a bowel obstruction and can be seen with sudden, life-threatening volvulus associated with the malrotation of the intestine.

The First Few Hours

Take a thorough history and perform a physical examination. Look for complications of GERD.

History

A goal is to separate GER, which requires no treatment, from GERD, which requires a more aggressive approach. In addition, you do not want to miss other cause of vomiting that can be mistaken for GERD (Table 16-1). The typical child with GER but not GERD is a "happy spitter" and has no signs of any illness. He or she seems to have effortless vomiting, and the gastric contents dribble down the chin. Projectile or forceful vomiting can occur in some infants with GER, but this increases the likelihood of a pathologic process. Projectile vomiting is a classic symptom of pyloric stenosis, for example, which tends to present at 4 to 6 weeks of age. Be sure to ask for other possible causes of obstruction, such as bilious vomiting—a clue to

TABLE 16-1
Causes of Vomiting

Obstructive
Pyloric stenosis
Malrotation with intermittent
  volvulus
Intermittent intussusception
Intestinal duplication
Hirschsprung disease
Antral/duodenal web
Foreign body
Incarcerated hernia
Superior mesenteric artery
  syndrome
Gastric bezoar

GI disorders
Achalasia
Gastroparesis
Gastroenteritis
Peptic ulcer disease
Gastroesophageal reflux
Eosinophilic esophagitis/
  gastroenteritis
Food allergy or intolerance
Inflammatory bowel disease
Pancreatitis
Appendicitis
Food intolerance or allergy

Neurologic
Hydrocephalus
Subdural hematoma
Intracranial hemorrhage
Mass lesion
Migraine headaches

Infectious
Sepsis
Meningitis
Urinary tract infection
Pneumonia
Otitis media
Hepatitis

Metabolic/endocrine
Galactosemia
Hereditary fructose intolerance
Urea cycle defects
Amino and organic acidemias
Congenital adrenal hyperplasia
Maple syrup urine disease
Hypercalcemia
Glycogen storage disease type 1
Fatty acid oxidation disorders

Renal
Obstructive uropathy
Renal insufficiency

Toxic
Lead poisoning
Iron
Vitamin A or D overdose
Medications that cause vomiting
Organophosphate exposure

Cardiac
Congestive heart failure

Other
Posttussive vomiting
Cyclic vomiting
Vestibular abnormality or
  inflammation

obstruction past the pylorus. Acute gastroenteritis may cause vomiting but is usually associated with diarrhea and, unlike GER, is short-lived. Some normal infants will spit up or vomit if they are overfed, so take a good feeding history. Most infants do not need more than 32 to 35 ounces of formula a day. Consider causes of vomiting that are outside of the gastrointestinal (GI) tract, such as increased intracranial pressure, which causes alterations in mental status or other neurologic abnormalities. A history of fever suggests an infectious cause of vomiting. Hematemesis suggests blood loss from the upper GI tract and could suggest esophagitis, among other diagnoses. If the vomiting or regurgitation starts after 6 months of life, it is less likely to result from simple GER. In the case of an infant, make sure that the newborn screen was normal. Some metabolic or endocrine diseases, such as galactosemia, maple syrup urine disease, and congenital adrenal hyperplasia, may cause vomiting. Inquire about problems in the respiratory tract such as asthma, wheezing, cough, hoarseness, apnea, and recurrent pneumonia. Other signs of GERD include feeding problems, poor weight gain, and irritability.

ALTEs associated with reflux typically occur while the child is awake and within an hour after feeding. The baby may arch its back and gag and choke during the episode. Because the apnea in this situation is usually obstructive in nature, the parents may give a history of their baby's struggle to breath during the episode but not being able to move air—"trying to breathe but can't." Take a developmental history, because developmentally delayed children are at high risk for reflux.

Physical Examination

The child with GER will have a normal physical examination, including normal growth and development. There will be no signs of increased intracranial pressure, such as a large head or bulging fontanelle. Patients with GERD may show signs of associated pathologic conditions such as wheezing or failure to thrive.

Labs and Tests to Consider

GER can be diagnosed by history and physical examination alone in most infants and older children. The case patient above had GER without GERD and required no further testing.

Key Diagnostic Labs and Tests

Esophageal pH Monitoring. This is considered a valid measure of the degree of esophageal exposure to acid and, therefore, to reflux. In this test, a microelectrode is placed through the nose into the lower esophagus. The device records the esophageal pH over an extended period (usually 24 hours, but at least 16 hours are required). Parents are asked to complete a symptom diary so that episodes of esophageal pH <4.0 can be correlated with symptoms. If the patient is on antacid therapy, the test may fail to detect reflux.

Multichannel Intraluminal Impedance (MII). This new technology measures changes in electrical impedance as a food bolus moves in the esophagus. When combined with esophageal pH monitoring, the test can determine the degree of both acid and nonacid reflux over a 24-hour period. Validated normal values for this test and correlations with GERD-related pathology in children are not available, but the use of MII might increase as we learn more.

Endoscopy. This procedure evaluates the presence and severity of esophagitis and can exclude conditions such as Crohn's disease, esophageal webs, or eosinophilic esophagitis. A biopsy is required because the esophagus can appear normal despite the presence of esophagitis.

Imaging

The primary imaging modalities include an upper gastrointestinal series and scintigraphy.

Upper Gastrointestinal Series (UGI). The primary value of an UGI is to diagnose anatomic abnormalities, such as malrotation or esophageal stricture. It does not take very long, so it can easily miss an episode of reflux in a child with GERD. Also, many normal children reflux intermittently, so the presence of reflux on a UGI is not diagnostic.

CLINICAL PEARL

The UGI is neither sensitive nor specific for the diagnosis of GERD.

Scintigraphy. This is a nuclear medicine test in which the patient is fed technetium-labeled food or formula. One then looks for evidence of aspiration into the lungs and reflux into the esophagus at periods of up to 24 hours after ingestion. The test can also assess gastric emptying time. As with the UGI, it is not very sensitive for GERD and there is a lack of normative data.

Treatment

Infants with GER without GERD require no treatment other than reassurance to the parents. However, if frequent spitting up with occasional emesis is bothersome, further intervention is sometimes needed. In the case of mild GERD, thickening of feedings has been found to reduce the quantity and frequency of regurgitation, although it has no significant effect on irritability or reflux as measured by pH probe studies. Most gastroenterologists use one teaspoon to one tablespoon of rice cereal per ounce of formula. Note that each teaspoon of rice cereal increases the caloric density by about 5 calories per ounce of formula. Also, it may be necessary to crosscut the nipple to make it easier for the infant to get the thickened feeding out of the bottle. Some prethickened infant formulas are available as well. Be aware that rice cereal will not thicken breast milk because it is quickly broken down by breast milk enzymes. A commercially available thickener (called Simplythick) may work with pumped breast milk.

Positioning, in particular the prone position and the left lateral decubitus position, is also effective in reducing reflux, but these positions are not recommended in infants because they are associated with sudden infant death syndrome. The "back to sleep" program, which recommends a supine position for infants, applies to babies with reflux as well. Many pediatricians ask parents to hold the child upright on a shoulder for 20 to 30 minutes after feeding, although reports of the effectiveness of this strategy are largely anecdotal. Elevating the head of the crib does not seem to work in the supine position. Infant seats, including car seats, tend to worsen reflux.

Formula changes may also be considered for GER or GERD. A minority of infants appear to have an intolerance to cow's milk protein and respond to a trial of protein hydrolysate–based hypoallergenic formula. For breast-fed infants, taking the mother off cow's milk and other dairy products may be reasonable. A trial of these changes in the diet is usually given for 2 to 4 weeks. Older children with GERD should avoid caffeine, tobacco, and perhaps spicy foods. For infants with reflux, exposure to secondhand smoke should be reduced.

For patients with GERD, such as older children with heartburn and infants with respiratory symptoms, esophagitis, or failure to thrive, pharmacotherapy is recommended in addition to the above measures. Proton pump inhibitors, such as lansoprazole, omeprazole, and esomeprazole, are more effective than histamine-2 receptor antagonists such as ranitidine, cimetidine, or nizatidine. Aluminum-containing antacids, such as aluminum hydroxide, which is often combined commercially with magnesium hydroxide, are not routinely used in infants because of concerns about aluminum toxicity. This can lead to neurologic abnormalities, anemia, and osteopenia. Sucralfate is a surface-active agent that is helpful in a minority of cases of esophagitis but also contains aluminum. These agents should be used only as temporizing or rescue agents. Prokinetic drugs such as metoclopramide are available, but side effects are a problem and the results of controlled trials have yielded conflicting results. They are no longer routinely used in GERD.

Surgery is the final option for treatment. The Nissen fundoplication, in which part of the stomach is wrapped around the lower esophagus, is the most popular procedure. It can be performed either as an open procedure through a laparotomy or laparoscopically. Most candidates have failed medical treatment or experienced serious complications from GERD, such as recurrent aspiration pneumonia. Many have neurologically based oropharyngeal dysfunction. Reoperation rates range from 8% to 16% in centers of excellence, with the highest rates of reoperation occurring in the first 1 to 2 years after surgery. Postfundoplication complications are more common in neurologically impaired children.

Admission Criteria and Level-of-Care Criteria

Evaluation for GERD does not necessarily require admission because pH probes and UGIs are routinely performed as outpatient procedures. Admission is sometimes needed for patients with complicated GERD, especially for those with aspiration pneumonia, ALTE, status asthmaticus, or failure to thrive that has not responded to outpatient treatment. Admission may also be required when the cause of the vomiting is unclear and the patient is unable to tolerate oral feedings.

EXTENDED IN-HOSPITAL MANAGEMENT

When the complications of GERD cannot be controlled, some patients may be treated with continuous nasogastric or gastrostomy tube feedings. Continuous feedings allow the smallest volume of feeding per hour and yet maintain required intake for growth. Patients who are poor candidates for Nissen fundoplication are sometimes fed with nasojejunal, gastrojejunal, or jejunal tube feedings. When the feeding tube is placed past the pyloric sphincter, regurgitation or emesis is greatly reduced.

DISPOSITION

Patients should be followed up with by their physician and monitored for symptoms of GERD. Because GERD can improve with age, a trial off medication is warranted as symptoms resolve. The long-term safety of protein pump inhibitors (PPIs) in children has not been well studied. However, most studies to date have found that these medications are safe in both the short and long term. Although validation of these observations is needed, there have been some recent reports of an increased risk of *Clostridium difficile* infections in patients on PPIs as well as of osteopenia in adults.

Discharge Goals

Hospitalizations for diagnosis or management are typically brief. Patients undergoing Nissen fundoplication or nasogastric or gastrostomy tube placement should be able to tolerate a full feeding regimen before discharge.

Outpatient Care

Most children with GERD can be managed in the outpatient setting. The parents of the case patients were appropriately reassured as to the benign nature of GER by the child's pediatrician. They chose not to start any medications but did thicken her feeds with 1 tablespoon of rice cereal per ounce of formula. They also kept her head elevated for 20 to 30 minutes after feeds. This combination reduced but did not eliminate the number of spit-ups.

 WHAT YOU NEED TO REMEMBER

- Physiologic gastroesophageal reflux (GER) is common in infants, peaks at 4 to 6 months, and usually resolves by 12 months of age.
- In some cases of GER and mild GERD, thickened feedings, changes in position after feedings, and a trial of a hypoallergenic formula may be helpful.
- Gastroesophageal reflux disease (GERD) may cause respiratory symptoms, poor weight gain, feeding resistance, esophagitis, and heartburn.
- Even though GER improves in the prone position, infants should still sleep on their backs to reduce the risk of sudden infant death syndrome.
- PPIs are the most effective medications for treating esophagitis.

SUGGESTED READINGS

Michail S. Gastroesophageal reflux. *Pediatr Rev* 2007:28:101–109.

Nelson SP, Chen EH, Syniar GM, et al. Prevalence of symptoms of gastroesophageal reflux during infancy. A pediatric practice-based survey. Pediatric Practice Research Group. *Arch Pediatr Adolesc Med* 1997;151:569–572.

Nelson SP, Chen EH, Syniar GM, et al. Prevalence of symptoms of gastroesophageal reflux during childhood: a pediatric practice-based survey. Pediatric Practice Research Group. *Arch Pediatr Adolesc Med* 2000;154:150–154.

North American Society for Pediatric Gastroenterology and Nutrition. Pediatric GE reflux clinical practice guidelines. *J Pediatr Gastroenterol Nutr* 2001;32(Suppl 2): S2–S29.

Winter HS. Gastroesophageal reflux in infants. *UpToDate* 2007.

Yadlapalli K, Sarvananthan R. Gastro-oesophageal reflux in children. *BMJ Clin Evid* 2008;10:310.

Henoch-Schönlein Purpura

PAMELA F. WEISS

THE PATIENT ENCOUNTER

A 6-year-old boy was taken to his pediatrician with a 4-day history of sore throat, fever, joint pains, and a rash. His temperature was 38.6°C (101.5°F) and the rest of his vitals signs, including blood pressure, were normal. Physical examination revealed pharyngitis, a left ankle effusion, and purpura on his buttocks and the backs of his legs. A rapid streptococcal test was positive. His platelet count and urinalysis were normal. He was started on oral amoxicillin for strep throat and acetaminophen for symptomatic relief of his arthritis, which was presumed to be secondary to Henoch-Schönlein purpura (HSP). Over the next 3 days, his fever resolved but he developed severe abdominal pain and bloody stools. He presented to the ER with a pulse of 120 beats per minute and a blood pressure of 160/90 mm Hg. His abdomen was rigid and his stool guaiac-positive. A repeat urinalysis showed 2+ protein and casts.

OVERVIEW

Definition

Vasculitis is defined as inflammation of the blood vessels. It is classified according to the size of the affected vessels and the presence or absence of granuloma. This chapter focuses on HSP, a small-vessel, nongranulomatous vasculitis, which is defined by palpable purpura plus one or more of the following: diffuse abdominal pain, arthritis or arthralgias, or a biopsy demonstrating IgA deposition. In the majority of children, HSP is a relatively benign and self-limited disease. However, it can be complicated by severe abdominal pain, gastrointestinal bleeding, intussusception, hypertension, pulmonary hemorrhage, carditis, orchitis, encephalopathy, nephrotic or nephritic syndrome, and acute renal failure.

Pathophysiology

HSP is a leukocytoclastic vasculitis associated with IgA deposition. Circulating IgA forms immune complexes and activates the alternative complement pathway. IgA is then deposited in affected organs and small vessels, resulting in inflammation and, in some cases, end-organ damage. Skin biopsy, although usually not required for diagnosis, demonstrates small-vessel involvement and accumulation of neutrophils and monocytes. Other serologic factors hypothesized to play a role in pathogenesis include transforming growth factor β (which stimulates IgA production), tumor necrosis factor α, decreased factor XIII levels, and decreased prostaglandin I synthesis.

While HSP most commonly presents in otherwise healthy children, certain autoimmune risk factors may predispose a child to the development of this vasculitis. HSP occurs more commonly in children with complement deficiencies and hereditary fever syndromes, such as familial Mediterranean fever syndrome.

Epidemiology

HSP, the most common childhood vasculitis, accounts for more than 50% of all childhood vasculitis in the United States. The annual incidence of HSP is 8 to 20 per 100,000 children. Unlike most vasculitides, HSP occurs more commonly in males than in females (1.5:1.0). The peak age of onset is 6 years, with most cases occurring between 3 and 15 years of age. Up to 40% of affected children require hospitalization for management of the acute disease manifestations. Familial occurrence and an association with genetic polymorphisms have been described.

Etiology

Most cases occur in winter or spring. The prominent seasonal variation suggests that antecedent infections may be important in the pathogenesis of disease. Triggers that have been associated with HSP are listed in Table 17-1.

ACUTE MANAGEMENT AND WORKUP

The acute management and workup of HSP should identify the children with severe disease who require more intensive inpatient management than the majority of children, who can be safely and successfully treated as outpatients.

The First 15 Minutes

In the majority of HSP cases, immediate intervention is not necessary and the clinician can proceed to the history and physical examination. Rare situations in which immediate clinical care should precede a thorough history and examination include hypertensive crisis, hemodynamic instability secondary to severe gastrointestinal or pulmonary hemorrhage, or intestinal perforation.

The First Few Hours

A thorough history, physical examination, and the appropriate use of laboratory tests and imaging studies are important in devising an appropriate care plan.

TABLE 17-1
Triggers for Henoch-Schönlein Purpura

Bacterial infections	Group A β–hemolytic *Streptococcus*, *Staphylococcus aureus*, *Kingella kingae*, *Bartonella henselae*, *Helicobacter pylori*, *Bordetella pertussis*, *Mycobacterium avium intracellular complex*, *Salmonella*, *Shigella*, *Campylobacter*, *Mycoplasma pneumoniae*
Viral infections	Epstein–Barr virus, hepatitis A, hepatitis B, human immunodeficiency virus, parvovirus B-19, adenovirus, varicella, Coxsackie virus, herpes simplex virus
Immunizations	Influenza, MMR, hepatitis B, meningicoccus, BCG, tetanus–diphtheria, smallpox
Drug exposure	Nonsteroidal anti-inflammatory drugs, thiazide diuretics, ACE inhibitors, macrolide antibiotics, vancomycin, fluoroquinolones

ACE, angiotensin converting enzyme; BCG, bacille Calmette–Guérin; MMR, measles, mumps, rubella.

History

Children with HSP typically have a purpuric rash and nonspecific systemic symptoms, such as fever and malaise. Additionally, abdominal and joint complaints are often present. In as many as 25% of patients, the joint and abdominal symptoms may precede the appearance of the typical rash by up to 2 weeks, making the diagnosis more challenging. Gastrointestinal complaints may include spasmodic, colicky pain; nausea; vomiting; diarrhea; and bleeding. HSP-associated arthritis typically affects the knees and ankles.

Physical Examination

Purpura is present in 100% of children with HSP. The rash may consist of petechiae, larger purpuric lesions, or bullous lesions. The rash is classically located on the buttocks and lower extremities, but it can also be found on the face, behind the ears, or in any dependent area (including below the elbows and on the lower back). Subcutaneous edema or deep bruising may also occur. Arthritis, the second most common disease manifestation, occurs in two-thirds of these children. Effusions may be present in any joint; however, the knees and ankles are most common.

> ### CLINICAL PEARL
>
> *Guarding or rebound on abdominal examination should raise concern for intussusception or intestinal perforation; both are rare but serious complications.*

Labs and Tests to Consider

There are no diagnostic labs for HSP. However, the judicious use of laboratory tests and imaging studies will help to evaluate for acute complications such as gastrointestinal hemorrhage, intussusception, intestinal perforation, and acute renal failure.

Key Diagnostic Labs and Tests

Laboratory studies should include a complete blood count (thrombocytopenia would indicate an alternate diagnosis), electrolytes (to detect renal insufficiency), and urinalysis (to assess for hematuria and proteinuria). The erythrocyte sedimentation rate (ESR) is usually normal or only slightly elevated in HSP, so a very elevated ESR may indicate another diagnosis or intestinal perforation. A rectal exam and Hemoccult test should be performed to evaluate for gastrointestinal bleeding. Tests for streptococcal infection (rapid strep, throat culture, antistreptolysin-O titers) are positive in 10% to 50% of patients. If the diagnosis is unclear, an autoimmune workup—including an antinuclear antibody (ANA) panel, antinuclear cytoplasmic antibody (ANCA), and serum complement levels—should be obtained.

The patient in the case illustrated above had a peripheral white count of 15,000/μL, a hemoglobin level of 12 g/dL, and a platelet level of 450,000/μL. His electrolytes were significant for a blood urea nitrogen (BUN) level of 40 mg/dL and a creatinine measure of 1.2 mg/dL. His C-reactive protein (CRP) level was 3 mg/dL and ESR was 35 mm/hr. His stool guaiac was positive. His elevated blood pressure, proteinuria, and elevated BUN and creatinine levels confirmed renal involvement. His abdominal examination and stool guaiac raised concern for intestinal ischemia and possible intussusception. All the studies were consistent with the initial diagnosis of HSP.

Imaging

Ultrasonography is required in cases of suspected intussusception. The patient's abdominal ultrasound is presented in Figure 17-1. Barium enema

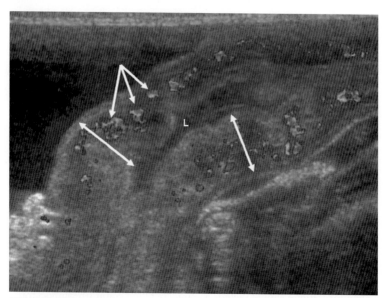

FIGURE 17-1: Doppler ultrasound of a 6-year-old child with bowel edema and inflammation from Henoch-Schönlein purpura. The ultrasound shows thickened bowel walls (double-headed arrows) and increased blood flow in the intestinal walls (single-headed arrows).

may also be useful but can miss ileoileal intussusception, which is a common location for HSP-associated intussusception. If testicular pain or swelling is noted on physical examination, ultrasonography and technetium radionuclide scanning will help to exclude testicular torsion. A chest radiograph is required if hemoptysis or severe respiratory symptoms are present. If further definition of pulmonary involvement is required, then computed tomography (CT) of the chest should be obtained.

Treatment

The current literature supports the notion that early use of corticosteroids is associated with better outcomes in HSP. In complicated cases that require admission, pulse methylprednisolone (30 mg/kg up to 1 g) is warranted. The optimal dose and duration of pulse corticosteroid therapy has not been well studied. In milder cases, doses of 2 mg/kg divided twice daily may be sufficient. If the course of corticosteroids is too short or the dose is tapered too rapidly, a recurrence of symptoms may be precipitated. A 2- to 3-week corticosteroid taper is reasonable. In life-threatening cases, plasmapheresis followed by intravenous cyclophosphamide is warranted. Antihypertensive therapy may be required during and after hospitalization. Nonsteroidal anti-inflammatory agents for symptomatic treatment should be administered with care, given the possibility of renal dysfunction, but they are usually not needed if corticosteroids are given.

Admission Criteria and Level-of-Care Criteria

Absolute criteria for admission include evidence of a hypertensive crisis, acute renal failure or renal insufficiency, pulmonary hemorrhage or hypoxia, intussusception or intestinal perforation, ischemia, or hemorrhage. Admission should be considered for patients with mild to moderate dehydration, inability to walk secondary to arthritis, a need for intravenous pain medication, or an unreliable social situation.

Patients can usually be managed on a general pediatric floor. However, consider admission to the intensive care unit for patients with massive gastrointestinal bleeding or an oxygen requirement above 50% to 60% FiO_2. Patients who require surgical reduction of intussusception or management of intestinal perforation may be managed on a surgical floor.

EXTENDED IN-HOSPITAL MANAGEMENT

The presence of intussusception, poorly controlled hypertension, or acute renal failure may lead to prolonged hospitalization. As in the illustrative case, renal biopsy may be performed to better delineate the extent of renal involvement.

DISPOSITION

Discharge Goals

Consider discharge when patients are clinically improved and able to tolerate oral intake. If gastrointestinal or pulmonary hemorrhage prompted the admission, hemoglobin values should be stable. Blood pressure and urinary output should be normal.

Outpatient Care

The onset of renal involvement may be delayed for weeks or months. A normal urinalysis and renal function at disease onset should not be reassuring; 75% to 90% of renal disease is detectable within 4 weeks of disease onset. During active disease, urinalysis should be performed and blood pressure checked weekly. If there is evidence of renal involvement, BUN and creatinine should be followed. After the acute manifestations have resolved, a urinalysis should be performed and blood pressure checked monthly for 3 months and then again at 6 months, along with BUN and creatinine if renal disease was present. Up to one third of children will have a recurrence of HSP; recurrences typically occur within 90 days.

WHAT YOU NEED TO REMEMBER

- Abdominal symptoms and arthritis may precede the development of purpura by 2 weeks.
- Intussusception and intestinal perforation are rare but life-threatening complications.
- Blood pressure, urinalysis, and BUN (creatinine if appropriate) should be followed for several months after hospital discharge, as renal involvement can be delayed and HSP can progress to chronic renal failure.
- Early corticosteroid therapy for complex inpatient cases is recommended.

SUGGESTED READINGS

Dedeoglu F, Sundel RP. Vasculitis in children. *Pediatr Clin North Am* 2005;52(2): 547–575.

Hattori M, Ito K, Konomoto T, et al. Plasmapheresis as the sole therapy for rapidly progressive Henoch-Schönlein purpura nephritis in children. *Am J Kidney Dis* 1999;33(3):427–433.

Ronkainen J, Koskimies O, Ala-Houhala M, et al. Early prednisone therapy in Henoch-Schonlein purpura: a randomized, double-blind, placebo-controlled trial. *J Pediatr* 2006;149(2):241–247.

Saulsbury FT. Clinical update: Henoch-Schonlein purpura. *Lancet* 2007;369(9566): 976–978.

Tarshish P, Bernstein J, Edelmann CM Jr. Henoch-Schönlein purpura nephritis: course of disease and efficacy of cyclophosphamide. *Pediatr Nephrol* 2004;19(1): 51–56.

Tizard EJ, Hamilton-Ayres MJ. Henoch Schönlein purpura. *Arch Dis Child Educ Pract Ed* 2008;93(1):1–8.

Weiss PF, Feinstein JA, Luan X, et al. Effects of corticosteroid on Henoch-Schönlein purpura: a systematic review. *Pediatrics* 2007;120(5):1079–1087.

Hypertension

SANDRA AMARAL

THE PATIENT ENCOUNTER

A 6-year-old boy is taken to the emergency department (ED) because he is "acting funny." The parents report that the boy had complained of a headache for the past 2 days. On the day of admission, he was agitated and became combative. In the ED, his blood pressure (BP) is 152/107 mm Hg. His heart rate is 125 beats per minute and his respiratory rate is 20 breaths per minute. On examination, the boy has no gross focal neurologic deficits but remains combative and agitated. He has mild pretibial edema bilaterally. His urine is tea-colored. In the ED, the child experiences a generalized tonic–clonic seizure.

OVERVIEW

Definition

Hypertension in children and adolescents is defined as an average systolic and/or diastolic BP reading that is ≥95th percentile for gender, age, and height on at least three occasions. BP between the 90th and 95th percentiles is considered "prehypertension." If a patient is truly hypertensive, the hypertension is then staged. Stage 1 refers to a BP that is 95th to 99th percentile plus 5 mm Hg. Stage 2 refers to a BP that is above the 99th percentile plus 5 mm Hg. BP normative charts can be found in The Fourth Report on the Diagnosis, Evaluation and Treatment of High Blood Pressure in Children and Adolescents (1). Although the true classification of pediatric hypertension includes three elevated BP readings on separate occasions, this is not possible in an acute setting.

Pathophysiology

BP is the product of cardiac output and total peripheral vascular resistance. Thus, hypertension occurs when either cardiac output and/or total peripheral vascular resistance is increased. Cardiac output may be increased by such factors as fluid overload or increased sympathetic outflow. Increased peripheral resistance may be mediated by activation of the renin–angiotensin system.

Epidemiology

Hypertension occurs in 2% to 5% of all children and adolescents. Estimates vary widely depending on how hypertension is defined and what the ethnic and body mass index distribution is within the designated population. There is some evidence to suggest that the incidence of pediatric hypertension is on the rise, coincident with increases in pediatric weight. Hypertension is a leading cause of chronic disease in children, after asthma and obesity.

Hypertension is often underrecognized because normal BP values vary by age, height, and gender. In a chart review of 14,187 children and adolescents who were seen for well-child care in Texas, 507 (3.5%) had hypertension, but only 131 (26%) had the diagnosis of high BP documented in the medical record (2).

Etiology

Hypertension may be primary or secondary. *Primary hypertension* refers to hypertension with no identifiable cause. Common causes of secondary hypertension by age grouping are detailed in Table 18-1. In general, the younger the patient and the higher the BP, the more likely is the existence of a secondary cause.

ACUTE MANAGEMENT AND WORKUP

The acute management and workup of hypertension should confirm the diagnosis and identify patients who will benefit immediately from treatment versus those who may be harmed by acute treatment.

The First 15 Minutes

The bladder cuff width should be approximately 40% of the circumference of the arm measured midway between the olecranon and acromion processes and should cover about two-thirds the length of the arm from the olecranon to the acromion. The bladder cuff length should cover 80% to 100% when it is wrapped around the arm.

> **CLINICAL PEARL**
>
> *Because it is challenging to obtain an accurate BP reading in pediatric patients, the first thing to do is repeat the BP by auscultation, using the appropriate size BP cuff.*

Once an elevated BP reading is confirmed, the severity and degree of hypertension should be assessed. *Hypertensive emergency* refers to an elevation of systolic or diastolic BP with acute end-organ damage, including cerebral infarct or hemorrhage, pulmonary edema, or hypertensive encephalopathy. *Hypertensive urgency* is defined as an elevation in BP without evidence of

TABLE 18-1

Etiologies of Secondary Hypertension in Children and Adolescents by Age

	Neonates and Infants	1–10 Years of Age	11 Years of Age and Older
Most common causes	Renal artery stenosis Renal artery or venous thrombosis Congenital renal anomalies Aortic coarctation Bronchopulmonary dysplasia	Glomerulonephritis Obstructive uropathy Chronic pyelonephritis Renal dysplasia Aortic coarctation Renovascular disease	Renal parenchymal disease Essential hypertension Aortic coarctation
Other possible causes	Medications Patent ductus arteriosus Intraventricular hemorrhage Tumor	Endocrine causes Tumor Pain, anxiety, "white coat" hypertension Obstructive sleep apnea Essential hypertension Medications, heavy metals Obesity	Endocrine causes Tumor Preeclampsia Renal artery stenosis Pain, anxiety, "white coat" hypertension Sleep apnea Medications or ingestions Obesity

end-organ damage. The patient's full set of vital signs should be reviewed. The physical exam should include a thorough neurologic examination. Patients with increased intracranial pressure (ICP) may present with Cushing's triad: hypertension, bradycardia, and respiratory depression; but these findings may present late in the course. Headache may be the earliest sign. A normal examination does not rule out increased ICP. If there is concern of increased ICP, a head CT should be obtained immediately. Lowering the BP acutely in a patient with increased ICP may decrease cerebral perfusion and lead to herniation.

The patient described in this encounter had altered mental status and seizures. He was promptly treated for seizure activity and then sent for a head CT. The head CT was normal.

The First Few Hours

The history and physical exam should focus on identifying any signs or symptoms of hypertension. The differential diagnosis is broad but can be narrowed by a good history and thorough physical examination. The workup may be tailored to the suspected cause of hypertension. The narrowed differential will also help indicate the appropriate treatment.

History

Children with hypertension are often asymptomatic. Hypertensive urgency may be associated with complaints of headache, blurred vision, and nausea. If there is glomerulonephritis, the patient will likely have tea-colored urine and mild edema. There may be a history of pharyngitis or impetigo several weeks earlier. A good history of estimated urine output is important. Patients with renal insufficiency or urinary obstruction may present with decreased urine output. History of frequent pyelonephritis suggests renal scarring. An evaluation of the patient's growth and development is helpful. Patients with chronic kidney disease will often have impaired growth. Systemic symptoms, such as joint pain or butterfly facial rash, suggest systemic lupus erythematosus (SLE). Flushing, tachycardia, and palpitations might suggest pheochromocytoma. History of medication use is also important. Medications, such as corticosteroids, often cause hypertension. If the patient is an infant, the history of an umbilical artery catheter presents a risk factor for renal artery thrombosis. It is also important to obtain a family history of hypertension, renal disease, and autoimmune diseases.

Physical Examination

In patients with pediatric hypertension, the physical exam is often normal. However, various secondary causes of hypertension may have clinical manifestations. Abdominal bruits may be heard in patients with renovascular disease. Four-extremity pulse and BP measurements should be performed to rule out aortic coarctation. An abdominal mass may be present, with severe urinary obstruction or tumor. Patients with hyperthyroidism may demonstrate exophthalmos or goiter. Café-au-lait spots might be present if the patient has neurofibromatosis. If the patient is cushingoid, there may a history of corticosteroid use and/or there may be adrenal problems. The patient's body mass index should also be calculated to assess obesity.

Labs and Test to Consider

Basic labs can rule out many causes of hypertension and narrow the differential diagnosis. Imaging is also helpful in identifying the etiology.

Key Diagnostic Labs and Tests

The basic workup of hypertension includes a comprehensive metabolic panel, complete blood count, and urinalysis. If a patient has acute or chronic renal failure, the patient's creatinine level will be elevated and there may be electrolyte abnormalities. A urinalysis that reveals numerous red blood cells and associated red blood cell casts is consistent with glomerulonephritis. C3 and C4 should also be checked if glomerulonephritis is suspected. In post-infectious glomerulonephritis, C3 is low in more than 90% of patients. Anemia may indicate chronic kidney disease. Other tests to consider include thyroid function studies to diagnose hyperthyroidism and urine catecholamines to diagnose pheochromocytoma. Serum renin and aldosterone levels are helpful to diagnose endocrine-mediated hypertension. In obese patients, a sleep study may be helpful. If a patient has an altered mental status and there is concern about ingestion, a toxicology screen is appropriate. In all patients with true hypertension, a fasting lipid panel is important to assess cardiovascular risk.

The patient in this case had severely elevated hypertension for age with mild edema and tea-colored urine. He also had manifestations of hypertensive emergency. His seizure activity was treated promptly and his head CT was negative. His initial workup with complete blood count (CBC), comprehensive metabolic panel, and urinalysis revealed renal insufficiency, gross hematuria, and mild proteinuria. His C3 level was also low. The working diagnosis was post-infectious glomerulonephritis.

Imaging

Patients with hypertension should undergo renal ultrasound with Doppler to assess renal anatomy. Ultrasound can rule out urinary obstruction and hydronephrosis. If kidney disease is present and of long standing, the kidneys may appear small and echogenic on ultrasound. Doppler examination is important to rule out main renal artery stenosis; however, a negative test does not rule out renal vascular disease. In a very young patient with very high BP, magnetic resonance imaging or a computed tomography angiogram of the abdomen may be indicated. If the angiogram is negative and suspicion for renovascular disease is high, renal arteriography is the next step.

Arteriography, an invasive study, is the gold standard for identifying reno-vascular disease.

Treatment

If increased ICP is not a concern, but the patient has stage 2 or symptomatic hypertension, then BP should be lowered slowly and promptly. BP should be lowered by no more than 10% initially, with a goal of 25% reduction over 8 hours of treatment. Hypertensive emergency is treated with intravenous medication, most commonly by continuous infusion. Pharmacologic therapy for asymptomatic stage 1 hypertension may be delayed while further evaluation and dietary or lifestyle changes are implemented. Current medications that are approved for hypertension treatment in children are detailed in Table 18-2.

If a patient has a secondary cause of hypertension, treatment also includes treatment of the primary disorder. The patient in this encounter had post-infectious glomerulonephritis. Treatment was supportive care and BP management. Hypertension and gross hematuria generally resolve over several weeks.

Admission Criteria and Level-of-Care Criteria

A hypertensive emergency warrants admission to the intensive care unit (ICU) and continuous infusion of antihypertensive medication. Generally, patients with stage 2 hypertension will be admitted for further workup and treatment. Patients with less severe hypertension may be treated as outpatients if close follow-up is ensured.

EXTENDED IN-HOSPITAL MANAGEMENT

The length of hospitalization for hypertension depends greatly on the underlying cause. If hypertension can be reasonably controlled medically, further workup of the etiology may be performed on an outpatient basis.

DISPOSITION

Discharge Goals

Goal BP is <95th percentile, or <90th if a patient has intrinsic renal disease, diabetes mellitus, or heart failure. This goal may not be attained by the time of discharge. If the patient's BP is reduced to the level of stage 1 hypertension and the patient is asymptomatic, discharge may be appropriate. Good follow-up must be ensured.

Outpatient Care

Patients should be discharged with a home BP monitoring system. Parents should be instructed on how to use the BP monitor. BPs should be taken

TABLE 18-2

Summary of Antihypertensive Medications Used in Children

	Neonates and Infants	Older Children
Intravenous medications	Enalaprilat Hydralazine Labetalol Nicardipine Sodium nitroprusside	Enalaprilat Esmolol Fenoldopam Hydralazine Labetalol Nicardipine Nitroprusside
Oral medications	Amlodipine Captopril Chlorothiazide Hydralazine Hydrochlorothiazide Isradipine Labetalol Minoxidil Propranolol Spironolactone	ACE-inhibitors: benazapril, captopril, enalapril, fosinopril, lisinopril, quinapril, ramipril Aldosterone receptor antagonists: eplerenone, spironolactone Angiotensin II receptor blockers: candesartan, irbesartan, losartan, valsartan A and β blockers: labetalol, carvedilol β blockers: atenolol, metoprolol, propranolol, bisoprolol Calcium channel blockers: amlodipine, felodipine, isradipine, nifedipine Central α-agonists: clonidine, methyldopa Diuretics: chlorothiazide, hydrochlorothiazide, furosemide, spironolactone, triamterene, amiloride Peripheral α antagonists: doxazosin, prazosin, terazosin Vasodilators: hydralazine, minoxidil

daily and with any symptoms of headache or blurred vision. Follow-up with a physician should be obtained within 1 week of discharge.

 WHAT YOU NEED TO REMEMBER

- The younger the patient, the more likely is the existence of a secondary cause of hypertension.
- Cushing's triad indicates increased intracranial pressure, and BP should not be lowered acutely.
- Hypertensive emergency includes signs of end-organ damage, such as pulmonary edema, cerebral hemorrhage, or hypertensive encephalopathy, and should be treated promptly but gradually.

REFERENCES

1. National High Blood Pressure Education Program Working Group on High Blood Pressure in Children and Adolescents. The Fourth Report on the Diagnosis, Evaluation and Treatment of High Blood Pressure in Children and Adolescents. *Pediatrics* 2004;114(2):555–576.
2. Hansen ML, Gunn PW, Kaelber DC. Underdiagnosis of hypertension in children and adolescents. *JAMA* 2007;298(8):874–879.

SUGGESTED READINGS

Flynn JT, Neonatal hypertension: diagnosis and management. *Pediatr Nephrol* 2000;14:332–341.

Lande MB, Flynn JT. Treatment of hypertension in children and adolescents. *Pediatr Nephrol* 2007 Aug [Epub ahead of print].

Portman RJ, McNiece KL, Swinford RD, et al. Pediatric hypertension: diagnosis, evaluation, management and treatment for the primary care physician. *Curr Probl Adolesc Health Care* 2005;35:262–294.

Hypoglycemia

SARA E. PINNEY AND DIVA D. DE LEÓN

THE PATIENT ENCOUNTER

An 11-month-old boy presented to the emergency department (ED) with a history of a 5-minute seizure-like episode at home consisting of bilateral eye deviation to the left and shaking of the right extremity. He had been healthy prior to the morning of the seizure event, with no symptoms of respiratory or gastrointestinal illness. He had had nothing to eat or drink since the previous evening, in preparation for an ambulatory procedure to place pressure equalization tubes for recurrent episodes of otitis media. During the episode he was unresponsive. In the ED, his blood glucose was 37 mg/dL as measured by bedside glucose meter. He was afebrile with a temperature of 99.1°F (37.3°C), a heart rate of 143 beats per minute (bpm), a respiratory rate of 33 breaths per minute, 100% SaO_2 on room air. On exam, he was awake and fussy but consolable. He had no dysmorphisms, his neurologic exam was nonfocal, and the rest of the physical exam was normal.

OVERVIEW

Definition

Hypoglycemia is considered a sign but not a diagnosis; therefore the documentation of hypoglycemia should be followed by a complete diagnostic evaluation. The classic definition of hypoglycemia is referred to as "Whipple's triad" and includes (i) symptoms of hypoglycemia (jitteriness, shakiness, nausea, vomiting, sweating, seizures, hunger, tachycardia, lethargy, loss of consciousness); (ii) measured blood glucose <50 mg/dL; and (iii) relief of symptoms with treatment to raise the blood glucose to the normal range. As with adults, normal blood glucose values for infants and children are in the range of 70 to 90 mg/dL. Activation of glucose counterregulatory symptoms occurs when blood glucose is between 65 and 70 mg/dL and frank symptoms of hypoglycemia begin to occur at blood glucose levels between 50 and 55mg/dL. Cognitive dysfunction typically begins at blood glucose levels between 45 and 50 mg/dL. The threshold of 50 mg/dL is used to diagnose hypoglycemia because this is low enough to include only cases with a clearly identifiable disorder.

Pathophysiology

Hypoglycemia is due to a disruption of the hormonally induced counterregulatory mechanisms that are activated to maintain the blood glucose within a normal range; it can be analyzed with a "fasting system approach." Three metabolic systems—hepatic glycogenolysis, hepatic gluconeogenesis, and hepatic ketogenesis—are employed during periods of fasting to maintain the fuel supply to the brain, which does not have its own source of fuel. For the first 12 to 16 hours of fasting in normal infants, glucose from hepatic glycogenolysis is supplemented with hepatic gluconeogenesis derived from amino acids released from muscle protein turnover. After 12 to 16 hours in normal infants (24 to 36 hours in adults), hepatic glucose production declines. Once the glycogenolysis supply is depleted, the body transitions to using fat as the major source of fuel. Adipose tissue lipolysis, fatty acid oxidation, and ketogenesis are activated. Ketones become an alternative source of fuel for the brain at this stage of fasting because the brain cannot metabolize fatty acids directly.

As fasting proceeds, insulin secretion is suppressed while other endocrine hormones are activated to stimulate glycogenolysis, gluconeogenesis, and ketogenesis. Cortisol activates gluconeogenesis, while glucagon stimulates glycogenolysis and ketogenesis. Epinephrine stimulates glycogenolysis, gluconeogenesis, and ketogenesis and also suppresses insulin. Growth hormone stimulates ketogenesis by increasing adipose tissue lipolysis.

Hypoglycemia results when there is a disruption of one of the three metabolic systems or one of the hormonal responses to fasting. The integrity of the metabolic and hormonal systems is reflected in the plasma levels of critical fuels and hormones at the time of hypoglycemia; therefore the most important specimens for diagnosis are those obtained at the time of hypoglycemia, known as the "critical sample."

Epidemiology

The incidence of hypoglycemia varies with the definition, the etiology of the hypoglycemia, and the population being studied. Congenital hyperinsulinism is the most common cause of persistent hypoglycemia in infants and children, with an estimated incidence of 1:50,000 in the United States and as high as 1:3,700 in parts of Saudi Arabia.

Etiology

Table 19-1 provides the common causes of hypoglycemia separated into age of presentation.

ACUTE MANAGEMENT AND WORKUP

Hypoglycemia is considered a symptom but not a diagnosis. Therefore you should investigate documented hypoglycemia with a complete diagnostic workup. Up to one third of children evaluated in the ED for unsuspected hypoglycemia will have a significant metabolic or endocrinologic disorder. Plasma levels of critical fuels and hormones at the time of hypoglycemia are

TABLE 19-1

Causes of Hypoglycemia

Transient Neonatal Hypoglycemia	Prolonged Neonatal Hypoglycemia	Persistent Neonatal, Infantile, or Childhood Hypoglycemia
Developmental immaturity of fasting adaptation (first 12 to 24 hours of life in normal newborns):	Prolonged neonatal hyperinsulinism	Hormonal disorders
Prematurity	IUGR	Hyperinsulinism
Normal newborn	Prematurity	K_{ATP} channel hyperinsulinism
Due to maternal factors:	Birth asphyxia	Hyperinsulinism/hyperammonemia
Maternal diabetes	Maternal toxemia/ preeclampsia	Glucokinase hyperinsulinism
IV glucose administration during labor and delivery		SCHAD hyperinsulinism
Medications: oral hypoglycemics, terbutaline, propranolol		Congenital disorders of glycosylation
		Beckwith–Wiedemann syndrome
		Acquired islet cell adenoma
		Insulin administration (Munchausen by proxy)
		Oral sulfonylurea drugs
		Counterregulatory hormone deficiency
		Panhypopituitarism
		Isolated growth hormone deficiency
		Adrenocortotropic hormone deficiency
		Primary adrenal insufficiency
		Epinephrine deficiency

(continued)

TABLE 19-1

Causes of Hypoglycemia (Continued)

Transient Neonatal Hypoglycemia	Prolonged Neonatal Hypoglycemia	Persistent Neonatal, Infantile, or Childhood Hypoglycemia
		Glycogenolysis disorders
		GSD 0 – glycogen synthase deficiency
		GSD 3 – debranching enzyme deficiency
		GSD 6 – liver phosphorylase deficiency
		GSD 9 – phosphorylase kinase deficiency
		Gluconeogenesis disorders
		GSD 1a – glucose-6-phosphatase deficiency
		GSD 1b – glucose-6-phosphate translocase deficiency
		Fructose 1,6-diphosphase deficiency
		Pyruvate carboxylase deficiency
		Lipolysis disorder
		Propranolol
		Fatty acid oxidation disorder
		Carnitine transport deficiency
		Carnitine palmitoyl-transferase 1 deficiency
		Carnitine translocase deficiency
		Carnitine palmitoyl-transferase 2 deficiency
		Very long chain acyl-CoA dehydrogenase deficiency

crucial for determining the etiology of hypoglycemia and are referred to as the critical sample (discussed below under "Labs and Tests to Consider").

The First 15 Minutes

For symptomatic patients (e.g., seizing or lethargic), the immediate treatment of hypoglycemia is important to prevent long-term neurologic sequelae. Consider obtaining a critical sample only if it will not delay treatment. After obtaining the critical sample, you should treat the hypoglycemia initially by feeding the child if he or she is conscious enough to avoid pulmonary aspiration. Alternatively, you may treat the patient with an IV bolus of 10% dextrose (2 mL/kg) followed by a continuous IV dextrose infusion to provide at least 8 mg/kg/min of glucose (5 mL/kg/hr of 10% dextrose).

The First Few Hours

The main priority in the first few hours is to stabilize the patient's glucose level and begin to search for the underlying cause of the hypoglycemia. Initially, the blood glucose levels should be followed every 15 minutes until they have stabilized to values >70 mg/dL. The patient should remain on the IV dextrose infusion, and blood glucose should then be followed every 2 to 3 hours.

History

In obtaining a history from a child with hypoglycemia, it is important that you inquire about the acute episode. Ask about the signs or symptoms demonstrated by the child. Did he have jitteriness, shakiness, nausea, vomiting, sweating, seizures, hunger, tachycardia, lethargy, staring episodes, or loss of consciousness? What time of day did the incident occur? How long had the child fasted prior to the incident? If the child had just eaten, what was the composition of the meal? Did the child have any other sign of acute illness? What was the child's eating pattern over several days prior to the episode?

It is also important that you obtain an accurate birth history, because this can provide important clues in determining the etiology of the hypoglycemia. Were there any complications with the pregnancy, including gestational diabetes or toxemia of pregnancy? Was the infant born prematurely, with intrauterine growth retardation (IUGR), or was the infant large for gestational age? Did hypoglycemia present at birth, and if so, how was it treated? Has the child had a prior Nissen fundoplication surgery? Other helpful historical information may include whether there were any recent changes in diet or if the child had just begun to sleep through the night without waking to feed.

Physical Examination

Vital signs may show tachycardia or an increased respiratory rate. If an acute illness reveals a preexisting disorder of hypoglycemia, the child may be febrile or have signs of a viral illness. The presence of midline facial defects, including cleft palate or a single central incisor, or of bilateral nystagmus and microphallus may indicate hypopituitarism, which includes deficiencies of cortisol and growth hormone. Ambiguous genitalia may indicate a diagnosis of congenital adrenal hyperplasia and cortisol deficiency. Infants with hyper-insulinism are often born large for their gestational age and have a history of hypoglycemia presenting shortly after birth. Hepatomegaly suggests a form of glycogen storage disease. Hyperpigmentation of the skin could be a sign of primary adrenal insufficiency.

Labs and Tests to Consider

Plasma levels of critical fuels and hormones at the time of hypoglycemia are crucial for determining its etiology. The critical sample, informally referred to as *didja* tubes (i.e., did you remember to get . . .), should be obtained via a blood-drawing intravenous catheter or by venipuncture; but obtaining the critical sample should not delay treating the hypoglycemia.

Key Diagnostic Labs and Tests

In a normal infant or child fasted to hypoglycemia (occurring between 24 and 36 hours) with a measured plasma glucose level <50 mg/dL, you can expect the following:

- Exhaustion of glycogen stores (and therefore no glycemic response to glucagon)
- Modest suppression of gluconeogenic substrate levels compared with the fed state (lactate <1.5 mM)
- Tripling of free fatty acids (2 to 5 mM)
- Elevation of β-hydroxybutyrate approximately 50- to 100-fold
- Suppression of insulin to unmeasurable levels (<2 μM/mL).

By comparing the expected values from a normal fasting response to a critical sample collected from a patient with hypoglycemia, you can determine the etiology of the hypoglycemia by examining where in the pathway the patient failed to maintain a normal fasting metabolic profile.

In collecting the critical sample, you must first obtain a stat plasma glucose level (i.e., from the intensive care unit's lab) to confirm that the blood glucose is <50 mg/dL. Once hypoglycemia is confirmed, collect a critical sample that includes a basic metabolic panel (with serum bicarbonate), lactate, β-hydroxybutyrate, free fatty acids, insulin, C-peptide, cortisol, growth hormone, ammonia, IGFBP-1, acyl carnitine profile, total and free carnitine levels, urinary ketones, and urine organic acids. After the critical sample is collected, you should perform a glucagon stimulation test: Administer 1 mg of glucagon either IV or IM and measure the blood glucose level every 10 minutes for 40 minutes. A positive test is an increase of 30 mg/dL in blood glucose and indicates increased insulin action.

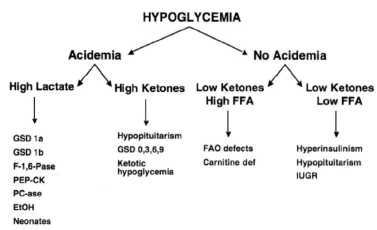

FIGURE 19-1: Evaluation of hypoglycemia. GSD 1a = glycogen storage disease type 1a (glucose-6-phosphatase deficiency); GSD 1b = glycogen storage disease type 1b (glucose-6-phosphate translocase deficiency); F-1,6-Pase = fructose-1,6-diphosphatase deficiency; PEP-CK = phosphoenolpyruvate carboxykinase deficiency; PC = pyruvate carboxylase deficiency; EtOH = ethanol exposure; GSD 0, 3, 6, 9 = glycogen storage disease types 0, 3, 6, 9 (defects of glycogenolysis); FAO defects = fatty acid oxidation defects; IUGR = intrauterine grow retardation. Adapted from: Stanley CA, Hypoglycemia. In: Radovicks S, MacGillivray MH, eds. *Pediatric endocrinology, a practical clinical guide.* New Jersey: Human Press, 2003, pp. 511–521.

As seen in Figure 19-1, the presence of acidemia is an easy way to initially segregate the disorders of hypoglycemia. The metabolic pattern that includes acidemia (defined as a HCO_3 <15 to 17 mEq/L) and elevated lactate levels is typical of defects in hepatic gluconeogenesis. These defects include GSD 1a (glucose-6-phosphatase) deficiency, GSD 1b (glucose-6-phosphate translocase) deficiency, and fructose-1,6-diphosphatase deficiency. This pattern is also typical of normal neonates on the first day of life and in ethanol intoxication. Other rare disorders, such as deficiencies of pyruvate carboxylase (PC) and phosphoenolpyruvate carboxykinase (PEP-CK), can present with acidemia and elevated lactate levels. Acidemia due to an increased amount of ketones typifies normal children with accelerate fasting profiles (often called ketotic hypoglycemia), hypopituitarism, and defects of glycogenolysis (GSD types 0, 3, 6, and 9).

The lack of acidemia (HCO_3 is >16 to 18 mEq/L) along with the absence of a rise in either ketones or free fatty acid levels is indicative of hyperinsulinism. Any measurable insulin level at the time of hypoglycemia is diagnostic of hyperinsulinism. The diagnosis of hyperinsulinism is often made based on findings that are consistent with increased insulin action, such as suppressed free fatty acids and ketones at the time of hypoglycemia. A positive glucagon stimulation test at the time of hypoglycemia indicates suppression of glycogenolysis by increased insulin action. Measurement of the C-peptide level is included in the critical sample for consideration of Munchausen by proxy in the case where an elevated insulin level is measured.

In young infants, the absence of acidemia along with low levels of ketones and free fatty acids also can indicate a diagnosis of hypopituitarism. A cortisol response <10 μg/dL at the time of hypoglycemia is inadequate. A growth hormone response <10 ng/mL at the time of hypoglycemia indicates an inadequate response; however, it may take up to 1 hour after an episode of hypoglycemia to elicit the maximum stimulation of growth hormone, which may not be represented in the critical sample value.

Hypoglycemia without acidemia but characterized by suppressed ketones and elevated levels of free fatty acids is a metabolic profile that is characteristic of disorders of fatty acid oxidation, the most common of which is medium-chain acyl-CoA dehydrogenase deficiency. Children with this disorder can present with acute life-threatening episodes of illness provoked by fasting more than 8 to 12 hours.

Late-dumping syndrome or postprandial hypoglycemia, a frequent complication of Nissen fundoplication, differs from the forms of hypoglycemia described above in that the hypoglycemia occurs postprandially rather than during periods of fasting. The mechanism involves accelerated gastric emptying with a rapid rise in blood glucose levels, which triggers an exaggerated insulin response and subsequent hypoglycemia approximately 1 to 2 hours after a meal.

Imaging

The utility of imaging studies is also dependent on the etiology of the hypoglycemia. For example, magnetic resonance imaging (MRI) of the brain with pituitary imaging is helpful in identifying forms of congenital absence or malformation of the pituitary gland. A positron emission tomography (PET) scan with the 18F-dopa radioisotope may be useful in certain forms of hyperinsulinism.

Treatment

Untreated hypoglycemia can result in severe neurodevelopmental sequelae, brain damage, and death; therefore, the initial treatment of hypoglycemia should aim at stabilizing blood glucose levels.

CLINICAL PEARL

Initial treatment should include either feeding the child if he or she is conscious enough to avoid aspiration and/or administering an IV bolus of 10% dextrose at 2 mL/kg followed by a continuous infusion of 10% dextrose to supply 8 mg/kg/min of glucose (5 mL/kg/hr).

After treating the hypoglycemia, you should initially follow blood glucose values every 15 minutes to ensure that they have stabilized at values >70 mg/dL. You should then check the patient's blood glucose levels every 2 to 3 hours once he or she is stabilized on the continuous infusion of dextrose. Infants with congenital hyperinsulinism will require glucose infusions rates as high as 20 to 25 mg/kg/min. In the case of an emergency or if no IV access can be obtained, glucagon 1 mg, by IV or IM injection, can be given and may treat the hypoglycemia if the underlying cause is a form of hyperinsulinism.

The remaining treatments of hypoglycemia depend on the underlying etiology of the disorder. If a diagnosis of hyperinsulinism is made, treatment with diazoxide, octreotide, or partial pancreatectomy may be indicated. In hypopituitarism, cortisol and growth hormone deficiencies can cause hypoglycemia and their replacement must be initiated. If adrenal insufficiency is found to be the cause of hypoglycemia, you should treat the patient with hydrocortisone replacement therapy. For children with hypoglycemia due to glycogen storage diseases and fatty oxidation defects or those with ketotic hypoglycemia, the treatment consists of avoiding prolonged fasting. For children with glycogen storage diseases, the consumption of cornstarch prolongs the fasting tolerance. For children with postprandial hypoglycemia after Nissen fundoplication, feeding manipulations and/or the use of medications that slow down the absorption of carbohydrates is required.

Admission Criteria and Level of Care

The admission of children with hypoglycemia is often required to ensure that their blood glucose levels can be maintained in the normal range while a diagnosis is made. Diagnosis of the etiology of hypoglycemia may involve a formal fasting systems evaluation, which should be performed after the placement of a blood-drawing IV. Central lines may be required in children needing high-concentration dextrose infusions to maintain their blood sugars at a level >70 mg/dL.

EXTENDED IN-HOSPITAL MANAGEMENT

Children with newly diagnosed hypoglycemia often require extended hospitalizations. When glucose levels have been stabilized after the initial presentation, diagnostic testing must be conducted and may include a formal fasting systems evaluation. After the etiology of hypoglycemia is determined, corrective therapy must be implemented, which may include medications, surgery, and or implementation of specific feeding regimens. During the hospitalization, the child's family must receive instruction about home blood glucose monitoring and how to administer emergency treatment for hypoglycemia, depending on the etiology (i.e., glucagon injection or Solucortef injection).

DISPOSITION

Discharge Goals

Before discharge, it is important that the child be able to maintain his blood glucose level in a normal range over a time period equivalent to his home regimen of fasting, which is usually overnight. A safety fast must be conducted prior to discharge after the child has returned to his or her baseline state with several days of adequate calorie intake. This fast does not require the extensive blood draw of the critical sample if hypoglycemia occurs, only confirmatory repeated bedside glucose meter checks approximately every 3 hours to see that the child is maintaining the blood glucose in the safe range (>70 mg/dL). Because most children typically sleep 8 to 10 hours overnight, a child is considered to pass a safety fast when he or she is able to maintain a blood sugar level of >70 mg/dL for 10 to 12 hours while fasting.

Outpatient Care

Families of patients with hypoglycemia must be taught how to check blood glucose levels with a home glucose meter prior to discharge. Initially after discharge, they should check and record morning fasting and prefeeding blood glucose levels. The frequency of blood glucose monitoring should be increased at times of illness.

WHAT YOU NEED TO REMEMBER

- Hypoglycemia is a sign and not a diagnosis. The documentation of hypoglycemia must be followed by an appropriate diagnostic test, as about one-third of cases may have a severe metabolic or endocrinologic disorder. Normal blood glucose levels are the same for infants, children, and adults: 70 to 90 mg/dL.
- Clues from the patient history and physical exam that may help with the diagnosis include a history of LGA (large for gestational age), IUGR (intrauterine growth retardation), or being an infant of diabetic mother; the length of fasting preceding the hypoglycemia; the presence of midline facial defects; hepatomegaly; or symptoms of an acute illness.
- The critical sample at time of hypoglycemia (plasma glucose <50 mg/dL) consists of a basic metabolic panel (with a serum bicarbonate), lactate, β-hydroxybutyrate, free fatty acids, insulin, C-peptide, cortisol, growth hormone, ammonia, IGFBP-1 (insulin-like growth factor binding protein-1), acyl carnitine profile, total and free carnitine levels, urinary ketones, and urine organic acids.

- Untreated hypoglycemia can result in severe neurodevelopmental sequelae, brain damage, and death. Therefore the immediate treatment of hypoglycemia is critical: an IV bolus of 10% dextrose (2 mL/kg) followed by a continuous IV dextrose infusion to provide at least 8 mg/kg/min of glucose (5mL/kg/hr of 10% dextrose).

SUGGESTED READINGS

De León DD Stanley CA. Mechanism of disease: advances in diagnosis and treatment of hyperinsulinism. *Nature Clin Pract Endocrinol Metab* 2007;3:57–58.

De León DD, Stanley CA, Sperling MA. Hypoglycemia in neonates and infants. In Sperling MA ed. *Pediatric Endocrinology*, 3rd ed. Philadelphia: Saunders/Elsevier Science, 2008:165–197.

Stanley CA. Hypoglycemia. In Radovick S, MacGillivray MH, eds. *Pediatric Endocrinology: A Practical Clinical Guide*. Totowa, NJ: Humana Press, 2003:511–521.

Thornton PS, Finegold DN, Stanley CA, et al. Hypoglycemia in the infant and child. In Sperling MA, ed. *Pediatric Endocrinology*, 2nd ed. Philadelphia: Elsevier Science, 2002:367–384.

Idiopathic Thrombocytopenic Purpura

MICHELE SAYSANA

THE PATIENT ENCOUNTER

A 5-year-old otherwise healthy male presents to his pediatrician's office with complaints of a rash for 2 days and a nosebleed today at school. He had an upper respiratory tract infection approximately 2 weeks ago. His other history and review of symptoms is unremarkable. His physical exam is remarkable for scattered petechiae and purpura. He does not have any lymphadenopathy or hepatosplenomegaly on examination. His pediatrician orders a complete blood count (CBC), which shows a hemoglobin level of 12.5g/dL, a white blood cell (WBC) count of 7,000/μL with a normal differential, and a platelet count of 5,000/μL.

OVERVIEW

Definition

In children, idiopathic thrombocytopenic purpura (ITP) is characterized by thrombocytopenia with a sudden onset of petechiae and purpura, or mucosal bleeding in a previously healthy child. Acute ITP is a self-limited disorder and lasts ≤6 months. Chronic ITP is defined as thrombocytopenia for >6 months following diagnosis.

Pathophysiology

ITP is an acquired disorder that causes isolated thrombocytopenia. Many children may have a history of a recent viral infection or, much less commonly, immunization with a live virus vaccine such as measles, mumps, and rubella, or varicella vaccines. The thrombocytopenia results from platelet destruction due to antiplatelet antibodies. These antibodies bind to the platelet surface and augment the destruction by Fc receptor–mediated phagocytosis in the liver and spleen.

Epidemiology

ITP is the most common cause of thrombocytopenia in healthy children and occurs in 5 of 100,000 children <15 years of age per year. It affects males and females equally and usually occurs in children 2 to 6 years old. Almost 80% of children with ITP will recover completely in 6 to 12 months after diagnosis; the remainder of those with ITP develop chronic ITP (1).

Etiology

More than 50% of cases of ITP are preceded by a viral infection, such as Epstein–Barr virus or varicella zoster. A history of recent vaccination with live virus vaccine has also been linked to ITP. Approximately 1 in 25,000 children who receive the measles-mumps-rubella (MMR) vaccine develop ITP (2).

ACUTE MANAGEMENT AND WORKUP

The acute management and workup help to identify those patients with severe or life-threatening bleeding due to severe thrombocytopenia and to exclude other causes of thrombocytopenia.

The First 15 Minutes

In an ill-appearing child, the initial assessment helps to determine whether to intervene immediately or to proceed with the history and physical examination. About 3% of patients will have severe bleeding and need to be identified early so that they can be treated aggressively (3). The majority of children will present with purpura and bruising alone. Although intracranial hemorrhage is rare in ITP, you should consider it in a child with severe headache, acute mental status changes, or focal neurologic findings combined with thrombocytopenia.

The First Few Hours

A good history, thorough physical exam, and appropriate use of labs are important in making the diagnosis and excluding other causes of bleeding, bruising, and thrombocytopenia.

History

Children with ITP typically present with bruising and purpura that develop over 24 to 48 hours. In addition, children may have a history of epistaxis, menorrhagia, or other mucous membrane bleeding. Viral symptoms may precede the onset of bruising and purpura. Children may have a history of receiving a live virus vaccine a few weeks prior. Those with ITP are usually otherwise healthy children without other signs or symptoms, such as fatigue, weight loss, fever, or pain.

Physical Examination

On physical examination, petechiae and purpura are the most common findings. Bruising in the oral cavity, especially on the buccal mucosa, may be present. If the patient has had prolonged epistaxis, clots may be seen in the nares as well. Because petechiae and purpura can be signs of more serious illnesses, such as leukemia, nonaccidental trauma, meningococcemia, or aplastic anemia, you should perform a thorough exam. Special attention should be paid to the abdominal exam to evaluate for hepatomegaly and/or splenomegaly. The patient should be examined thoroughly for lymphadenopathy as well. Lymphadenopathy in combination with hepatosplenomegaly, petechiae, and purpura should raise suspicion for leukemia.

Labs and Tests to Consider

The patient's history and physical exam should help guide the laboratory evaluation. The most important test to obtain is a CBC with a peripheral blood smear. If children have other physical findings or symptoms other than bleeding or purpura, you should consider additional testing, such as bone marrow aspiration and coagulation studies such as prothrombin time (PT), partial thromboplastin time (PTT), and international normalized ratio (INR).

Key Diagnostic Labs and Tests

The CBC in a child with ITP will usually show isolated thrombocytopenia with a platelet count often <30,000/μL. Occasionally, the platelet count falls below 5,000/μL. The hemoglobin, hematocrit, and red cell mean corpuscular volume (MCV) are normal, as are the WBC count and differential. However, in cases of significant bleeding, anemia may be present as well. The peripheral blood smear should be evaluated by a pathologist. The characteristic finding on the smear is large, sparse platelets with normal-appearing red and white blood cells. The peripheral blood smear is instrumental in ruling out leukemia and aplastic anemia. In children who either have other signs or symptoms or do not respond to therapy, bone marrow aspiration and coagulation studies may be necessary to further evaluate thrombocytopenia.

The patient in the case illustrated earlier has a peripheral white blood cell count of 7,000/μL, a hemoglobin level of 12.5 g/dL, and a platelet count of 5,000/μL with a differential of 20% lymphocytes and 70% segmented neutrophils. The peripheral smear reveals scant, large platelets with normal RBCs and WBCs. His isolated thrombocytopenia in combination with his history and physical exam findings are consistent with the diagnosis of ITP.

Imaging

Imaging is not usually employed to make the diagnosis of ITP. However, computed tomography (CT) of the brain without contrast may be indicated in children who have symptoms of intracranial hemorrhage, such as an acute onset of severe headache, mental status changes, or other focal neurologic findings.

Treatment

The treatment of ITP is based on guidelines developed by the American Society of Hematology. Treatment is based on clinical findings and the platelet count of each patient. If the child does not have any significant bleeding and the platelet count is >30,000/μL, no treatment or hospitalization may be required. Parents should be counseled to avoid giving their child ibuprofen and aspirin, to have the child avoid contact sports, and to limit any of the child's physical activities that might lead to bleeding. You should reassure parents that most children will recover spontaneously (including our case patient) and that the incidence of intracranial hemorrhage is exceedingly low.

Three treatments have been shown to be successful in raising the platelet count: oral corticosteroids, intravenous immunoglobulin (IVIG), and anti-Rh_0D therapy. Oral prednisone is the easiest and least expensive at a dose of 1 to 2 mg/kg/day and will increase the platelet count within a few days after treatment. However, the platelet count may decline as prednisone is tapered. IVIG and anti-Rh_0D immunoglobulin are very expensive and must be given intravenously. These two treatments are usually reserved for patients with significant bleeding. Both IVIG and anti-Rh_0D immunoglobulin are blood products and have some adverse effects, such as headache, nausea, vomiting, fever, and chills. Children with severe bleeding should be treated with IVIG or anti-Rh_0D immunoglobulin and steroids and should also be hospitalized and given supportive care, such as blood transfusions.

CLINICAL PEARL

Platelet transfusion is usually not necessary because the platelets are quickly destroyed by the antiplatelet antibody and are not effective at preventing bleeding. It is usually reserved for life-threatening hemorrhage, such as intracranial hemorrhage.

Children who develop chronic ITP as defined by thrombocytopenia lasting >6 months usually respond to therapy for short periods of time. However, some may undergo splenectomy to treat chronic ITP. As many as 60% to 80% of patients undergoing splenectomy recover completely and have a normal platelet count. About 10% to 15% of patients have some improvement in platelet count, and 5% to 10% show no improvement at all (2). Patients who undergo splenectomy should be immunized against pneumococcus and *Haemophilus influenzae* type b prior to surgery because of the risk of overwhelming septicemia due to encapsulated bacteria. Rituximab (anti-CD20 monoclonal antibody) may also be used to treat patients with chronic ITP.

Admission Criteria and Level-of-Care Criteria

Absolute criteria for admission include evidence of severe or life-threatening hemorrhage. Depending on the severity of the hemorrhage, patients may need admission to the pediatric intensive care unit. If the diagnosis of ITP is uncertain or another diagnosis is likely, such as leukemia, meningococcemia, or aplastic anemia, then the child needs admission for further evaluation and management. You will usually need to admit children with a platelet count of 5,000 to 10,000/μL or who are <2 months of age.

EXTENDED IN-HOSPITAL MANAGEMENT

Patients with continued significant bleeding will require prolonged hospitalization. Those patients with intracranial hemorrhage will also require additional care in the hospital, including platelet transfusion, drug therapy, and neurosurgical intervention. Some of these patients may also need an emergent splenectomy to help control the bleeding. If a patient does not respond to therapy and bleeding continues, further evaluation will be required, which may include a bone marrow aspirate and coagulation studies.

DISPOSITION

Discharge Goals

You may consider discharging the patient from the hospital when bleeding has ceased and the patient's platelet count is on the rise. Patients should be able to tolerate adequate oral intake. The parent should be comfortable caring for the child at home and should have close follow-up with their primary care doctor and, if needed, a pediatric hematologist.

Outpatient Care

After discharge from the hospital, patients should have prompt follow-up with their primary care doctor. Patients should have follow-up CBCs to monitor the platelet count, and parents need to be educated about the usual course of ITP. These children must avoid ibuprofen and aspirin as well as contact sports until the platelet count normalizes. Patients should also limit activities in which they are at risk for falls and injuries.

WHAT YOU NEED TO REMEMBER

- Isolated thrombocytopenia in a child with purpura and bruising is characteristic of ITP.
- The majority of children with ITP will have resolution of the disease within 6 months of onset.
- Platelet transfusion is not helpful in disease treatment.
- Drug therapy with steroids, IVIG, and anti-Rh_0D therapy are beneficial in patients with significant bleeding.
- Splenectomy is usually reserved for patients with chronic ITP.

REFERENCES

1. Fogarty PF, Segal JB. The epidemiology of immune thrombocytopenic purpura. *Curr Opin Hematol* 2007;14:515–519.
2. Buchanan GR. Thrombocytopenia during childhood: what the pediatrician needs to know. *Pediatr Rev* 2005;26:401–409.
3. Tarantino MD, Bolton-Maggs PH. Update on the management of immune thrombocytopenic purpura in children. *Curr Opin Hematol* 2007;14:526–534.

SUGGESTED READINGS

Geddis AE, Balduini CL. Diagnosis of immune thrombocytopenic purpura in children. *Curr Opin Hematol* 2007;14:520–525.

George JN, Woolf SH, Raskob GE, et al. Idiopathic thrombocytopenic purpura: a practice guideline developed by explicit methods for the American Society of Hematology. *Blood* 1996;88:3–40.

Kuhne T, Blanchette V, Buchanan GR, et al. Splenectomy in children with idiopathic thrombocytopenic purpura: a prospective study of 134 children from the Intercontinental Childhood ITP study group. *Pediatr Blood Cancer* 2007;49:829–834.

Inflammatory Bowel Disease

ANDREW B. GROSSMAN AND PETAR MAMULA

THE PATIENT ENCOUNTER

A 13-year-old boy presents to the emergency department with a 4-day history of progressively increasing abdominal pain and 1 day of tactile fever. He also has had 3 to 4 episodes of bloody, loose bowel movements daily for the past 2 days. His past medical history is significant for his having been diagnosed, approximately 4 years earlier, with Crohn's disease, which affects his stomach, small bowel, and colon. His current medications include an anti-inflammatory medication, mesalamine; an immunomodulator, 6-mercaptopurine; and an antibiotic, metronidazole. He has an oral temperature of 39.2°C (102.6°F) and moderate tachycardia. His abdomen is diffusely tender to palpation, most prominently at the right lower quadrant. He has no perianal lesions or any discomfort on rectal examination, although his stool is Hemoccult-positive.

OVERVIEW

Definition

Chronic inflammatory bowel disease (IBD) represents one of the most common inflammatory disorders to affect children and adolescents. The two most common forms of IBD include ulcerative colitis (UC), characterized by inflammation that extends continuously from the rectum and typically involves only the colon, and Crohn's disease, characterized by inflammation and ulceration that can affect the entire gastrointestinal tract in a noncontinuous distribution.

Pathophysiology

IBD is thought to be the result of an environmental trigger in a genetically predisposed individual. Crohn's disease results in chronic inflammation that affects any component of the gastrointestinal tract in a noncontinuous distribution (i.e., "skip lesion distribution"). In contrast, UC always involves the rectum, with contiguous involvement extending proximally to include the descending colon in 50% of cases and the entire colon in 10% of cases. The location and extent of the disease determines the clinical presentation. When the small bowel in Crohn's disease is affected, patients often present with evidence of malabsorption, including diarrhea, abdominal pain, weight loss, or growth deceleration. When the colon is involved in either Crohn's disease or UC, symptoms of colitis, such as abdominal cramping and bloody diarrhea, are common.

The inflammation in Crohn's disease can affect the entire thickness of the gastrointestinal wall, which has multiple implications. When the entire thickness of the bowel is involved, enteric fistulas can form and communicate with another area of bowel, the skin, or even the bladder or vagina. Additionally, patients with Crohn's disease are at risk for bowel perforation and abscess/phlegmon formation. Inflammation can also result in narrowing and fibrotic stricturing of the bowel, which places the patient at risk for an obstruction.

Epidemiology

Approximately 30% of patients with Crohn's disease and 20% of patients with UC first manifest symptoms in childhood or adolescence.

Incidence

The incidence of IBD is 2 to 7 cases per 100,000 per year.

Prevalence

The prevalence of pediatric Crohn's disease is estimated to be 43 cases per 100,000, while the prevalence of UC ranges from 50 to 75 per 100,000.

Etiology

The pathogenesis of IBD is thought to be multifactorial. The current theory is that a triggering event occurs in an individual with a genetic predisposition, resulting in chronic inflammation. Although the etiology of the precipitating event is unclear, environmental triggers, such as specific antigens and luminal bacteria, are probably involved. Other proposed triggers include early childhood use of antibiotics or nonsteroidal anti-inflammatory drugs.

ACUTE MANAGEMENT AND WORKUP

The acute management and workup of a patient who presents with a potential exacerbation of IBD requires that you obtain a concise history that characterizes the patient's prior clinical course and current presentation. You should follow the history with a physical examination and possibly laboratory and radiologic testing with a goal of determining if the patient requires immediate inpatient medical treatment.

The First 15 Minutes

There are several serious complications for you to consider in the early evaluation of an IBD patient who presents with an acute exacerbation. They include:

- Sepsis
- Abscess (intra-abdominal or perirectal)

- Intestinal obstruction
- Pancreatitis
- Fulminant colitis and toxic megacolon (much less common in Crohn's disease than in UC)

To evaluate for these complications, immediately obtain a focused history, probing for details of fever, severe bloody diarrhea with any reported shock-like symptoms, and bilious emesis or other evidence of intestinal obstruction. You should begin the physical examination by focusing on any abnormality in the patient's vital signs (e.g., fever, tachycardia, hypotension). You should perform a comprehensive abdominal examination; concerning findings include hypoactive or absent bowel sounds, which suggests obstruction, guarding, or severe tenderness with the presence of a discrete mass, which could be due to an abscess. A perirectal and internal rectal examination will reveal tenderness and possibly drainage, fluctuance, or erythema in the case of a perirectal abscess.

The First Few Hours

Once an emergent clinical scenario has been ruled out, a thorough history and physical exam and appropriate laboratory and radiologic testing are essential to developing an appropriate assessment and plan.

History

Children with an exacerbation of IBD can present with myriad symptoms, depending on the site of inflammation. The most common symptoms include abdominal pain, diarrhea, weight loss, gastrointestinal (GI) bleeding, fatigue, and nausea/vomiting. It is important to elicit the patient's presenting complaint and focus on the duration, location, nature, and severity of the abdominal pain, and whether concomitant emesis is present. The frequency and texture of bowel movements and the presence of GI bleeding must be characterized and compared with the patient's baseline status. Distinguishing between a flare of Crohn's disease and infectious gastroenteritis can be difficult; the presence of sick contacts suggests an acute infection. A history of common extraintestinal manifestations of Crohn's disease, including oral aphthous ulcers, arthritis, fatigue, fevers, perianal skin tags, fissures/fistulas, or rashes such as erythema nodosum or pyoderma gangrenosum, should be sought.

It is often instructive to ascertain whether the patient's current symptoms are representative of his or her "typical flare." Many children with IBD are treated with immunosuppressive medications, such as 6-mercaptopurine, azathioprine, methotrexate, infliximab, or adalimumab. The use of these medications should increase suspicion for the possibility of an infectious complication, especially for a febrile patient. It is also essential for you to determine the past surgical history, as previous abdominal surgery is an additional risk factor for intestinal obstruction.

Physical Examination

The patient's general appearance can often reflect the severity of illness. Fever could be due to chronic illness or an acute infection. Evidence of dehydration should be sought, including dry mucous membranes, prolonged capillary refill, or tachycardia. Tachycardia could also be indicative of fever or anemia. Pallor may be indicative of anemia. The patient's height and weight should be carefully plotted and compared with previous measurements to determine if weight loss has occurred.

You should perform a focused abdominal examination, including auscultation, palpation, and percussion, to help determine the location and severity of pain. Diminished or absent bowel sounds could indicate severe inflammation or obstruction. Fullness in the right lower quadrant is a common finding indicative of an inflamed bowel, while a discrete tender mass might be indicative of an abscess.

A visual perirectal and internal rectal examination with testing for occult blood is a necessary component of the evaluation of an acutely ill patient with Crohn's disease. Erythema, induration, fluctuance, and severe tenderness suggest the presence of a perianal abscess. Other perianal findings can include large skin tags, perianal fissures, and perianal fistulas with or without active drainage.

CLINICAL PEARL

Extraintestinal manifestations of IBD include uveitis, hepatobiliary disease, arthritis, spondylitis, erythema nodosum, and renal stones.

Labs and Tests to Consider

Pertinent laboratory studies can provide information regarding the acute presentation as well as the recent chronic course of the patient's disease. Based on the presenting complaint, you may have to use imaging studies to help delineate the nature of the problem and to rule out the presence of emergent complications.

Key Diagnostic Labs and Tests

Table 21-1 lists pertinent laboratory and microbiology testing that might be helpful in the evaluation of an acutely ill IBD patient. Stool cultures should be performed when there has been an acute change in bowel pattern or texture that could be due to infection. Blood culture is only rarely necessary when there is high suspicion for sepsis or an abscess.

Imaging

An abdominal x-ray is typically warranted in the evaluation of an IBD patient with acute abdominal pain. Dilated loops of bowel or air–fluid levels

TABLE 21-1

Laboratory Testing for an Acute Exacerbation of Inflammatory Bowel Disease

Test	Findings	Notes
Complete blood count with differential	Anemia, thrombocytosis, leukopenia, leukocytosis	*Anemia:* Acute versus chronic, could indicate acute blood loss, chronic blood loss, chronic iron deficiency. *Thrombocytosis:* Acute-phase reactant, can indicate ongoing inflammation, active bleeding, or iron deficiency anemia. *Leukopenia:* Medication effect (6-MP, azathioprine, methotrexate) or sepsis. *Leukocytosis:* Medication effect (corticosteroids) or infection/inflammation.
ESR and CRP	Elevation	Nonspecific markers of inflammation, elevated with increased disease activity, also with infection, other sources of inflammation.
Comprehensive metabolic panel	Elevated transaminases, elevated alkaline phosphatase/GGT, hypoalbuminemia	*Transaminases:* Acute hepatitis, reaction to medications. *Alkaline phosphatase/GGT:* Cholelithiasis, primary sclerosing cholangitis, reaction to medications. *Albumin:* Inflamed small bowel can result in protein-losing enteropathy; good marker of chronic small bowel disease activity.

Test	Finding	Notes
Amylase, lipase	Elevation	Acute pancreatitis (incidence increased with Crohn's disease with upper GI inflammation; 3% of patients treated with 6-MP/azathioprine).
Stool cultures	*Escherichia coli* (0157), *Salmonella, Shigella, Clostridium difficile* toxins, *Yersinia, Campylobacter*	Sources of infectious colitis, which can mimic an IBD flare.
Blood culture	Bacteremia	Bacteremia is uncommon during a flare of Crohn's disease.
Urinalysis	Hematuria	Patients with affected terminal ileum are at increased risk for nephrolithiasis.

CRP, C-reactive protein; ESR, erythrocyte sedimentation rate; GGT, gamma glutamyl transferase.

can indicate an obstruction, while pneumoperitoneum is a sign of intestinal perforation. A computed tomography (CT) scan with oral and intravenous contrast is the cross-sectional imaging modality most commonly employed to assess patient's for acute complications, such as abscesses, and can demonstrate obstruction or fistulas. At some centers, magnetic resonance imaging (MRI) is replacing CT, particularly in evaluating for the extent of perianal disease. MRI has the benefit of reducing exposure to ionizing radiation; however, the duration of the study sometimes necessitates sedation for pediatric patients. Ultrasound can also demonstrate bowel wall thickening, evidence of obstruction, or the presence of an abdominal abscess. Sonography is increasingly being utilized because of the relative ease of the exam and the lack of radiation, although an experienced operator is necessary.

Treatment

Table 21-2 lists the medications most commonly prescribed for the treatment of IBD. The treatment algorithm for an acute exacerbation of IBD will vary depending on whether the patient has Crohn's disease or UC, the specific etiology of the current symptoms, and whether the patient is experiencing a disease flare, infectious complication, medication toxicity, or a surgical emergency.

Admission Criteria and Level-of-Care Criteria

Absolute criteria for admission include a perianal or intra-abdominal abscess, concern for sepsis, vomiting and abdominal pain caused by suspected partial small bowel obstruction that requires possible surgical intervention, hemodynamic instability, fulminant colitis with significant ongoing GI blood loss, or symptomatic acute pancreatitis. Otherwise you should determine whether the patient is stable enough to be discharged and the feasibility of response to outpatient management. If outpatient management of the acute flare has failed (e.g., oral prednisone), inpatient hospitalization and treatment (e.g., intravenous corticosteroids) is indicated.

Most patients can be admitted to a regular pediatric or pediatric gastroenterology floor. A pediatric gastroenterologist should either be managing or consulting in the patient's care. You should obtain early surgical consultation when there is any concern about obstruction or abscess that might require surgical drainage.

EXTENDED INPATIENT MANAGEMENT

The patient referenced earlier presented with acute abdominal pain, most prominent in the right lower quadrant, a change in the character of bowel movements, and high fever. He was managed with 6-MP, an immunomodulator that increases his risk of infection. A CT scan did not reveal an intra-abdominal abscess. Laboratory studies revealed no evidence of pancreatitis and

TABLE 21-2
Common Medications for the Treatment of IBD

Medication	Notes
Aminosalicylates	
Mesalamine (PO and PR) Sulfasalazine Balsalazide Olsalazine	Exhibit modest local anti-inflammatory effect; used for treatment of mild to moderate IBD and maintenance of remission; various formulations release in different locations in the GI tract.
Corticosteroids	
Prednisone Methylprednisolone	Potent and fast-acting anti-inflammatory effect; used to treat acute flares of disease; not indicated for maintenance therapy due to multiple adverse effects and loss of effect.
Budesonide	Special ileal controlled-release formulation, effective for ileocolonic Crohn's disease; decreased systemic absorption results in fewer side effects.
Antibiotics	
Metronidazole Ciprofloxacin	First-line therapy for perianal involvement, other infectious complications (e.g., abscess); some anti-inflammatory effect.
Immunomodulators	
Azathioprine 6-Mercaptopurine	Daily maintenance immunosuppressive therapy indicated for treatment of moderate to severe disease, to treat steroid-dependent or steroid-refractory disease, and to maintain remission. Require 2 to 4 months to achieve efficacy. Increased risk of pancreatitis, hepatitis, leukopenia, and infection.

(continued)

TABLE 21-2

Common Medications for the Treatment of IBD (Continued)

Medication	Notes
Immunomodulators	
Methotrexate	Same indications as azathioprine and 6-mercaptopurine; administered once weekly either PO or SQ. Increased risk of hepatitis, leukopenia, and infection. Nausea is a common side effect. Concomitant folic acid supplementation recommended.
Biological therapies	
Infliximab	Treatment of severe active or fistulizing disease not responding to other therapies. Decreases inflammation by neutralizing proinflammatory cytokines (TNF-α). Intravenous infusion administered every 8 weeks after three loading doses. Suppresses the immune response. Risk of antibody formation, which leads to loss of efficacy or infusion reaction.
Adalimumab	Similar to infliximab, but 100% humanized, so less risk of antibody formation. Administered SQ once every other week.

TNF-α_2 tumor necrosis factor alpha.

stool cultures were negative; the patient was, therefore, determined to be suffering from a significant acute flare of his Crohn's disease without infectious complications. The patient received intravenous corticosteroids, which are the mainstay of treatment for an acute exacerbation of Crohn's disease because of their strong anti-inflammatory effect as well as the associated rapid response. The typical dosing for intravenous methylprednisolone is 1 mg/kg twice daily (maximum dose 24 mg twice daily). Treatment efficacy was assessed by overall patient clinical status, improvement in abdominal pain, a decrease in GI blood loss, and improvement in the frequency and texture of bowel movements. Daily hemoglobin monitoring might be required if GI blood loss is considerable, and blood transfusion should be considered if the hemoglobin decreases below 8 g/dL and/or the patient is hemodynamically unstable.

If corticosteroid therapy is not effective and abdominal pain or bloody diarrhea continues, you should reevaluate the patient for infectious complications. This reevaluation can include repeat stool cultures as well as flexible sigmoidoscopy with colonic tissue sent for polymerase chain reaction (PCR) testing for cytomegalovirus, which is a potential etiology for refractory colitis in a patient treated with immunosuppressive medications. Assuming no infectious etiology, the patient might require treatment with infliximab (see Table 21-2), a biologic agent that also has a rapid therapeutic response.

DISPOSITION

Discharge Goals

Prior to discharge, the patient's symptoms should improve but not necessarily abate. A child can be discharged even if abdominal pain has not completely resolved or the bowel movements have not quite yet normalized as long as tangible improvement has been documented and the patient is deemed stable for outpatient management. Continued significant GI blood loss, intolerance of oral feeding or medications, or refractory symptoms would prevent discharge. Once the patient is home, communication and close follow-up with the primary pediatric gastroenterologist is critical. You should consider postdischarge laboratory testing; for example, an anemic Crohn's disease patient who was experiencing GI blood loss should have a follow-up blood count.

Outpatient Goals

The outpatient management of this patient initially involves ensuring that the symptoms do not recur with outpatient management. For a patient discharged on oral corticosteroids, you should implement an appropriate weaning schedule as tolerated. For patients with GI bleeding, follow-up of laboratory evaluations is essential. Relapse of symptoms once antimicrobial therapy has been completed would warrant an investigation for repeat infection.

The second goal of outpatient management is to evaluate the patient's maintenance regimen and determine that it has been optimized. While an acute flare is not unexpected, severe or frequent Crohn's disease exacerbations might suggest that maintenance therapy is not adequate. Additionally, growth parameters must be carefully assessed on a regular basis. For the pediatric Crohn's disease patient, even in the absence of significant symptoms, poor weight gain or linear growth is evidence of therapeutic failure and might necessitate escalation of therapy. For the patient in the case study, the dose of 6-mercaptopurine might need to be increased, or, alternatively, methotrexate might be a better option.

WHAT YOU NEED TO REMEMBER

- A focused history and physical examination and judicious use of laboratory, microbiologic, and radiologic testing can help confirm the most common Crohn's disease complications, including pancreatitis, partial intestinal obstruction, and infections.
- Knowledge of the patient's location of disease, typical flare symptoms, and maintenance medications will help focus the diagnostic testing in the acute setting.
- An intra-abdominal or perianal abscess must be considered and ruled out in the febrile Crohn's disease patient, particularly one treated with immunosuppressive medications.

SUGGESTED READINGS

Escher JC, Taminiau JA, Nieuwenhuis EE, et al. Treatment of inflammatory bowel disease in childhood: best available evidence. *Infl Bowel Dis* 2003;9:34–58.

Griffiths AM, Hugot JP. Crohn disease. In Walker WA, Goulet O, Kleinman RE, et al, eds. *Pediatric Gastrointestinal Disease*, 4th ed. Hamilton, Ontario: BC Decker, 2004.

Grossman AB, Baldassano RN. Specific considerations in the treatment of pediatric inflammatory bowel disease. *Expert Rev Gastroenterol Hepatol* 2008;2:105–124.

Heyman MB, Kirschner BS, Gold BD. Children with early-onset inflammatory bowel disease (IBD): Analysis of a pediatric IBD consortium registry. *J Pediatr* 2005;146: 35–40.

Kugathasan S, Judd RH, Hoffmann RG, et al. Epidemiologic and clinical characteristics of children with newly diagnosed inflammatory bowel disease in Wisconsin: a statewide population based study. *J Pediatr* 2003;143:525–531.

Mamula P, Markowitz JE, Baldassano RN. *Pediatric Inflammatory Bowel Disease*. New York: Springer Science and Business Media, 2008.

Intussusception

THAO M. NGUYEN AND JEFFREY F. LINZER, SR.

THE PATIENT ENCOUNTER

A 9-month-old male is brought to the emergency department with a 1-day history of vomiting and intermittent irritability and crying. He has not had any fever. Vital signs were as follows: heart rate, 180 beats per minute; respiratory rate, 36 breaths per minute; blood pressure, 80/50 mm Hg; and temperature, 37.2°C (99°F). On physical examination, the patient draws in his legs when crying. A right-sided abdominal mass is palpated. A digital rectal exam reveals soft stool in the vault that is positive for occult blood.

OVERVIEW

Definition

Intussusception is the prolapse or telescoping of one portion of the bowel into an immediately adjacent segment, leading to acute intestinal obstruction.

Pathophysiology

Intussusception occurs most often at the terminal ileum into the colon (ileocolic), but ileoileal, jejunojejunal, jejunoileal, and colocolic types have also been described. It appears that an imbalance in the longitudinal forces along the intestinal wall results in the invagination of the proximal portion of bowel into the distal lumen. In the process, lymphatic return is impeded, which leads to venous congestion, bowel wall edema, and eventually results in infarction of the intestinal mucosa. The ischemic mucosa sloughs off, leading first to occult bleeding and then to the classic "currant jelly" stool (a mixture of frank blood and mucous). If untreated, the ischemic process progresses to bowel obstruction, necrosis, and perforation of the bowel wall.

Epidemiology

Intussusception is the most common cause of intestinal obstruction in early childhood. Most affected infants are 5 to 10 months of age; two-thirds present <1 year, while 80% are <2 years of age at presentation. Intussusception is extremely rare in the neonatal period and after 6 years of age. The estimated incidence is 1 to 4 per 1,000 live births. Globally, there is a male-to-female predominance of approximately 2:1.

Etiology

Most cases of intussusception do not have an identifiable pathologic lead point. Approximately 30% of patients with intussusception have a preceding viral illness. Viral infections can induce lymphoid hyperplasia in the intestinal tract, resulting in hypertrophied Peyer's patches in the terminal ileum, which then serve as potential lead point for ileocolic intussusception.

Older children, on the other hand, tend to have pathologic conditions associated with their intussusception. These conditions include Meckel diverticulum, duplication cyst, polyps, lymphoma, Henoch–Schönlein purpura, and cystic fibrosis. In the postoperative period, adhesions have been implicated in small bowel intussusception (i.e., ileoileal, jejunoileal, or jejunojejunal).

ACUTE MANAGEMENT AND WORKUP

The acute management and workup help to distinguish between children with surgical and nonsurgical abdominal conditions. A child with intermittent colicky abdominal pain, especially if <5 years of age, requires a high index of suspicion for intussusception. In the early presentation, patients typically appear normal between episodes of pain.

The First 15 Minutes

In addition to evaluating the ABCs (airway, breathing, and circulation), the initial "eyeball" assessment helps to determine if the patient is clinically stable. In patients who are comfortable at rest and do not appear to be in pain, a thorough directed history and exam may be performed. However, those patients who are actively in pain, are persistently vomiting, appear dehydrated, or have clinical evidence of peritonitis, shock, or sepsis should have their care directed to stabilization. Oral intake should be withheld until a surgical condition has been ruled out. Isotonic intravenous (IV) fluid resuscitation should be initiated to correct dehydration or shock.

The First Few Hours

In those relatively stable patients for whom there is a high index of suspicion for intussusception, an enema contrast study may be the only radiology study needed. However, all patients should have their pain and hydration well managed prior to obtaining the exam. In patients without signs of shock, small, frequent doses of short-acting IV opiates may be used for pain control. A nasogastric tube can be placed on intermittent suction to decompress the stomach in patients with bowel obstruction. A pediatric surgeon should be consulted and available prior to attempted reduction because of the risk for bowel perforation during the reduction procedure. Occasionally, surgical intervention may be necessary to correct the intussusception because of the failure of contrast reduction or in patients with peritonitis.

History

Patients with intussusception often lack the classic signs and symptoms, which can lead to an unfortunate delay in diagnosis. The triad of vomiting, colicky abdominal pain, and "currant jelly" stools occurs only in 15% to 30% of patients. One third of patients do not pass blood or mucous or develop an abdominal mass. Older children can have pain alone without other signs or symptoms.

The typical patient is usually an infant who presents with a sudden onset of intermittent, severe, and progressive abdominal pain accompanied by inconsolable crying and drawing up of the legs toward the abdomen, followed by nonbilious vomiting. Between the painful episodes, which usually occur at 15- to 20-minute intervals, the child may appear completely well and pain free. Initially, loose or watery stools present concurrently with vomiting and may be mistaken for gastroenteritis. Blood or mucous usually passes rectally within 12 to 24 hours of the onset of symptoms. Somnolence and decreased activity typically develop later in the process, along with bilious vomiting from increasing intestinal obstruction. Occasionally, altered consciousness may dominate the initial presentation and may be confused with sepsis.

Physical Examination

The pathognomonic physical findings in intussusception are a sausage-shaped mass in the right upper quadrant with an absence of bowel in the right lower quadrant (Dance sign). This is present in two thirds of cases yet is difficult to detect in practice, especially in crying infants. You can best palpate the mass when the infant is quiet, between spasms of colic.

CLINICAL PEARL

Occult blood in the stools is the first sign of impaired mucosal blood supply and is present in up to 75% of cases in infants who present without bloody stools. The classic "currant jelly" stools appear later in the disease process.

If obstruction is complete, the abdomen may be distended. Peritonitis secondary to intestinal infarction and perforation can be suggested by the findings of rigidity and involuntary guarding.

Labs and Tests to Consider

No specific laboratory tests can aid in making the diagnosis of intussusception. Laboratory studies should be directed at contributory or secondary issues as needed for a febrile, dehydrated, or unstable patient. Leukocytosis may be seen in the late stage of gangrenous bowel but is not specific for this condition. Dehydration may cause electrolytes abnormalities such as hypo- or hypernatremia.

The patient in the case illustrated previously had a peripheral white blood cell count of 14,000/µL with 5% bands and 70% segmented neutrophils, a hemoglobin count of 10.7 g/dL, a blood urea nitrogen (BUN) level of 24, and a creatinine level of 0.8. The platelet count and remainder of the electrolytes were within the range of normal values. The nonspecific findings of the white blood cell count and differential do not provide any additional guidance towards the underlying condition, while his elevated BUN and creatinine levels suggest prerenal azotemia.

Key Diagnostic Labs and Test

There are no key diagnostic labs for you to consider in assessing intussusception.

Imaging

If intussusception is strongly suspected and the patient does not have signs of peritonitis or shock, obtain a contrast enema study without delay. Such a study may be both diagnostic and therapeutic in the nonoperative reduction of intussusception. Both pneumatic (air contrast) and hydrostatic (saline, water-soluble iodinated radiopaque contrast medium barium), either under fluoroscopy or ultrasound guidance, have been used with good success. However, air contrast enema tends to be the method of choice. Although there have been no large comparison studies, air contrast enemas have had a higher success rates with lower radiation exposure. There is also no risk of a barium-induced peritonitis, which could occur from a rupture with a barium contrast enema. Perforation rates appear similar, <1%, with both techniques.

If the diagnosis is unclear at presentation or if the patient is not a candidate for nonoperative correction, the initial workup may include plain abdominal radiographs. These should include the following views: flat plate, cross-table lateral or upright if the patient is able to stand, and cross-table prone in infants. While the sensitivity (45%) is poor for the diagnosis of intussusception, abdominal radiographs serve an important role in assessing for possible complications, such as perforation or small bowel obstruction. Radiographic findings suggestive of intussusception may show an absence of bowel gas in the right upper quadrant. At times, a meniscus sign, which is a rounded soft-tissue mass protruding into the gas-filled lumen of the colon, may be present (Fig. 22-1).

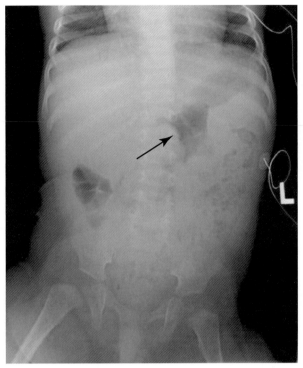

FIGURE 22-1: Plain x-ray of the abdomen showing mid-transverse colon intussusception with meniscus sign (*arrow*).

Abdominal ultrasonography serves as a reliable noninvasive screening tool, especially for children with atypical presentation or at low risk for intussusception. In the hands of an experienced operator, ultrasound approaches 100% accuracy in the detection of acute intussusception. The classic ultrasound image of intussusception, the target or pseudokidney sign, represents layers of intestine within intestine (Fig. 22-2). Furthermore, ultrasound can identify the presence of a pathologic lead point in intussusception and can help to predict which children are most likely to need surgical intervention.

Abdominal computed tomography (CT) should not be used as the primary detection method due to, radiation exposure, potential risks associated with sedation of an already ill young child, and cost. You should reserve this imaging modality for patients with an inconclusive or atypical ultrasound or when there is suspicion of oncologic disease.

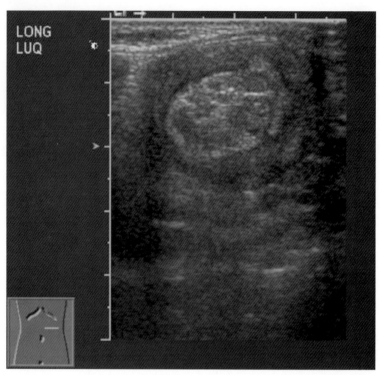

FIGURE 22-2: Abdominal ultrasound showing target sign (*transverse view*).

The case patient's abdominal radiograph was negative; however, the ultrasound was consistent with intussusception.

Treatment

Although intussusception can self-resolve on occasion, most cases require some intervention. In the stable patient, pneumatic or hydrostatic contrast enema is the treatment of choice. The longer signs and symptoms are present, the less likely it is that there will be a successful reduction.

You may attempt enema reduction with either hydrostatic barium contrast technique or pneumatic reduction with air under fluoroscopic or ultrasonographic guidance in clinically stable, well-hydrated patients who present without evidence of peritonitis. Successful reduction of ileocolic intussusception with contrast enema occurs in 60% to 90% of patients. Success is more likely to be achieved in patients with idiopathic intussusception who are >6 months of age and for whom an early diagnosis was made within 24 to 48 hours of symptom onset. In patients with an identifiable lead point or radiographic evidence of intestinal obstruction, you can attempt nonoperative reduction, but usually surgical reduction will be required.

A contrast enema study should always be done in consultation with a pediatric surgeon who is immediately available in case of any complications, including failure to reduce or bowel perforation. Most cases of intussusception that have failed reduction by enema can be reduced by retrograde manual reduction at the time of operative intervention.

With the success of early diagnosis, appropriate fluid resuscitation, and therapeutic intervention, the mortality rate from intussusception in children is currently <1%.

The patient in this case underwent pneumatic reduction with an air enema study under fluoroscopic guidance (Figs. 22-3).

Admission Criteria and Level-of-Care Criteria

Admission is indicated for all patients because the recurrence of intussusception after initial reduction is approximately 10% in patients with successful nonoperative reduction. Some 50% of children with recurrent intussusception will present within 48 hours, although recurrences have been reported up to 18 months later. After successful pneumatic reduction, the case patient was admitted for observation under the pediatric surgery service.

EXTENDED IN-HOSPITAL MANAGEMENT

Extended admission >24 hours after nonoperative reduction is not necessary unless there are complications such as perforation and peritonitis. Postoperative complications are more frequent with a delayed diagnosis of intussusception.

DISPOSITION

Discharge Goals

Patients should be pain-free and able to tolerate oral intake without vomiting.

Outpatient Care

Patients at low risk for intussusception and negative screening tests (i.e., Hemoccult, abdominal ultrasonography) may be sent home with appropriate discharge instructions and follow-up.

The case patient was discharged home after a 24-hour observation period with a caution to return if he had symptom recurrence (colicky pain, persistent vomiting, or bloody stools).

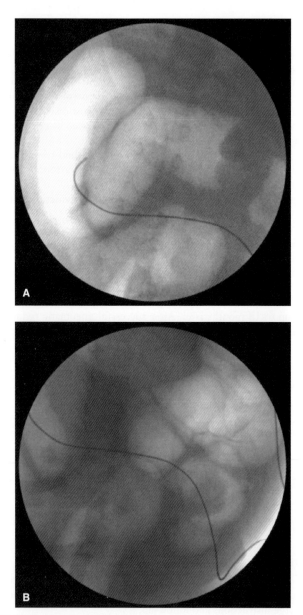

FIGURE 22-3: Air enema showing reduction of an ileocolic intussusception. **A.** Air enema showing ileocolic intussusception at hepatic flexure (*prone view*). **B.** Air enema showing reduction of the intussusception to the ileocecal valve (*prone view*).

WHAT YOU NEED TO REMEMBER

- The classic triad of vomiting, colicky abdominal pain, and "currant jelly" stools occurs in <30% of cases. Occult blood is present 75% of the time.
- All patients should be stabilized with pain control prior to any attempts at reduction.
- A contrast enema study is diagnostic as well as therapeutic; early intervention coupled with a high index of suspicion for intussusception improves the chance for a successful nonoperative reduction.
- Nonoperative reduction should always be done with a pediatric surgeon available in case of failure to reduce or complications such as perforation.

SUGGESTED READINGS

Applegate KE. Intussusception in children: imaging choices. *Semin Roentgenol* 2008;43:15–21.

Cox TD, Winters WD, Weinberger E. CT of intussusception in the pediatric patient: diagnosis and pitfalls. *Pediatr Radiol* 1996;26:26–31.

Daneman A, Navarro O. Intussusception. Part 1: A review of diagnostic approaches. *Pediatr Radiol* 2003;33:79–85.

Davis CF, McCabe AJ, Raine PAM. The ins and outs of intussusception: history and management over the past fifty years. *J Pediatr Surg* 2003;38:60–64.

Hadidi AT, El Shal N. Childhood intussusception: a comparative study of nonsurgical management. *J Pediatr Surg* 1999;34:304–307.

Harrington L, Connolly B, Hu X, et al. Ultrasonographic and clinical predictors of intussusception. *J Pediatr* 1998;132:836–839.

Kaiser AD, Applegate KE, Ladd AP. Current success in the treatment of intussusception in children. *Surgery* 2007;142:469–477.

Ko HS, Schenk JP, Tröger J, et al. Current radiological management of intussusception in children. *Eur Radiol* 2007;17:2411–2421.

Losek JD, Fiete RL. Intussusception and the diagnostic value of testing stool for occult blood. *Am J Emerg Med* 1991;9:1–3.

Parashar UD, Holman RC, Cummings KC, et al. Trends in intussusception-associated hospitalizations and deaths among US infants. *Pediatrics* 2000;106:1413–1421.

Sargent MA, Babyn P, Alton DJ. Plain abdominal radiography in suspected intussusception: a reassessment. *Pediatr Radiol* 1994;24:17–20.

Juvenile Idiopathic Arthritis

MEGAN K. YUNGHANS

THE PATIENT ENCOUNTER

A 6-year-old boy is taken to his pediatrician with a 4-day history of daily fevers ranging from 38.9°C to 39.4°C (102°F to 103°F). The fevers occur once daily in the early evening. The boy's parents describe him as ill-appearing when the fevers are present but well the rest of the day. His parents have also noted a nonpruritic rash on his trunk when he is febrile. On examination, he was afebrile and well-appearing. His exam was unremarkable. He was sent home with anticipatory guidance and instructions to return to clinic in 2 to 3 days if the fevers continued.

The boy and his parents return to clinic 2 weeks after his first visit. The family reports that he has had persistent once-daily fevers with rash during this time. However, because the boy otherwise looked well, his family did not bring him back for reevaluation. However, for the past 2 days the boy has been complaining of left knee pain, and his parents noticed that this knee was swollen. On physical examination, he was afebrile and had no rash. His left knee had obvious swelling with an effusion, decreased flexion, and pain with range-of-motion testing. His exam was also notable for hepatomegaly as well as axillary and cervical lymphadenopathy. The boy was then referred to the emergency department for further evaluation.

OVERVIEW

Definition

Arthritis is defined as joint swelling or a combination of joint warmth, tenderness, and limitation of movement or pain with movement. Juvenile idiopathic arthritis (JIA) is defined as persistent arthritis in one or more joints in a child younger <16 years of age that lasts for >6 weeks when all other causes of the arthritis have been excluded. These causes include infectious (septic arthritis, acute rheumatic fever), inflammatory (systemic lupus erythematous, inflammatory bowel disease), and neoplastic (leukemia, lymphoma) etiologies. JIA is currently divided into eight categories based on the clinical course during the first 6 months of illness (Table 23-1). The International League Against Rheumatism developed this classification, which now replaces the previously used juvenile rheumatoid arthritis (JRA) classification from the American College of Rheumatology. This chapter will focus on systemic-onset JIA.

TABLE 23-1
The Classification of Juvenile Idiopathic Arthritis

JIA Classification	Clinical Features
Systemic arthritis	Arthritis accompanied or preceded by daily fever for a minimum of 2 weeks with one or more accompanying findings (rash, lymphadenopathy, hepatosplenomegaly, or serositis) when other disorders have been excluded.
Oligoarthritis	Arthritis of 1 to 4 joints during the first 6 months of disease.
Persistent	Only 1 to 4 joints are affected throughout the disease course.
Extended	More than 4 joints are affected after the first 6 months of disease
Polyarthritis	
RF-negative	More than 4 joints are affected in the first 6 months of disease and tests for RF are negative.
RF-positive	More than 4 joints are affected in the first 6 months of disease and tests for RF are positive on two occasions a minimum of 2 months apart during the first 6 months of disease.
Enthesitis-related arthritis	Arthritis and/or enthesitis with at least two of the following: spinal/sacroiliac pain, HLA B27–positive, positive family history in a first- or second-degree relative of HLA B27–related disease, acute uveitis, or onset of arthritis in a boy >6 years of age.
Psoriatic arthritis	Arthritis with psoriasis or at least two of the following: dactylitis, nail abnormalities, or family history of psoriasis in a first-degree relative.
Other	Arthritis of unknown etiology for ≥6 weeks that does not fit in one of the previously listed categories or fulfills the criteria for more than one category.

Pathophysiology

Although the etiology and physiology of JIA are not well understood, the resultant pathology is well characterized. Active disease results in hypertrophy of the synovium and hyperplasia of the synovial lining in the affected joint, with infiltration of lymphocytes and plasma cells. This inflammation may lead to destruction of articular cartilage with contiguous bone erosion and destruction.

Epidemiology

The prevalence of JIA is estimated to be between 16 and 150 per 100,000 children, with an incidence of 10 to 20 cases per 100,000 children. Systemic-onset JIA accounts for approximately 10% of all cases of JIA, while oligoarthritis and polyarthritis account for approximately 40% and 25%, respectively. Oligoarthritis and polyarthritis both occur throughout childhood, with a peak between 1 and 3 years of age. In both oligoarthritis and polyarthritis, there is a female predominance. Systemic-onset JIA occurs throughout childhood with no peak age of onset. Males and females are equally affected.

Etiology

The etiology is not known, although JIA appears to be a mulitfactorial autoimmune disease. There is evidence that B cells, T cells, and inflammatory cytokines may all play a role in the disease. B cells appear to play a role in the creation of immune complexes, which have been isolated in children with JIA. These immune complexes activate an inflammatory cascade, resulting in joint inflammation and leukocyte recruitment. The exact mechanism of T-cell involvement is unknown; however, the presence of activated T cells and TH1 cytokines in the synovium of children with JIA supports their involvement. Inflammatory cytokines have also been found to be elevated in certain subtypes of JIA. For example, high levels of interleukin-6 (IL-6) have been found in systemic-onset disease. There may also be a hereditary basis for the disease, as research has uncovered increased human leukocyte antigen (HLA) genotypes associated with specific disease subtypes.

ACUTE MANAGEMENT AND WORKUP

The acute management and workup of a patient presenting with symptoms of systemic-onset JIA (high, spiking fever and rash, with or without signs of arthritis) help to identify those patients who have severe illness requiring immediate intervention and those who are stable enough to undergo a comprehensive evaluation on either an inpatient or outpatient basis.

The First 15 Minutes

The first few minutes of your patient encounter should determine if your patient is stable enough to continue with a thorough history and physical.

First, ensure that the patient has appropriate attention to the ABCs (airway, breathing, and circulation). Then assess the general demeanor of the patient. A sleepy patient or one who is difficult to arouse may indicate a serious bacterial infection or neurologic involvement. Next, assess the patient's vital signs. Heart rates, respiratory rates, and blood pressures that differ significantly from age-adjusted norms should be immediately addressed.

The First Few Hours

A thorough history and physical exam are essential components in patient care during the first few hours. Based on the information obtained, an assessment with a broad differential diagnosis and plan of care should be made.

History

Children with systemic-onset JIA classically present with daily or twice-daily spiking fevers accompanied by a macular salmon-colored rash. The fevers are characterized by a rapid rise in temperature, typically reaching >39°C (102.2°F), followed by a quick return to baseline. The fevers occur mostly in the evening or early morning but may occur at any time of the day. These children will often appear ill while the temperature is elevated, but appear healthy the rest of the day. The rash consists of discrete salmon-colored macules. It may occur anywhere on the body but is typically seen on the trunk and extremities. The rash usually appears when the child is febrile and fades as the fever resolves. The rash is rarely pruritic. In addition to being induced by fever, the rash may be precipitated by a hot bath or rubbing the skin (Koebner phenomenon). Hepatomegaly, splenomegaly, lymphadenopathy, and pericarditis are also common features of systemic-onset JIA. These extra-articular manifestations are of variable duration but may recur with acute exacerbations of the arthritis. In the majority of cases, these manifestations will resolve within 5 years of diagnosis.

The arthritis of systemic-onset JIA may present at the same time as the systemic features noted above, or it may appear several weeks or months later. The arthritis typically affects the wrists, knees, and ankles, but other joints (hands, hips, cervical spine) may also be affected.

Physical Examination

You must examine all joints (including the jaw, neck, fingers, and toes) for signs of arthritis. First, evaluate for any swelling. Compare the affected joint visually to its unaffected partner to see if there is any obvious swelling/asymmetry (in the case patient, the left and right knees should be looked at side by side). Then palpate the joint to check for warmth, tenderness, or an effusion. Next assess the range of motion for the joints, noting if there are any limitations or pain with this examination. Be sure to compare the findings in each joint with its partner joint if possible (this is not possible for the jaw and spine).

If there is concern for JIA or the diagnosis of JIA has been made, an ophthalmologist must examine the patient for any evidence of uveitis. Uveitis is most commonly found in patients with oligoarthritis who are antinuclear antibody (ANA)–positive. Uveitis is rarely found in systemic-onset JIA.

Labs and Tests to Consider

No laboratory or radiographic findings are pathognomonic for systemic-onset JIA. Because systemic-onset JIA is a diagnosis of exclusion and can be made only after arthritis has been present for 6 weeks, laboratory and radiologic tests should be used to exclude other disease processes that may have similar presentations.

Key Diagnostic Labs and Tests

In systemic-onset JIA, a complete blood count (CBC) typically reveals leukocytosis, thrombocytosis, and anemia. The white blood cell (WBC) count may be as high as 30,000 to 50,000/mm^3 with a predominance of granulocytes. The hemoglobin levels may range between 7 and 10 g/dL, and the platelet count is often >500,000/mm^3. The erythrocyte sedimentation rate (ESR) and C-reactive protein (CRP) are both characteristically elevated. The ESR is often >60 to 100 mm/hr. The ESR and CRP may be followed to monitor for improvement as well as the efficacy of therapy.

Additional laboratory studies that may be suggestive of systemic-onset JIA include mild elevation of the hepatic transaminases, hypoalbuminemia, and increased immunoglobulin levels. Ferritin levels may also be elevated. Urinalysis may show mild proteinuria during a febrile episode but otherwise should be normal. The WBC count in synovial fluid, if aspirated from a joint with active arthritis, is elevated, with counts ranging from 600 to 100,000/mm^3. The glucose in the synovial fluid is often low; however, a culture and Gram stain of the fluid will be negative.

CLINICAL PEARL

ANA may be positive in up to 10% of children with systemic-onset JIA. Rheumatoid factor (RF) is rarely positive in systemic-onset JIA.

The case patient had a WBC count of 27,000/mm^3, a hemoglobin level of 8 g/dL, and a platelet count of 450,000/mm^3. His ESR was 93 mm/hr and his ANA was negative. He had blood cultures drawn in the ER, which were negative. His left knee effusion was drained in the ER. The fluid had a WBC count of 50,000/mm^3, and the culture was negative.

Imaging

Plain radiographs, bone scans, and magnetic resonance imaging (MRI) are mainly used to exclude other diseases such as infection or malignancy. There are, however, radiographic changes in JIA that may support its diagnosis. Early in the course of JIA, radiographs may show soft tissue swelling, periosteal new bone formation, and osteoporosis of the bones near the affected joint. Later in the disease course, active joint involvement may cause either premature epiphyseal closure or increased development. Both may lead to limb-length discrepancy. If the cervical spine is involved, radiographs may reveal fusion of the cervical apophyseal joints.

Treatment

The immediate treatment goals for systemic-onset JIA are to control the symptoms, arrest the inflammatory process, preserve function, and prevent deformity. These goals are best achieved through a combination of pharmacologic therapy, physical and occupational therapy, and psychosocial support. Remission is ultimately defined as <15 minutes of morning stiffness, no joint effusion, no joint pain, and a normal hematocrit for 2 consecutive months (if the anemia was due to JIA).

Pharmacologic therapy should be initiated in a stepwise fashion, beginning with the simplest, least toxic treatment appropriate for the level of disease severity present. Additional medications may then be added or substituted as needed. Nonsteroidal anti-inflammatory drugs (NSAIDs) are typically the first-line therapy in all types of JIA. In many children with systemic-onset JIA, NSAIDs alone may induce remission. Glucocorticoids may be started in conjunction with NSAIDs for systemic-onset JIA if serious or life-threatening complications (e.g., pericarditis, pleuritis) are present. In this situation, intravenous pulse therapy with methylprednisolone should be administered. Oral glucocorticoids (prednisone) may also be utilized if the disease has caused marked disability (severe pain, refusal to walk) despite adequate NSAID therapy. In this case, glucocorticoids should be used as a bridging medication to control symptoms until a disease-modifying antirheumatic drug (DMARD) can be started. The glucocorticoids should then be weaned once adequate control has been achieved.

The most widely used DMARD is methotrexate. Other DMARDs that have been shown to be effective in systemic-onset JIA include sulfasalazine, intramuscular gold, cyclophosphamide, and azathioprine. It may take up to 6 weeks after methotrexate is initiated for a clinical response to be seen (hence the need for a bridging medication). If a child does not show improvement in symptoms after 4 to 6 weeks of oral methotrexate, the subcutaneous route should be employed. If a child fails to show improvement 4 to 6 weeks after this change, you should consider changing the DMARD or starting an anticytokine medication. These drugs are classified as biologics. Etanercept (an antagonist to the tumor necrosis factor–alpha receptor) is the most widely used biologic drug. Infliximab and adalimumab are also available for anticytokine therapy. If disease remission is not achieved after this stepwise approach, then you should consider autologous stem cell transplant.

If one or two joints have active arthritis, you can consider administering intra-articular glucocorticoid injections as a supplement to the systemic anti-inflammatory therapy. A good time to consider this is before the initiation of anticytokine therapy.

Once remission is achieved, the pharmacologic regimen that achieved the remission should be continued for approximately 12 additional months. At this point, the medications may be weaned and the patient monitored for any signs of disease reoccurrence.

Physical and occupational therapists are also an integral part of the treatment for systemic-onset JIA. They teach the use of heat therapy (to decrease pain and improve mobility) and cold therapy (to decrease inflammation). They fashion splints, which reduce stress on a joint and help prevent contractures. They also develop programs that teach patients range-of-motion and strengthening exercises. In addition, physical and occupational therapists can create assistive devices for activities of daily living that reduce both joint pain and stress.

Psychosocial support is equally as important in the treatment of JIA. This will address the patient's stresses from living with a chronic illness, provide appropriate education, and ensure that school-based and community resources are available to the patient.

Admission Criteria and Level-of-Care Criteria

Admission should be considered for patients who are first presenting with symptoms of systemic-onset JIA so that other etiologies (infectious, inflammatory, and neoplastic) may be evaluated and excluded. This evaluation can take place on the general pediatric floor. During the initial workup, it may be helpful to involve pediatric infectious disease, oncology, and rheumatology consultants.

Admission is also necessary for patients who develop life-threatening symptoms, such as pericarditis, large pericardial effusion, or macrophage activation syndrome (MAS). MAS typically is triggered by NSAIDs or other pharmacologic therapy; however, it can also be triggered by an infection or it can occur spontaneously. MAS presents with fever, altered mental status, elevated liver enzymes, and a sudden drop in hemoglobin, platelet count, and fibrinogen with a progression to disseminated intravascular coagulation. These patients often need to be stabilized and managed in the intensive care unit before they may be safely cared for on the general pediatric floor. An experienced rheumatologist should be involved in the care of these patients.

EXTENDED IN-HOSPITAL MANAGEMENT

Signs of serositis (pericarditis, large pericardial effusion) that do not respond quickly to pulse methylprednisolone or other therapeutic modalities may result in extended in-hospital management. MAS will result in prolonged hospitalization.

DISPOSITION

Discharge Goals

In the case study provided in this chapter, discharge should be considered once serious infectious, inflammatory, and neoplastic etiologies have been excluded and the patient is clinically stable. Prior to discharge, the patient should also have follow-up arranged with his primary care provider and a pediatric rheumatologist. His parents should receive education on what to expect after discharge and when they should seek immediate medical care.

When a patient is admitted because of one of the life-threatening situations, such as pericarditis or MAS, he or she would be ready for discharge once the precipitating symptom had resolved or was well controlled on a medical regimen that could be followed at home.

Outpatient Care

After discharge, patients should follow up with their primary care physician for routine care, drug monitoring, and to ensure proper coordination between the multidisciplinary team (e.g., rheumatologist, ophthalmologist, physical and occupational therapists, and psychologist) caring for the patient. Patients also need close follow-up with a pediatric rheumatologist who will monitor disease activity and make medication adjustments as needed. Patients also need close follow-up with an ophthalmologist to be monitored for signs of uveitis. For systemic-onset JIA, unless uveitis is found, only yearly ophthalmologic screening is needed.

The case patient was ultimately diagnosed with systemic-onset JIA after his arthritis was present for 6 weeks and other etiologies for the arthritis were excluded. His rheumatologist started him on an NSAID. He failed to show significant improvement after 4 weeks of therapy and therefore was started on methotrexate. After 4 weeks of methotrexate therapy, he was showing clinical improvement and therefore continued on this medication until approximately 12 months after the documentation of remission.

WHAT YOU NEED TO REMEMBER

- Systemic-onset JIA is a diagnosis of exclusion.
- The diagnosis of all classes of JIA can be made only after the arthritis has been present for 6 weeks.
- Labs and radiographs cannot assist in the diagnosis of JIA. They only support the diagnosis of JIA and help to exclude other diseases.
- Treatment for JIA involves a multidisciplinary approach.

SUGGESTED READINGS

Cassidy JT, Petty RE. Juvenile rheumatoid arthritis. In Cassidy JT, Petty RE, eds. *Textbook of Pediatric Rheumatology*, 4th ed. Philadelphia: Saunders, 2001.

Giannini EH, Ruperto N, Ravelli A, et al. Preliminary definition of improvement in juvenile arthritis. *Arthritis Rheum* 1997;40:1202–1209.

Goldmuntz EA, White PH. Juvenile idiopathic arthritis: a review for the pediatrician. *Pediatr Rev* 2006;27:e24–e32.

Ilowite NT. Current treatment of juvenile rheumatoid arthritis. *Pediatrics* 2002;109: 109–115.

Moore TL. Immunopathogenesis of juvenile rheumatoid arthritis. *Curr Opin Rheumatol* 1999;11:377–383.

Moorthy LN, Onel KB. Juvenile idiopathic arthritis: making the diagnosis and drug treatments. *J Musculo Med* 2004;11:581–588; 2004;12:634–638.

Sandborg CI, Wallace CA. Position Statement of the American College of Rheumatology Regarding Referral of Children and Adolescents to Pediatric Rheumatologists. *Arthritis Care Res* 1999;12:48–51.

Kawasaki Disease

CHRISTOPHER GAYDOS

THE PATIENT ENCOUNTER

A 4-year-old girl was taken to her pediatrician after having fever for 3 days, an erythematous rash, and a unilateral swollen cervical lymph node. She was diagnosed with strep throat and given amoxicillin. Her fever continued for the next 2 days and she developed swollen hands and feet and bilateral conjunctival injection. She was taken to the emergency department on day 5 of her fever, after her parents noticed that she was increasingly irritable and that her lips were red and swollen. On emergency department presentation, she had a fever of 40°C (104°F) and was mildly tachycardic. On examination, she was irritable, with nonpitting edema in her hands and feet and a diffuse erythematous rash that was desquamating over the perianal area. She had unilateral cervical lymphadenopathy; a strawberry tongue with red, cracked lips; and bilateral conjunctival injection.

OVERVIEW

Definition

Kawasaki disease is an acute, self-limited vasculitis that occurs predominantly in infants and young children and is the leading cause of acquired cardiovascular disease in children in the United States. It is defined by fever (>38.3°C or >101°F) for ≥5 days and at least four of the following:

- Bilateral conjunctival injection
- Polymorphous rash
- Oral mucosal changes
- Changes in the extremities
- Cervical adenopathy

These criteria are often but not always present at presentation, but it is important that at least four of five of the criteria be present during the acute phase (the first 7 to 10 days of fever).

In recent years, the concept of incomplete or atypical Kawasaki disease has emerged. Incomplete (formerly referred to as "atypical") Kawasaki disease is defined as fever for ≥5 days, at least two of the five criteria noted previously, and laboratory findings consistent with severe systemic inflammation. Coronary artery changes confirm the diagnosis of incomplete Kawasaki disease.

Pathophysiology

The signs and symptoms of Kawasaki disease are thought to be due to an inflammatory response to an as yet unidentified trigger. This immune response occurs during the acute phase and results in activation and increased proliferation of monocytes, macrophages, T cells, and B lymphocytes; it results in a cytokine cascade and endothelial cell activation. These events cause a microvasculitis, subsequent inflammation of medium-sized arteries, and eventual aneurysmal formation, especially of the coronary arteries.

Epidemiology

Kawasaki disease is found in people of all racial backgrounds but is markedly more prevalent in children of Japanese ancestry. It most often presents in children <5 years of age and is rare in children <6 months and >8 years of age. Boys are affected 1.5 times as often as girls. The incidence of Kawasaki disease in the United States ranges from 9.1 to 16.9 cases per 100,000 children <5 years. Siblings of children with Kawasaki disease have a higher incidence than do individuals in the general population, as do children of parents with a history of Kawasaki disease.

Etiology

The etiology of Kawasaki disease is still unknown and the subject of great debate in pediatric circles. The fact that there is a distinct seasonality (a predominance of cases in January and June/July) suggests an infectious trigger that causes the inflammatory cascade. The overrepresentation of Asians and increased incidence within families suggest that genetics plays a role as well. The epidemiology supports the hypothesis that Kawasaki's disease is caused by an as yet unknown infectious agent that leads to clinically apparent disease in those with a specific genetic predisposition to this disorder.

ACUTE MANAGEMENT AND WORKUP

The acute management and workup is geared toward elucidating the necessary criteria to diagnose Kawasaki disease. It is also important to investigate and rule out other similarly presenting illnesses that can be dangerous if missed, such as toxic shock syndrome, Rocky Mountain spotted fever, Stevens-Johnson syndrome, and juvenile idiopathic arthritis.

The First 15 Minutes

It is important to make sure that the patient is stable before beginning a detailed history and physical. Review the patient's vital signs to look for tachycardia—which may be present due to fever—and hypotension, which could indicate shock or sepsis.

The First Few Hours

A detailed history and physical are key to diagnosing Kawasaki disease. There is usually plenty of time to secure the diagnosis before starting treatment to avoid long-term sequelae.

History

Because there is no specific test for Kawasaki disease and some of the physical exam features may no longer be evident on presentation, a detailed history is crucial in making the diagnosis. Do not get distracted by prior diagnoses, as it is common for Kawasaki disease to be misdiagnosed in the first few days before the complete constellation of findings appears. The exact date of fever onset is important not only in the diagnosis but also in establishing where the patient is in the natural history of the disease. Be sure to ask specifically about each of the five major criteria if this information was not volunteered during the history. Other relevant features associated with Kawasaki disease but not part of the diagnostic criteria include:

- Arthritis and/or arthralgia
- Diarrhea/vomiting
- Myocarditis
- Urethritis
- Hepatic dysfunction
- Hydrops of gallbladder

Physical Examination

Children usually present as ill-appearing, uncomfortable, but nontoxic. The conjunctivitis occurs soon after the start of fever and can resolve spontaneously. It is nonpurulent and often does not completely reach the iris, leaving a thin ring of unaffected sclera (perilimbic sparing). The rash can take many forms but is typically erythematous and maculopapular and involves the trunk and extremities. It also often begins in the groin area and can be limited to that. Desquamation sometimes occurs several days after the rash appears. Oral mucosal changes include diffuse erythema of oral mucosa, dry cracked lips, strawberry tongue, and injected pharynx. The extremity changes common to Kawasaki disease include edema of the hands and feet, erythema of the palms and/or soles, and periungual desquamation. The cervical adenitis is typically unilateral and >1.5 cm. It is also the most likely criterion to be absent on examination. The cardiac exam is usually normal during the acute phase, as cardiac sequelae do not present until later. Tachycardia is common but is usually due to fever or dehydration.

CLINICAL PEARL

Uveitis is detected in up to 85% of children with Kawasaki disease but is rarely present in children with systemic onset juvenile idiopathic arthritis.

Labs and Tests to Consider

Although there is no specific test for Kawasaki disease, certain lab values can help support the clinical diagnosis.

Key Diagnostic Labs and Tests

A complete blood count and C-reactive protein (CRP) can be helpful in following the progression of the illness and the effectiveness of treatment. In cases of incomplete Kawasaki disease, the following lab findings can help to support the diagnosis:

- Elevated CRP and erythrocyte sedimentation rate (ESR)
- Leukocytosis
- Normochromic/normocytic anemia
- Hyponatremia
- Sterile pyuria
- Hypoalbuminemia

CSF pleocytosis may be seen if a septic workup is done prior to the diagnosis, but lumbar puncture is unnecessary to make the case for Kawasaki disease. During the second week of illness, thrombocytosis is often seen, with platelet counts ranging from 500,000 to >1 million. Thrombocytopenia can be seen on presentation and places the patient at higher risk for a coronary artery aneurysm.

Imaging

Coronary artery aneurysms develop in 20% to 25% of untreated cases and ≤5% of treated patients. Echocardiography is necessary at diagnosis not only to look for coronary artery changes or enlargement (aneurysm is uncommon in the acute phase) but also as a baseline study. Repeat echocardiography is needed 6 to 8 weeks after the onset of symptoms to confirm the efficacy of treatment. Myocarditis, pericarditis, and valvulitis are uncommon but possible complications and should be examined during echocardiography as well.

Treatment

Treatment for Kawasaki disease is directed toward the inflammatory response that causes the clinical manifestations. Intravenous immune globulin (IVIG) is the mainstay of treatment. Although the exact mechanism is unknown, it appears to have general anti-inflammatory effects, with reduction of fever and inflammatory markers. A single dose of 2 g/kg is given over 10 to 12 hours. Studies have found that those treated with IVIG <10 days after fever onset had significantly reduced chances of developing a coronary artery aneurysm. In addition, high-dose aspirin is also used both for its antiplatelet properties and as an anti-inflammatory medication, although it appears to have no effect on aneurysm formation. A total of 80 to 100 mg/kg/day divided into four doses is used in the acute phase. Once the patient has been afebrile for 3 to 7 days, the dose is decreased to 3 to 5 mg/kg once a day. This dose is continued for 6 to 8 weeks until inflammatory markers have normalized and no coronary artery damage has been noted on repeat echocardiogram.

The child in the case presentation met the criteria for Kawasaki disease; no other cause of her signs and symptoms could be found. She received IVIG on the second day of hospitalization with prompt resolution of fever. She did not subsequently develop coronary artery abnormalities.

Admission Criteria and Level-of-Care Criteria

You should admit all patients diagnosed with Kawasaki disease and treat them with IVIG and high-dose aspirin therapy. An echocardiogram should be ordered, but treatment should not be delayed for this. You should also consider admitting patients with early signs of Kawasaki disease (those having the criteria but who have been febrile for <5 days) based on the level of suspicion. If you are uncertain, treatment can be delayed up until day 10 of fever without an increased risk of coronary artery disease. Most patients can be managed on the general pediatric floor, but those rare cases with congestive heart failure or cardiac shock may require admission to the intensive care unit.

EXTENDED IN-HOSPITAL MANAGEMENT

Although most patients defervesce within 24 hours after IVIG therapy, 10% to 15% will continue to be febrile or have their fever return. If this occurs, first reconsider the diagnosis. If Kawasaki disease remains likely, a second dose of IVIG should be administered at the same dosage at least 36 to 48 hours after the first infusion. Two thirds of nonresponders will respond to the second dose of IVIG. Once a patient has failed two doses, the evidence for further treatment is less established. A third dose is often given, and studies are currently under way to examine the efficacy of steroids, plasma exchange, and immunomodulators, but no clear guidelines have been established. Those who do not respond to a single IVIG dose have an increased risk of developing a coronary artery aneurysm.

DISPOSITION

Discharge Goals

Consider discharge in patients who have defervesced and remained afebrile and who have shown clinical signs of improvement. Following inflammatory markers like CRP and ESR can help determine that the systemic inflammation is decreasing. The average hospital stay for those with an uncomplicated course is 2 to 3 days. A baseline echocardiogram should be completed prior to discharge.

Outpatient Care

Instruct patients to follow up with their pediatrician within a few days of discharge. They should be given instructions to call their pediatrician or come back to the hospital if their fever returns or symptoms worsen. They should continue high-dose aspirin for 3 to 7 days after defervescence and then switch to low-dose aspirin.

A repeat echocardiogram should be scheduled at 6 to 8 weeks after discharge. Studies have shown that patients with normal echocardiograms at diagnosis and at 6 to 8 weeks are typically clinically asymptomatic for at least 10 to 20 years. However, new studies have suggested that some patients develop subtle endothelial dysfunction, which might put them at risk for early adult atherosclerosis.

Those with coronary artery changes will need continued monitoring by a cardiologist. They will typically be kept on low-dose aspirin to prevent thrombosis and myointimal proliferation, which can lead to coronary artery stenosis.

Live virus vaccines, such as measles and varicella, should be postponed for at least 11 months in children treated with IVIG. Passive immunity from the IVIG may reduce the immunogenicity of the vaccines. Anyone on long-term aspirin therapy requires yearly influenza vaccination because of the risk of Reye syndrome.

 WHAT YOU NEED TO REMEMBER

- Kawasaki disease is defined as fever for at least 5 days and four of the following: conjunctivitis, rash, extremity changes, cervical adenitis, and oral mucosal changes.
- Atypical Kawasaki disease is possible if the patient is febrile, has increased inflammatory markers, and has two of the criteria for Kawasaki disease.
- A coronary artery aneurysm is the most dangerous sequela of the disease.
- IVIG therapy and high-dose aspirin are the preferred treatment.
- Serial echocardiograms are needed to assess for coronary artery changes.

SUGGESTED READINGS

Burns JC, Glode MP. Kawasaki syndrome. *Lancet* 2004;364(9433):533–54

Falcini F. Kawasaki disease. *Curr Opin Rheumatol* 2006;18(1):33–38.

Newburger JW, Takahashi M, Gerber MA, et al. Diagnosis, treatment, and management of Kawasaki disease: a statement for health professionals Committee on Rheumatic Fever, Endocarditis, and Kawasaki Disease, Co Cardiovascular Disease in the Young, American Heart Association. *Cir* 2004;110:2747.

Satou GM, Giamelli J, Gewitz MH. Kawasaki disease: diagnosis, managemen long-term implications. *Cardiol Rev* 2007;15(4):163–169.

Wang CL, Wu YT, Liu CA, et al. Kawasaki disease: infection, immunity and ge ics. *Pediatr Infect Dis J* 2005;24(11):998–1004.

25

Leukemia

GLEN LEW

THE PATIENT ENCOUNTER

A 4-year-old girl presents in the clinic for evaluation of leg pain that she has experienced during the past month. She has already been seen several times in the past month at her pediatrician's office for the same complaint, but no specific diagnosis has been rendered. The pain is vague, not localized to a consistent area, and occurs throughout the day. Over the past week, she developed a low-grade fever. Her physical examination reveals pallor, mild cervical lymphadenopathy, but no focal extremity pain or joint swelling.

OVERVIEW

Definition

The overwhelming majority of childhood leukemia cases are "acute." Acute lymphoblastic leukemia (ALL) represents 75% of cases of pediatric leukemia, acute myeloid leukemia (AML) represents 20% of cases, but chronic myeloid leukemia (CML) accounts for only 5%. CML is not discussed further in this chapter. Chronic lymphocytic leukemia (CLL) does not occur in childhood.

Acute leukemia is usually defined as the occurrence of at least 25% bone marrow replacement with leukemia cells ("blasts"). Leukemia is then subclassified based on the origin of the malignant cells—for example, either ALL or myeloid/monocytic leukemia. The distinction between leukemia types is initially made by microscopic characteristics (French–American–British [FAB] classification system; e.g., L1-L3 or M0-M7) and confirmed by flow cytometric immunophenotyping, which has essentially replaced the use of special microscopic stains to determine cell lineage. Flow cytometry can accurately distinguish between B- and T-precursor ALL and AML subtypes.

Pathophysiology

Acute leukemia arises through genetic alterations to a hematopoietic cell, resulting in a preleukemic cell and, after multiple genetic events, a true leukemic blast. Once a leukemic clone is established and multiplies, it eventually replaces normal hematopoietic function in the marrow and often spreads to sites outside the marrow, such as the lymphatic system, and even potentially to "sanctuary" sites such as the central nervous system or testes. Soft tissue infiltrates ("chloromas") and/or gingival infiltration may be seen, especially in monocytic AML. The symptoms and signs of acute leukemia result from all of these factors, often producing symptomatic anemia and thrombocytopenia (e.g., pallor, bruising, petechiae) and vague systemic symptoms such as fever. Musculoskeletal pain is frequently seen in acute leukemia, particularly ALL, as a result of leukemic growth and inflammatory response in the bone marrow; if present, the musculoskeletal pain from ALL can mimic both rheumatologic and infectious causes.

Epidemiology

Acute leukemia, particularly ALL, is the most common pediatric malignancy, affecting approximately 3 to 4 of 100,000 children. ALL is almost four times more frequent than AML in childhood. ALL incidence peaks in pre–school-age children, while the incidence of AML rises slowly with age.

CLINICAL PEARL

Certain genetic syndromes, particularly Down syndrome (trisomy 21), and immunodeficiency states, predispose to acute leukemia.

Etiology

The etiology and sequence of genetic mutations that lead to leukemic transformation of a hematopoietic precursor is largely unknown. The timing of the initial preleukemic genetic change is often an in utero event in many cases of ALL, as described in Greaves' research on neonatal blood spots and the subsequent development of leukemia. Epidemiologic studies implicate population shifts and infectious events as likely important in leukemogenesis, particularly in ALL. However, specific infectious agents are not usually implicated. A few environmental exposures (e.g., ionizing radiation) have been linked to subsequent development of leukemia.

ACUTE MANAGEMENT AND WORKUP

The initial management of a child with suspected leukemia includes evaluating and stabilizing the patient as well as confirming the diagnosis and preparing for treatment.

The First 15 Minutes

In your initial evaluation of a child with suspected acute leukemia, you should primarily focus on potentially life-threatening signs or symptoms.

These are more likely to occur in patients with extreme hyperleukocytosis on presentation. Patients with significant adenopathy and/or a mediastinal mass are at risk for airway compromise, especially if they require sedation/anesthesia. Some patients may present with severe anemia and cardiovascular compromise, which requires immediate resuscitation with crystalloids followed by a blood transfusion. Neurologic symptoms, if present, can be caused by extreme hyperleukocytosis (with subsequent hypoperfusion to the brain), central nervous system (CNS) hemorrhage, or direct CNS involvement with leukemia. Because many children present with severe neutropenia, bacterial sepsis may also be present, and septic shock should be considered in the febrile, unstable patient with new-onset acute leukemia.

The First Few Hours

Initially, a thorough history and physical examination are obviously important. Even if the patient's diagnosis of leukemia has not yet been confirmed and the patient has not yet been seen by a pediatric hematologist/oncologist, many families prefer to know that leukemia is a consideration.

History

Acute leukemia typically presents with a combination of generalized symptoms plus specific symptoms related to pancytopenia. The duration of symptoms is highly variable, with some patients enduring months of symptoms (and often multiple physician visits and referrals), and others having symptoms that last no more than a day or two. Common symptoms are summarized in Table 25-1. Bone/joint pain, if present, broadens the differential

TABLE 25-1
Common Signs and Symptoms in Acute Leukemia and Their Incidence

Hepatosplenomegaly	60%–70%
Fever	40%–60%
Pallor	50%
Petechiae, purpura, bleeding	50%
Lymphadenopathy	50%
Bone/joint pain	30%
Fatigue	30%
Weight loss, anorexia	25%

diagnosis to include rheumatologic disorders, infections (e.g., septic arthritis or osteomyelitis), and even common problems such as growing pains. The presentation can be highly variable, and the absence of any of these symptoms does not rule out leukemia. A history of any recent corticosteroid administration should be elicited. If steroids have been given, making a definitive diagnosis may be more challenging, and the patient's potential risk group assessment and eligibility for clinical trials may be altered.

Physical Examination

The signs of acute leukemia are related to marrow dysfunction and leukemic proliferation; common signs are summarized in Table 25-1. Lymphadenopathy, often generalized and/or supraclavicular, is frequently noted, and massive adenopathy should raise concern for potential airway or cardiovascular compromise (superior vena cava [SVC] syndrome). In males, testicular enlargement may be present, especially in ALL. For patients with musculoskeletal complaints, often no specific physical findings are noted; however, true arthritis or focal pain can also be noted. It is important to note that the presence or absence of any of these findings does not definitively include or exclude leukemia as the final diagnosis.

Labs and Tests to Consider

Most patients with leukemia will show an abnormal complete blood count (CBC), as illustrated in Table 25-2. Chemistries are usually sent to screen for tumor lysis syndrome (elevated uric acid, potassium, phosphorus, and decreased calcium), which, even before the onset of treatment, may lead to renal insufficiency or failure. Lactate dehydrogenase (LDH) is often elevated as a nonspecific finding caused by rapid cell turnover. Inflammatory

---

TABLE 25-2
Common CBC Findings in Acute Leukemia

WBCs (PER/µL)	<10,000	50%
	10,000–50,000	30%
	>50,000	20%
Hemoglobin (g/dL)	<7	45%
	7–11	45%
	>11	10%
Platelets (PER k/µL)	<20,000	25%
	20,000–100,000	50%
	>100,000	25%

markers such as C-reactive protein (CRP) and erythrocyte sedimentation rate (ESR) are often elevated. Coagulation studies may show signs of disseminated intravascular coagulation, particularly in the promyelocytic (M3) subtype of AML.

Key Diagnostic Labs and Tests

In the case patient, laboratory studies revealed pancytopenia with WBCs of 3,900/μL, a hemoglobin count of 7.4 g/dL, and a platelet count of 54,000/μL. The laboratory technician is concerned about large, immature WBCs with scant cytoplasm and nucleoli present on the blood smear.

The majority of patients will show leukemia cells ("blasts") on manual differential. Blasts are usually described as large, immature, mononuclear WBCs with scant cytoplasm, sometimes with nuclear clefting or nucleoli present. ALL blasts tend to be smaller and less complex than AML blasts, which are usually larger and often have more cytoplasmic granules or Auer rods. Note that even for experienced hematologists or pathologists, it may be difficult to truly differentiate blasts from reactive/atypical lymphocytes and also to differentiate the blasts of ALL from those of AML.

Bone marrow aspiration (BMA) is the gold standard to confirm a diagnosis of acute leukemia, in which normal marrow is replaced by blasts (at least 25% by most classification schemes). Immunophenotyping by flow cytometry is used not only to confirm that abnormal cells are blasts but also to delineate their exact lineage (i.e., B or T precursor or myeloid). This can also be done on peripheral blood before BMA is obtained to help direct which studies should be sent from the marrow.

In patients with acute leukemia, bone marrow is usually also sent for chromosome analysis, which helps reveal the "signature" behind the patient's leukemia cells; different cytogenetic abnormalities in the otherwise "same" disease can impart significant differences in prognosis and treatment. Additionally, the majority of pediatric leukemia patients are treated as part of cooperative-group research studies, and extra bone marrow is often obtained for specific research-related questions.

Imaging

Most children with acute leukemia do not require imaging studies to finalize their diagnosis or staging. All patients should undergo a chest x-ray to ensure that there is no mediastinal adenopathy or tracheal compression. Patients who present with significant musculoskeletal symptoms often do undergo multiple radiographic studies. Plain radiographs may show osteopenia, vertebral compression fractures, lytic lesions, or metaphyseal bands ("leukemic lines"). Bone scan and/or magnetic resonance imaging (MRI) may show diffuse bone or bone marrow signal abnormalities, even in asymptomatic sites.

Treatment

Children with acute leukemia require multiagent chemotherapy directed by a pediatric oncologist, usually as part of a multidisciplinary team. Adolescent patients have been shown to have superior outcomes when treated by pediatric as opposed to adult oncologists and warrant referral to a pediatric tertiary care center. The majority of children with acute leukemia are offered participation and enrolled in a cooperative group research study (such as those from the Children's Oncology Group). These studies have dramatically improved outcomes, especially in ALL, in which >80% of children will be cured. Unfortunately, progress has been slower against AML, in which only 40% to 50% will achieve a long-term cure.

The details of chemotherapy for either ALL or AML are beyond the scope of this text. In general, patients receive initial multiagent chemotherapy to establish remission—that is, the eradication of overt leukemia, which allows the return of normal hematopoietic function. The intensity of therapy is often risk-based, with higher-risk subtypes receiving more intensive chemotherapy. In general, treatment for ALL is protracted ($\geq$2 years) but often only moderately intensive, occurring primarily in the outpatient setting. AML therapy is highly intensive and usually delivered in the hospital, but it is also of shorter duration (<1 year). Prophylaxis for CNS leukemia is given for both types of leukemia via intrathecal chemotherapy and sometimes via adjunctive radiation therapy.

Admission Criteria and Level-of-Care Criteria

Most children with acute leukemia are hospitalized for their initial stabilization, workup, and initiation of therapy. You should refer children who present with acute leukemia to a center experienced in pediatric cancer treatment.

EXTENDED IN-HOSPITAL MANAGEMENT

Beyond chemotherapy administration, management is aimed primarily at preventing and treating complications related to therapy and the primary disease. Patients are at risk of tumor lysis syndrome (as mentioned above) and are typically given vigorous hydration, *allopurinol* or *rasburicase* to prevent hyperuricemia, and close monitoring of electrolyte and fluid status to prevent complications, including renal failure. These patients are immunocompromised and are at risk of sepsis associated with neutropenia. Broad-spectrum antibiotics (such as *ceftazidime*, *cefepime*, or other antibiotics, based on institutional resistance patterns) are empirically indicated for febrile neutropenia. Prolonged fever that presents with neutropenia may indicate invasive fungal infection and may warrant the addition of broad-spectrum antifungal coverage.

DISPOSITION

Discharge Goals

Patients are usually discharged after the initiation of chemotherapy, when afebrile, clinically stable, and without evidence of tumor lysis syndrome or other complications. However, induction regimens for AML, as well as many newer regimens for ALL including dexamethasone, are highly intensive and more likely to result in serious infection. Some clinicians recommend empiric hospitalization (even without fever) until evidence of marrow recovery is present. For AML in particular, this may result in prolonged hospitalization (>1 month).

Outpatient Care

Patients have frequent follow-up visits in the outpatient setting to receive continued chemotherapy, especially for childhood ALL (most subsequent chemotherapy for AML is given in hospital). Continued evaluation of the disease status is also followed, especially during the first month, in which patients have repeat BMAs to assess for remission and also the rapidity of remission entry. Many newer chemotherapy protocols also include monitoring of minimal residual disease (MRD), the subclinical level of residual leukemia; higher MRD levels often impart a worsened prognosis and require more intensive treatment.

After therapy has been completed, most children continue to be followed, not only for potential relapse of leukemia but also late side effects of chemotherapy. These may include cardiotoxicity, growth and endocrine issues, secondary malignancies, and cognitive dysfunction. However, the long-term prognosis is still excellent in ALL and is improving in AML.

 WHAT YOU NEED TO REMEMBER

- Acute leukemia is the most common malignancy of childhood.
- Leukemia usually presents with signs and symptoms of bone marrow failure along with generalized systemic symptoms and may include musculoskeletal complaints.
- The CBC usually reveals pancytopenia (with variable leukopenia versus leukocytosis), often with blasts present on the blood smear.
- Bone marrow aspiration (and flow cytometry) help confirm the diagnosis and to determine the risk grouping and intensity of subsequent therapy.
- Patients, including adolescents, should be referred to a tertiary care center that has experience in treating pediatric cancers.
- The prognosis for ALL is good (>80% cure rate), while AML remains more of a challenge (40% to 50% cure rate).

SUGGESTED READINGS

National Cancer Institute. Childhood acute lymphoblastic leukemia treatment (PDQ). Available at: http://www.cancer.gov/cancertopics/pdq/treatment/childALL/HealthProfessional Accessed March 7, 2008.

National Cancer Institute. Childhood acute myeloid leukemia/other myeloid malignancies treatment (PDQ). Available at: http://www.cancer.gov/cancertopics/pdq/treatment/childAML/HealthProfessional Accessed March 7, 2008.

Golub TR, Arceci RJ. Acute myelogenous leukemia. In: Pizzo PA, Poplack DG, eds. *Principles and Practice of Pediatric Oncology*, 4th ed. Philadelphia: Lippincott Williams & Wilkins, 2002.

Margolin FJ, Steuber CP, Poplack DG. Acute lymphoblastic leukemia. In: Pizzo PA, Poplack DG, eds. *Principles and Practice of Pediatric Oncology*, 4th ed. Philadelphia: Lippincott Williams & Wilkins, 2002.

Pieters R, Carroll WL. Biology and treatment of acute lymphoblastic leukemia. *Pediatr Clin North Am* 2008;55:1–20.

Rubnitz JE. Acute myeloid leukemia. *Pediatr Clin North Am* 2008;55:21–51.

Meningitis

STEPHEN C. EPPES AND JAMES J. REESE, JR.

THE PATIENT ENCOUNTER

A 6-month-old full-term baby boy was taken to the emergency room department because of fever and fussiness for the past 24 hours. His past medical history was reportedly unremarkable, but the baby's parents had declined to give him immunizations. On examination, he was fussy but consolable; his temperature was 38.6°C (101.5°F) and his respiratory rate 30 breaths per minute. His anterior fontanelle was full; otherwise he had no focal signs of infection. A complete blood count (CBC) showed an elevated level of white blood cells (WBCs). A blood culture and lumbar puncture (LP) were performed.

OVERVIEW

Definition

Meningitis is defined as inflammation involving the membranes surrounding the brain. The term *encephalitis* refers to an infection within the parenchyma of the brain. The term *meningoencephalitis* refers to a disorder in which patients present with evidence of infection in both the meninges and brain parenchyma. This chapter focuses on acute meningitis and its significant complications, including hearing loss, cortical damage, and death.

Pathophysiology

The pathophysiology of meningitis depends on the etiologic agent. After invading the body, viruses may spread through the blood and reach the central nervous system (CNS) through the blood–brain barrier (BBB), which consists of the arachnoid membrane, choroid plexus epithelium, and cerebral microvascular endothelium. Less commonly, viruses reach the CNS by direct extension through either peripheral or cranial nerves (examples include herpes simplex virus [HSV] and rabies).

Bacteria have a different pathogenetic mechanism. Those species that tend to cause meningitis first colonize the nasopharynx. They can then invade the mucosal barrier to enter the blood. Next, they will spread through the bloodstream to the BBB, where they pass into the cerebrospinal fluid (CSF). The ensuing inflammatory response causes increased BBB permeability and both cytotoxic and vasogenic edema. The auditory system is especially sensitive to this inflammation. Brain damage may result from a variety of mechanisms, but the most important is a reduction in cortical blood perfusion with resultant ischemia.

Bacterial infection may also be introduced by head trauma or neurosurgical procedures. Focal infections, such as brain abscess, epidural empyema, and subdural empyema, may occur as complications from infection in the paranasal sinuses, the middle ear, and mastoid air cells and may occasionally result from hematogenous deposition of bacteria in the brain (classically seen in children with right-to-left shunts or endocarditis; Fig. 26-1).

Epidemiology

Pediatricians used to see many patients with meningitis, mostly because of the high incidence of *Haemophilus influenzae* type b (Hib) meningitis. Nowadays, thanks to effective immunizations, pediatric residents rarely diagnose a child outside of the neonatal age range with bacterial meningitis. Still, this is a serious medical condition that requires urgent and meticulous care.

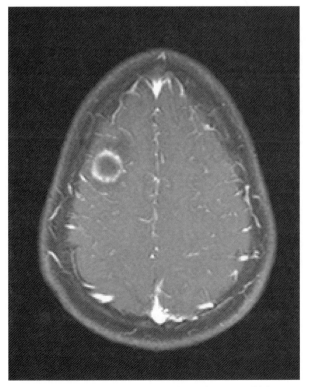

FIGURE 26-1: Ring-enhancing abscess in the right parietal lobe.

Most forms of meningitis are transmitted from person to person. Bacteria such as *Streptococcus pneumoniae* (also known as pneumococcus), Hib, and *Neisseria meningitidis* (also known as meningococcus) are respiratory pathogens. Enteroviruses are transmitted by feces and saliva. Neonatal pathogens are frequently passed from mother to infant in utero or via the peripartum. Some viruses that cause meningoencephalitis are transmitted from mosquito bites, while Lyme disease occurs as the result of tick attachments.

Several epidemiologic clues can help determine the most likely causative pathogen. First, there is a seasonal variation to many of these pathogens. Enterovirus activity peaks in late summer to early autumn but is more common around the year in warm climates. *S. pneumoniae* is more common in winter. Infection with *N. meningitidis* is most common around influenza season and may occur in outbreaks. Vector-borne infections, such as Lyme disease, occur during the warmer months.

The patient's travel history is important. For example, meningococcal disease is hyperendemic in sub-Saharan Africa, while West Nile virus is now mostly seen in the western United States and northern Mexico. Lyme disease is seen mainly in the coastal Northeast, the mid-Atlantic states, and the upper Midwest of the United States. The demographics of the patient may also hold important clues. As noted below, etiologies are often age-related. The immunization status of the patient (and the community) can influence the development of meningitis.

Incidence

The Centers for Disease Control and Prevention estimate that 30,000 to 75,000 cases of enteroviral meningitis occur yearly in the United States (although the true incidence may be much higher because of underreporting). In 1995, the incidence of bacterial meningitis was 0.2 per 100,000 in the United States, although that number continues to fall because of effective immunization. Bacterial meningitis was once most common in childhood but now is more common among adults.

Etiology

Meningitis can have many different etiologies: bacterial, viral, fungal, or parasitic. Most meningitis is acute, but chronic meningitis (i.e., meningitis that presents with symptoms for ≥4 weeks) caused by *Mycobacterium tuberculosis*, *Cryptococcus neoformans*, and other pathogens may also occur. *Aseptic meningitis* refers to those cases with CSF pleocytosis but without bacteria detected by either Gram stain or culture. Most cases of aseptic meningitis in children are caused by viruses (e.g., enteroviruses).

For bacterial meningitis, the patient's age helps to narrow the range of causative agents. In neonates, group B streptococci, enteric gram-negative bacilli (especially *Escherichia coli*, less commonly *Klebsiella* spp., *Enterobacter* spp., and *Citrobacter* spp.) and *Listeria monocytogenes* predominate. Among infants, older children, and adolescents, *S. pneumoniae* and *N. meningitidis* are most common. Immunization against Hib has made this organism extremely uncommon in vaccinated populations. Several clinical clues can also help to narrow the etiology. Immunocompromised patients are at risk for *S. pneumoniae* (with hypogammaglobulinemia, HIV infection, and asplenia), *N. meningitidis* (with terminal complement deficiencies), and *L. monocytogenes* (with abnormal cell-mediated immunity). Basilar skull fractures predispose patients to *S. pneumoniae*. Penetrating head trauma increases the risk of meningitis caused by *S. aureus*, coagulase-negative staphylococcal species, and gram-negative bacilli. Persons living in close quarters (e.g, military recruits, college students) are at risk for *N. meningitidis*.

In children, viruses are now the most common identifiable cause of meningitis, and enteroviruses (including echo- and Coxsackie viruses) are by far the most common. Younger children, including infants, are most frequently affected. Arboviruses, including those causing St. Louis and Lacrosse encephalitis, should be considered in the right geographic settings. West Nile virus may cause a polio-like syndrome with an asymmetric flaccid paralysis. Herpesviruses can cause meningoencephalitis in normal hosts, but more severe disease may result if the child is immunocompromised.

Borrelia burgdorferi is the etiologic agent for Lyme disease. The central nervous system (CNS) may be involved in more than 10% of patients with Lyme disease, usually within 3 months of the tick bite.

The microbiology of brain abscesses depends on the origin of the abscess, but frequent pathogens include streptococci, staphylococci, anaerobes, and sometimes gram-negative bacilli.

ACUTE MANAGEMENT AND WORKUP

The initial workup is usually performed in the emergency department. A key task is differentiating bacterial from aseptic meningitis.

The First 15 Minutes

If the patient has an altered level of consciousness, unstable vital signs, or respiratory depression, address these issues immediately. An IV can be started at the time blood work is being obtained so that antibiotics can be given promptly. If the patient appears stable, proceed with your history and physical so that you can figure out the diagnosis.

The First Few Hours

Even after early administration of antibiotics, patients need a lot of care and attention until you can feel confident that they will be medically stable throughout their recovery. Some patients will have sepsis with shock, multiorgan failure, and coagulopathy. Early complications of meningitis can include seizures and the syndrome of inappropriate antidiuretic hormone (SIADH).

History

The presence and severity of symptoms depends on the patient's age, immune function, and the pathogen involved. Classic symptoms include fever, headache, stiff neck, and confusion or behavioral changes. The symptoms may progress over hours to days, but a rapid progression from perfectly well to seriously ill over a few hours may also be seen. Younger infants may have fever, excess crying, irritability, decreased feeding, and a decreased activity level. About one fourth of patients with meningitis will have a seizure before diagnosis.

Specific points in the history may help to define the likelihood of the responsible pathogen. Enteroviral infection often shows a pattern with fever and nonspecific signs that resolve and then return with meningeal signs, as well as headache, myalgias, and vomiting or diarrhea. Meningococcal infection is the most likely cause of fulminant disease. When a patient has symptoms of CNS infection and a history of severe middle-ear disease or sinusitis, this should suggest the possibility of intracranial extension from these structures.

Physical Examination

The physical exam should help differentiate nonspecific febrile illnesses from meningitis. Remember that younger infants are less likely to show the classic signs of meningitis, such as nuchal rigidity. A bulging fontanelle indicates increased intracranial pressure (ICP) and is frequently observed with meningitis. A full or pulsatile fontanelle, however, is less specific and may simply be due to the infant's crying during the exam.

Older children are more likely to have classic findings, such as Kernig's and Brudzinski's signs. However, the absence of these signs does not reliably exclude the possibility of bacterial meningitis, as these findings are present in fewer than one fourth of patients with bacterial meningitis. A thorough neurologic exam should be done to establish the likelihood and location of neurologic damage and will serve as a baseline while the child is followed during hospitalization. You should try to look for papilledema and focal neurologic findings, which, if present, should prompt you to order imaging to look for abscess, empyema, tumor, hydrocephalus, or a venous sinus thrombosis. Ataxia is frequently seen with meningitis in older children. Cranial nerve abnormalities may be present, either from inflammation or increased ICP.

Other findings may lead you to consider specific pathogens. Meningococcemia is strongly associated with a petechial rash that often develops into purpura. The finding of CSF leaking from the ear or nose suggests the possibility of pneumococcal infection. A facial nerve palsy in the setting of meningitis is suggestive of Lyme disease. Viruses may present with a myriad of findings, depending on the effects of the virus on other body sites. Many viruses cause a diffuse maculopapular rash (as opposed to a petechial rash).

Labs and Tests to Consider

Although the diagnosis may be made clinically, it is still important to find the causative agent to help define treatment. You should have a low threshold for performing an LP because of the danger of missing the diagnosis of meningitis. However, some patients may be too sick for an immediate LP, including those with cardiovascular instability, respiratory distress, or florid sepsis with disseminated intravascular coagulation (DIC).

Key Diagnostic Labs and Tests

Because blood cultures are often positive for the same organism that is infecting the CNS, they should be obtained routinely when bacterial meningitis is being considered. A CBC may reveal leukocytosis. Serum electrolytes should be measured, as SIADH may occur.

In performing the LP, remember to check the opening pressure. Enough fluid should be obtained to perform the basic tests (cell count and differential, protein, glucose, Gram's stain and culture), and extra fluid should be obtained if nonpyogenic etiologies are being considered (e.g., enteroviral polymerase chain reaction [PCR]). Table 26-1 shows the laboratory findings that help differentiate bacterial meningitis from aseptic meningitis.

TABLE 26-1
CSF Parameters for Differentiating Among Causes of Meningitis

Lab Test	Aseptic Meningitis	Bacterial Meningitis
Gram stain	Negative	Positive in 75% of cases
Culture	Viral culture may be positive	Bacteria grow within 48 hours
WBC	Usually 50 to 500/mm^3	Usually >500/mm^3
Differential	Usually lymphocytic (though may initially have neutrophils)	Neutrophil predominance
Glucose	Often normal	Low

Pretreatment with antibiotics can lead to a negative Gram's stain and culture results but should not immediately change the other parameters. PCR testing allows the accurate detection of enteroviruses and HSV. For enteroviruses, cultures are time-consuming and do not provide information in a meaningful time frame. For HSV, the sensitivity of PCR-based tests is substantially higher than that of cultures.

CLINICAL PEARL

CSF HSV PCR remains positive in patients with HSV for 7 or more days despite acyclovir therapy. Therefore, empiric acyclovir therapy does not typically affect the yield of HSV PCR.

The LP in the case patient revealed CSF with a protein count of 80 mg/dL, a glucose concentration of 30 mg/dL, a RBC count of 3/mm³, and a WBC count of 453/mm³ with 86% neutrophils. The Gram stain on the CSF revealed gram-positive diplococci. These findings were consistent with bacterial meningitis. *S. pneumoniae* was subsequently isolated from the CSF culture, confirming the diagnosis.

Imaging

Imaging is not required to make the diagnosis of meningitis but can be useful to identify complications. A computed tomography (CT) scan should be performed in all patients with papilledema, focal neurologic deficits, or any other signs of increased intracranial pressure (ICP). Magnetic resonance imaging (MRI) permits better differentiation of infarcts that occur in the context of cerebritis.

Treatment

If bacterial meningitis is suspected, treatment should commence as quickly as possible. The administration of antibiotics should not be delayed for the purposes of intracranial imaging. However, the blood culture should still be drawn first. The recommendation for children outside the neonatal age range is to use a combination of vancomycin and a third-generation cephalosporin (e.g., ceftriaxone). While the cephalosporin has excellent CNS penetration and will treat the majority of pathogens, vancomycin is added to cover the possibility of a resistant pneumococcus. Narrow-spectrum coverage may be warranted if an organism is identified and antibiotic susceptibility information is available.

If a brain abscess is suspected, the combination of ceftriaxone, vancomycin, and metronidazole is typically used. For infected ventricular shunts, vancomycin is standard; cephalosporin may be added if there is a suspicion of a gram-negative organism and rifampin is frequently added to provide synergistic activity with vancomycin against staphylococci. Lyme meningitis is usually treated with ceftriaxone.

Because the inflammatory response in the CNS is largely responsible for neurologic damage in the setting of meningitis, it should be evident that reducing inflammation could improve outcomes. The corticosteroid dexamethasone has been studied in a number of trials of bacterial meningitis. Adjuvant corticosteroid therapy leads to reduced mortality in adults with pneumococcal meningitis. As a result, some experts recommend adjuvant corticosteroid therapy in children with suspected bacterial meningitis. However, the benefit in children with bacterial meningitis caused by bacteria other than haemophilus influenzae remains unproven. When used, dexamethasone should be administered with or just prior to the initial dose of antibiotics.

Therapy for viral meningitis is mainly supportive. Acyclovir is used to treat meningoencephalitis caused by HSV.

Admission Criteria and Level-of-Care Criteria

Most patients with meningitis will be admitted to the hospital. Selected cases of aseptic meningitis in older children may be managed in the ambulatory setting with close follow-up.

EXTENDED IN-HOSPITAL MANAGEMENT

Intensive care for bacterial meningitis should include therapies to maintain cerebral perfusion, such as blood pressure support, and measures to reduce ICP, such as elevating the head of bed, slight hyperventilation for intubated patients, fever control, and sometimes the administration of mannitol and barbiturates.

All patients should be watched very closely for the development of new neurologic findings or other complications. Among infants with bacterial meningitis, a rapidly increasing head circumference may signify the development of subdural effusion or hydrocephalus; in these situations, neuroimaging is necessary. Complications from bacterial meningitis include seizures, motor and cognitive impairment, and hearing loss. Fatal outcomes still occur in 10% to 20% of cases, depending on the pathogen.

The duration of intravenous (IV) antibiotic therapy depends on the pathogen(s) and the disease process identified. Meningitis due to pneumococcus is generally treated for 14 days and meningococcal disease for 7 days. A brain abscess is frequently treated for 6 weeks. Lyme meningitis usually responds to 2 to 4 weeks of therapy.

DISPOSITION
Discharge Goals

Patients with bacterial CNS infections are generally treated in the hospital for the full antibiotic course. The use of outpatient IV antibiotic therapy may be considered in selected patients, such as in a stable patient with a brain abscess. A minority of patients may have complications that require more prolonged hospitalization, as for intensive inpatient rehabilitation.

Children who are admitted with aseptic meningitis can usually be discharged after the blood and CSF bacterial cultures are negative for 48 hours or when CSF enterovirus PCR is positive.

Outpatient Care

Prophylactic antibiotics are recommended for family members and other close contacts of patients with bacterial meningitis caused by Hib or meningococcus. Rifampin can be given as chemoprophylaxis, although ceftriaxone and ciprofloxacin are also options for meningococcal exposure.

The greatest success with respect to bacterial meningitis has been its prevention by immunization. Twenty years ago, Hib was extremely common, but its incidence has declined by more than 95% in the United States since the introduction of effective vaccines almost two decades ago. A vaccine to protect against the seven most common of the >90 subtypes of *S. pneumoniae* has been in widespread use since 2000, and rates of invasive disease have declined dramatically. The past several years have seen increasing use of a vaccine that protects against serogroups A, C, Y, and W-135 of *N. meningitidis*. The vaccine is currently recommended for teenagers and high-risk children. Population data over the next few years will reveal if it will lead to a widespread decrease in incidence.

WHAT YOU NEED TO REMEMBER

- Bacterial meningitis is a medical emergency.
- Viral meningitis in childhood is very common and is usually associated with a good outcome.
- Infants with meningitis often lack the classic clinical findings.

SUGGESTED READINGS

Mongelluzzo J, Mohamad Z, Ten Have TR, et al. Corticosteriods and mortality in children with bacterial meningitis. *JAMA* 2008;299:2048–2055.

Nigrovic LE, Kuppermann N, Macias CG, et al. Clinical prediction rule for identifying children with cerebrospinal fluid pleocytosis at very low risk of bacterial meningitis. *JAMA* 2007;297(1):52–60.

Tunkel AR, Scheld WM. Acute meningitis. In Mandell GL, Bennett JE, Dolin R, eds. *Principles and Practice of Infectious Diseases*, 6th ed. Philadelphia: Elsevier, 2005.

van de Beek D, de Gans J, McIntyre P, et al. Corticosteroids for acute bacterial meningitis (review). *Cochrane Database Syst Rev* 2007;(1):CD004405.

Neonatal Hyperbilirubinemia

STACEY ROSE

THE PATIENT ENCOUNTER

A 3-day-old boy presents to the emergency department for worsening jaundice. The baby was born at term by spontaneous vaginal delivery to a 30-year-old mother with blood type AB-positive. Jaundice was noted at 20 hours of life and a transcutaneous bilirubin (TcB) at that time was 9 mg/dL. The serum bilirubin was not checked. He was discharged home from the hospital with his mother at 38 hours of life. At home, he is exclusively breast-feeding every 2 to 3 hours with good urine output and a normal stooling pattern. Upon evaluation in the ER, his weight is 8% lower than his birth weight. His exam was significant only for scleral icterus and jaundice involving the entire body.

OVERVIEW

Neonatal hyperbilirubinemia is extremely common and affects most infants. Although mild elevations in bilirubin are usually benign and resolve without intervention, serum bilirubin levels >25 mg/dL have been associated with permanent neurologic sequelae. This devastating outcome is usually preventable.

Definition

Physiologic jaundice refers to the mild elevation in unconjugated bilirubin levels (approximately 5 to 7 mg/dL) that occurs in the first week of life as a result of the increased bilirubin load and impaired clearance mechanisms occurring in most infants. *Acute bilirubin encephalopathy* refers to the neurologic changes seen in the first days to weeks of life as bilirubin crosses the blood–brain barrier and causes neuronal injury. *Kernicterus* is the chronic form of bilirubin encephalopathy and is characterized by sensorineural hearing loss, cerebral palsy, and gaze disturbances.

Pathophysiology

Bilirubin is released from hemoglobin during the breakdown of red blood cells (RBCs). In normal bilirubin metabolism, unconjugated bilirubin is taken up by hepatocytes in the liver and is conjugated to its more water-soluble and easily excretable form by the enzyme uridine diphosphate glucuronosyltransferase (UGT). Conjugated bilirubin then enters the gallbladder and intestine, where it is further metabolized and excreted.

Neonatal hyperbilirubinemia results from the increased bilirubin load and decreased clearance mechanisms that occur in most neonates:

- *Increased Bilirubin Production.* Increased bilirubin production results from the high RBC turnover in neonates. Bilirubin production is further increased in infants with hemolysis due to ABO incompatibility, glucose-6-phosphate dehydrogenase (G6PD) deficiency, or RBC membrane abnormalities such as hereditary spherocytosis.
- *Impaired Clearance Mechanisms.* Impaired clearance mechanisms result from the low levels of UGT activity found in infants. Clearance is reduced even further in infants with Gilbert syndrome or Crigler–Najjar types I and II.
- *Increased Enterohepatic Circulation.* Neonates experience a marked increase in enterohepatic circulation. Infants have beta-glucuronidase in the intestinal mucosa, which deconjugates the conjugated bilirubin, allowing it to be reabsorbed and to reenter the bloodstream. Due to minimal intake in the first few days of life, this process is exaggerated in breast-fed infants, a phenomenon termed *breast-feeding jaundice.*

The terms *direct* and *indirect* bilirubin are often used interchangeably with the terms *conjugated* and *unconjugated.* The former terms (direct/indirect) derive from the van den Bergh reaction, in which the conjugated bilirubin component is measured *directly* (by colorimetric analysis after reaction with a diazo compound). The subsequent addition of methanol allows for a measurement of total bilirubin, after which the unconjugated fraction is determined *indirectly*, by subtracting the conjugated bilirubin level from the total bilirubin level. The conjugated and direct bilirubin measurements are equivalent *except* that the direct component also measures "delta" bilirubin, which forms when conjugated bilirubin seeps retrograde into the serum and binds covalently to albumin. Because of the delta component's long half-life, the direct fraction can remain paradoxically elevated even as the conjugated hyperbilirubinemia improves.

Epidemiology

About 60% of infants will develop jaundice during the first week of life (1). Approximately 4% of term and near-term infants require inpatient treatment with phototherapy either before discharge from the nursery or during readmission to the hospital (2).

Etiology

Although most infants who present with jaundice have a functional etiology, pathologic causes should also be considered, particularly in cases of severe hyperbilirubinemia or hyperbilirubinemia that does not respond to treatment. Additionally, conjugated hyperbilirubinemia, defined as a conjugated bilirubin level >1.0 mg/dL or >15% of the total serum bilirubin, is always pathologic and requires further evaluation. The most common causes of conjugated and unconjugated hyperbilirubinemia are listed in Table 27-1.

TABLE 27-1
Common Causes of Neonatal Jaundice

Unconjugated Hyperbilirubinemia	Conjugated Hyperbilirubinemia
Increased production	Anatomic
• ABO incompatibility	• Biliary atresia
• G6PD deficiency	• Choledochal cyst
• Cephalohematoma or significant bruising	• Alagille syndrome
• Other hemoglobinopathies or RBC membrane defects	Metabolic
	• Tyrosinemia
Reduced clearance	• Galactosemia
• Gilbert syndrome	• Hypothyroidism
• Crigler–Najjar types I and II	Infectious
• Hypothyroidism	• Urinary tract infection
Increased enterohepatic circulation	• Sepsis
	• TORCH infections
• Breast-feeding jaundice	Other
• Breast-milk jaundice	• Idiopathic neonatal hepatitis
• Ileus	• Parenteral nutrition–related cholestasis
• Intestinal obstruction	

G6PD, glucose-6-phosphate dehydrogenase; RBC, red blood cell; TORCH, toxoplasmosis, other infections, rubella, cytomegalovirus, herpes simplex virus.

ACUTE MANAGEMENT AND WORKUP

The acute management and workup should focus on identifying patients with severe hyperbilirubinemia, those with nonphysiologic causes of jaundice, and those who are either septic or severely dehydrated. Phototherapy should be initiated as soon as reasonably possible.

The First 15 Minutes

On initial assessment, it is crucial to look for signs of acute bilirubin encephalopathy or kernicterus, such as poor feeding, lethargy, hypotonia, opisthotonus (a backward arching of the trunk), or retrocollis (a backward arching of the neck). If these are present, the baby is at risk of permanent neurologic damage and it is a medical emergency. The infant should be admitted to the hospital for immediate therapy.

The First Few Hours

You should perform a detailed history and physical exam, concentrating on risk factors for the presence or development of severe hyperbilirubinemia.

History

The history should focus on assessing the major risk factors associated with severe hyperbilirubinemia. On birth history, these include a gestational age <38 weeks, the presence of a cephalohematoma or significant bruising, and maternal factors such as being East Asian or having a blood type that is incompatible with that of the infant. A family history of a sibling who required phototherapy or who developed jaundice also places the infant at an increased likelihood of developing severe jaundice. Events during the nursery stay, such as the presence of jaundice within the first 24 hours of life or a predischarge serum or transcutaneous bilirubin above the 75th percentile for age, are also strong risk factors. Additionally, breast-fed infants are more likely to experience jaundice.

Physical Examination

Tachycardia may be caused by dehydration in the context of poor oral intake. Other findings that suggest dehydration include a sunken fontanelle and dry mucous membranes. Jaundice is most easily detected in the sclera and sublingual regions. The skin exam is less reliable in detecting jaundice, particularly in darkly pigmented infants. Pressing on the skin may be helpful in making the yellow skin discoloration more evident. Jaundice proceeds in a cephalocaudal direction, with the face and upper body being affected at lower bilirubin levels than the trunk and extremities; however, the extent of jaundice does not reliably correlate with the degree of hyperbilirubinemia. Hepatomegaly is associated with pathologic etiologies such as metabolic disorders, biliary atresia, viral hepatitis, and TORCH infections (toxoplasmosis, other infections, rubella, cytomegalovirus, herpes simplex virus). In a neurologic exam, the presence of hypotonia, opisthotonus, or retrocollis should raise immediate concerns for acute bilirubin encephalopathy or kernicterus.

Labs and Tests to Consider

Generally most infants who present with jaundice have a physiologic cause and extensive laboratory testing beyond a total serum bilirubin (TSB) or translutaneous bilirubin (TcB) is unnecessary. Imaging is not warranted in most cases.

Key Diagnostic Labs and Tests

Most babies have a bilirubin measurement prior to discharge from the newborn nursery. TcB measurements are a reasonable screening tool and have the advantage of being painless and immediately available. However, they are not always accurate at higher levels. If the bilirubin level is found to be greater than the 75th percentile, a TSB and direct bilirubin should be measured and a complete blood count, blood typing, and Coombs testing should be performed to evaluate for hemolysis. The infant's blood may contain maternal IgG antibodies that bind to antigens on the infant's RBC surface membrane. Complement proteins may subsequently bind to the bound antibodies, predisposing to RBC hemolysis. The **direct Coombs test** detects these antibodies or complement proteins, which are bound to the surface of RBCs.

When the bilirubin level is excessively elevated or is not responding to phototherapy, a reticulocyte count and G6PD test should be done and the albumin level measured. Most circulating bilirubin is bound to albumin; only the unbound or loosely bound fraction can cross the blood–brain barrier and cause neuronal toxicity.

CLINICAL PEARL

Infants with low levels of albumin or infants who are sick or premature and have impaired albumin binding may be at greater risk for developing kernicterus. In these cases, the bilirubin-to-albumin ratio should be used in conjunction with the TSB level to determine the optimal intervention.

In the presence of conjugated hyperbilirubinemia, a urinalysis and urine culture should be performed and a complete sepsis evaluation considered. Additionally, thyroid function testing and a galactosemia screen should be done if the newborn screen is not available.

In the case patient, the TSB level was 18.3 mg/dL at 70 hours of life. The patient was admitted to the hospital and started on phototherapy.

Imaging

Imaging is rarely needed in infants with unconjugated hyperbilirubinemia. However, infants with conjugated hyperbilirubinemia require a liver ultrasound to detect structural abnormalities and a hepatobiliary (DISIDA) scan to evaluate for causes of neonatal cholestasis, such as biliary atresia.

Treatment

Several treatment modalities have been used in severe hyperbilirubinemia. Phototherapy has long been the preferred primary treatment and should be initiated at the levels listed in Figure 27-1 to prevent kernicterus. Phototherapy converts bilirubin into a more soluble form that can be excreted without conjugation. To optimize phototherapy, wavelengths of light in the range of 460 to 490 nm should be used, lights should be placed

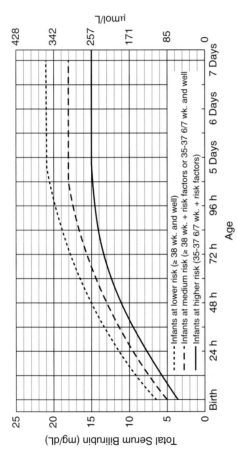

- Use total bilirubin. Do not subtract direct reacting or conjugated bilirubin.
- Risk factors = isoimmune hemolytic disease, G6PD deficiency, asphyxia, significant lethargy, temperature instability, sepsis, acidosis, or albumin < 3.0g/dL (if measured)
- For well infants 35-37 6/7 wk. can adjust TSB levels for intervention around the medium risk line. It is an option to intervene at lower TSB levels for infants closer to 35 wks and at higher TSB levels for those closer to 37 6/7 wk.
- It is an option to provide conventional phototherapy in hospital or at home at TSB levels 2-3 mg/dL (35-50 mmol/L) below those shown but home phototherapy should not be used in any infant with risk factors.

FIGURE 27-1: Guidelines for phototherapy in hospitalized infants of 35 or more weeks' gestation. From: American Academy of Pediatrics Subcommittee on hyperbilirubinemia. American Academy of Pediatrics Clinical Practice. *Pediatrics* 2004;114:297–316, with permission.

10 to 15 cm from the infant's body, and a maximal body surface area should be exposed. Bilirubin levels should fall within 4 to 8 hours; a 30% to 40% decrease can be expected within the first 24 hours.

Breast-feeding should be encouraged to continue during treatment with phototherapy. If intake is inadequate, consider increasing the frequency of feeds, consulting a lactation specialist, or supplementing with formula. Intravenous fluids are usually not needed but should be initiated if the infant is dehydrated and is unable to feed well.

For more severe hyperbilirubinemia, exchange transfusion may be necessary. A double-volume exchange transfusion removes both bilirubin and circulating antibodies that may cause hemolysis from the serum. Although this therapy is the most effective in lowering bilirubin levels, it is associated with a number of severe complications—including apnea, bradycardia, thrombosis, acidosis, thrombocytopenia, and hypocalcemia—and should be reserved for infants at high risk for developing kernicterus. For detailed guidelines about initiating exchange transfusions, please refer to the American Academy of Pediatrics' clinical guideline listed in the suggested readings, below.

Admission Criteria and Level-of-Care Criteria

Like the baby in the vignette, infants should be admitted to the hospital if the total bilirubin level is greater than the recommended range for beginning phototherapy (see Fig. 27-1). Additional criteria for admission include dehydration and poor feeding, a concern for sepsis, or a urinary tract infection. Phototherapy may be administered on the general pediatrics service, newborn nursery, or intensive care nursery. Infants with severe hyperbilirubinemia who have significant hemolysis, are exhibiting signs of bilirubin encephalopathy, or require exchange transfusion should be treated in an intensive care nursery.

EXTENDED IN-HOSPITAL MANAGEMENT

Most infants with neonatal hyperbilirubinemia will respond to phototherapy in the first 24 hours. If the infant does not respond and bilirubin levels continue to rise, the infant should be admitted to the intensive care unit to begin exchange transfusion and undergo further evaluation for the less common pathologic causes of hyperbilirubinemia. Additional laboratory and imaging studies should be considered. A liver biopsy may be necessary if the jaundice is severe and persistent.

DISPOSITION
Discharge Goals

The American Academy of Pediatrics recommends that all infants should be evaluated for the clinical risk factors associated with neonatal hyperbilirubinemia and/or have a serum or transcutaneous bilirubin level prior to discharge from the newborn nursery. All parents should receive education about the risk of hyperbilirubinemia before discharge from the nursery.

Hospitalized infants may be discharged when the total serum bilirubin levels fall below 13 to 14 mg/dL and the infant is feeding well with adequate hydration. It is not necessary to check a rebound bilirubin level after discontinuation of phototherapy prior to discharge. If hemolysis was present, verify that the hemoglobin level is stable and the reticulocyte count is appropriate.

Outpatient Care

Close outpatient follow-up is essential to avoid possible neurologic sequelae. Since early hospital discharge has been linked with a rise in cases of kernicterus, it is recommended that all infants discharged before 72 hours of life be followed up with within 24 to 72 hours of discharge from the hospital. Earlier follow-up may be necessary if clinical risk factors are present or the infant has a TSB greater than the 75th percentile for age.

The follow-up exam after discharge from the nursery or inpatient unit should include weight; an assessment of intake, urination, and stooling patterns; and the presence of jaundice. Because the physical exam may be unreliable in determining the degree of hyperbilirubinemia, a TSB or TcB should be obtained if there is any concern for jaundice.

 WHAT YOU NEED TO REMEMBER

- Neonatal hyperbilirubinemia is usually a benign, self-limited condition due to increased production and decreased clearance of bilirubin.
- Kernicterus is permanent neurologic damage related to severe hyperbilirubinemia.
- Jaundiced infants require close monitoring and careful follow-up to prevent kernicterus.
- Phototherapy and exchange transfusion are effective treatments in neonatal hyperbilirubinemia.

REFERENCES

1. Maisels MJ, McDonagh AF. Phototherapy for neonatal jaundice. *N Engl J Med* 2008;358:920–928.
2. Bhutani VK, Johnson LH, Schwoebel A, et al. A systems approach for neonatal hyperbilirubinemia in term and near-term newborns. *J Obstet Gynecol Neonatal Nurs* 2006;35:444–455.

SUGGESTED READINGS

American Academy of Pediatrics Subcommittee on Hyperbilirubinemia. American Academy of Pediatrics Clinical Practice Guideline: management of hyperbilirubinemia in the newborn infant 35 or more weeks of gestation. *Pediatrics* 2004;114: 297–316.

Bhutani VK, Johnson L, Sivieri EM. Predictive ability of a predischarge hour-specific serum bilirubin for subsequent significant hyperbilirubinemia in healthy term and near-term newborns. *Pediatrics* 1999;103:6–14.

Dennery PA, Seidman DS, Stevenson DK. Neonatal hyperbilirubinemia. *N Engl J Med* 2001;344:581–590.

Keren R, Luan X, Friedman S, et al. A comparison of alternative risk-assessment strategies for predicting significant neonatal hyperbilirubinemia in term and near-term infants. *Pediatrics* 2008;121:170–179.

Maisels MJ. Neonatal jaundice. Pediatrics in Review; 2006;27:443–453.

Nephrotic Syndrome

JENNIFER J. JACKSON AND LARRY A. GREENBAUM

THE PATIENT ENCOUNTER

A 4-year-old boy was taken to his pediatrician's office for eye swelling, which was more noticeable in the morning. He was prescribed diphenhydramine for allergic symptoms. Two days later, he presented to the emergency department with worsening eye swelling and abdominal distension. On exam, he was afebrile and in no distress. He had periorbital edema, ascites, scrotal edema, and pitting edema of his legs. A urinalysis revealed the following results: a specific gravity of 1.025, a pH level of 7, significant protein (i.e., 4+ protein, which corresponds to a urine protein concentration of approximately 2,000 mg/dL), and no gross or microscopic hematuria.

OVERVIEW

Definition

The four classic features of nephrotic syndrome (NS) are proteinuria ($>1,000$ mg/m^2/day), edema, hypoalbuminemia (≤ 2.5 g/dL), and hyperlipidemia. This chapter focuses on idiopathic NS, which is usually characterized by responsiveness to corticosteroids and a relapsing course. Complications of NS can include acute renal failure, infections, and thromboembolic events.

Pathophysiology

The glomerulus, which is the filtering unit of the kidney, allows water and small molecules to pass from the bloodstream into Bowman's space but restricts the transit of large molecules, such as proteins. In NS, the normal barrier function of the glomerulus is defective and proteins enter Bowman's space, leading to proteinuria. Hypoalbuminemia due to urinary albumin losses causes the intravascular oncotic pressure to decrease, which results in movement of water into the interstitial space. The consequent intravascular volume depletion leads to sodium retention by the kidneys. The combination of the interstitial movement of water and renal sodium retention causes edema. The hyperlipidemia in NS is secondary to decreased hepatic lipid metabolism and increased synthesis.

The etiology of the hypercoagulable state in NS is complex and includes a loss of anticoagulants (antithrombin III, protein C, and protein S) and a decreased intravascular volume. Similarly, a variety of immunologic defects predispose patients to infections, with ineffective opsonization playing a role in the increased risk of infections by encapsulated organisms such as *Streptococcus pneumoniae*.

Epidemiology

In the United States, the estimated incidence of childhood NS is 2 to 7 per 100,000. Idiopathic NS occurs approximately twice as often in males, with the majority of cases presenting between 1 and 6 years of age.

Etiology

The most common etiology of NS during childhood (Table 28-1) is minimal change disease (MCD), which is usually characterized by responsiveness to corticosteroids and a fairly normal-appearing biopsy by light microscopy. Focal segmental glomerulosclerosis (FSGS), the second most common cause of NS during childhood, typically does not respond to corticosteroids, and there is a significant risk for progression to kidney failure. Less common causes of childhood idiopathic NS are membranoproliferative glomerulonephritis (MPGN) and membranous nephropathy. While many cases of nephrotic syndrome are idiopathic, the cause can sometimes be determined. For example, obesity, human immunodeficiency virus (HIV) infection, and genetic disorders may be associated with FSGS, hepatitis C may be associated with MPGN, and hepatitis B infection and malignancy may be associated with membranous nephropathy.

During adolescence, MCD remains an important cause of NS, but other etiologies become more common. There is an increased risk of FSGS, membranous nephropathy, and secondary causes (lupus nephritis). Hence, biopsy is recommended before empiric corticosteroids are administered.

Nephrotic syndrome in the first 3 months of life usually has a genetic basis, with most cases due to mutations in the gene encoding the protein nephrin. Patients with this autosomal recessive disorder, often called congenital NS of the Finnish-type, typically have a history of premature birth and a large placenta. Mutations in WT1, the Wilms' tumor-suppressor gene, cause Denys–Drash syndrome, which is characterized by the triad of NS during the first 2 years of life, Wilms' tumor, and pseudohermaphroditism. Congenital infections, such as hepatitis B or syphilis, may also cause early-onset NS.

ACUTE MANAGEMENT AND WORKUP

The acute management and evaluation identifies children with complications of NS and children with secondary causes of NS.

The First 15 Minutes

Respiratory status can be compromised by large pleural effusions. Assess the patient for signs of increased respiratory effort, such as tachypnea or

TABLE 28-1
Causes of Pediatric Nephrotic Syndrome

Disease	Comments
Idiopathic Nephrotic Syndrome	
Minimal change disease	Most common etiology in children.
Focal segmental glomerulosclerosis (FSGS)	Usually resistant to steroids; important cause of pediatric kidney failure.
Membranoproliferative glomerulonephritis (MPGN)	Unusual before 6 years. C3 usually low; C4 low in some cases; nephritic features often present.
Membranous nephropathy	Uncommon in childhood; high risk of thrombosis.
Secondary Causes	
Lupus nephritis	Often concurrent with nephritic syndrome.
HIV associated nephropathy	FSGS most common finding.
Hepatitis B	Usually associated with membranous nephropathy.
Hepatitis C	Usually associated with MPGN.
Morbid obesity	FSGS.
Syphilis	Rare complication of congenital infection.
Sickle cell disease	FSGS most common finding.
Henoch–Schönlein purpura	Prominent extrarenal manifestations; nephrotic syndrome is less common than asymptomatic hematuria and proteinuria.
Poststreptoccocal glomerulonephritis	Nephritic features prominent; C3 low.
IgA nephropathy	Nephrotic syndrome is less common than asymptomatic hematuria and proteinuria.

TABLE 28-1

Causes of Pediatric Nephrotic Syndrome (Continued)

Disease	Comments
Medications	Penicillamine, nonsteroidal anti-inflammatory drugs (rare), others.
Malignancy	Rare complication of lymphoma or leukemia.
Genetic Causes	
Finnish-type congenital nephrotic syndrome	Autosomal recessive; usually presents in first 3 months.
Denys–Drash syndrome	Nephrotic syndrome due to diffuse mesangial sclerosis; may have male pseudohermaphroditism and/or Wilms' tumor.
Podocin gene mutations	Autosomal recessive cause of steroid resistant FSGS.
Alport syndrome	Nephrotic syndrome not common at presentation; hematuria invariable; deafness.
Nail–patella syndrome	Patients may have isolated proteinuria or nephrotic syndrome; autosomal dominant; nail, knee, and elbow abnormalities.
Frasier syndrome	FSGS; male pseudohermaphroditism.

retractions, and auscultate for decreased breath sounds consistent with pleural effusions at the lung bases. Initiate oxygen therapy for hypoxic patients. A pulmonary embolus, though rare, may also lead to respiratory distress or hypoxia.

The patient's blood pressure should be compared with normal values for age, gender, and height. Hypertension, while unusual in MCD, can be severe in other causes of NS (lupus nephritis, poststreptococcal glomerulonephritis [PSGN]).

You should assess patients with NS for serious infections such as sepsis, spontaneous bacterial peritonitis, pneumonia, and cellulitis. Patients with peritonitis usually have abdominal pain, with peritoneal signs such as guarding and rebound tenderness. Crampy abdominal pain, perhaps due to bowel wall edema, is common in children with NS but is usually transient and not associated with peritoneal signs or fever.

The First Few Hours

The initial assessment should utilize the history and laboratory testing to confirm the diagnosis of NS and determine the likelihood that the patient has MCD.

History

Edema is the most common presenting symptom. Patients typically have periorbital edema in the morning and this decreases during the day. Because extravascular fluid settles in dependent areas, periorbital edema decreases with ambulation. The fluid mobilizes to other areas where the edema is less obvious, although increased leg swelling in the evening may be noticeable. Other manifestations of edema include abdominal distention, weight gain, tight socks or shoes that do not fit, and labial or scrotal swelling. Decreased urine output may accompany worsening edema. The urine may be frothy owing to the elevated protein content. The edema in NS is usually obvious, although occasionally patients have minimal or undetectable edema; such patients present with a complication of NS or with an incidental finding of proteinuria on a urinalysis.

Visible hematuria is uncommon in MCD and should prompt consideration of other glomerular diseases (e.g., PSGN, lupus nephritis). The information in the history should allow you to evaluate the likelihood of secondary causes of NS. Ask about risk factors for infections (hepatitis B and C, HIV) and manifestations of lupus (rash, joint pain, mouth ulcers, hair loss). A family history of NS suggests a possible genetic etiology.

Physical Examination

Edema, the most prominent physical exam feature, can be assessed by examining the periorbital area, the face, the hands, the sacral area, the pretibial region, and the genitals. Females may develop labial edema and males may develop scrotal edema. Abdominal ascites may cause distention, a fluid wave, and shifting dullness. Rebound tenderness or guarding suggests spontaneous bacterial peritonitis. Pleural effusions are typically bilateral and can be identified by auscultation, with decreased breath sounds at the bases, a pleural friction rub, dullness to percussion, and egophony. Assess for respiratory distress caused by pleural effusions by noting tachypnea, nasal flaring, retractions, and grunting.

CLINICAL PEARL

A urinalysis is a rapid and sensitive test for nephrotic syndrome in a child with edema.

Labs and Tests to Consider

Lab tests determine whether NS is the etiology of edema. Lab tests and imaging studies are also important in determining the etiology of the NS and to investigate potential complications of NS.

Key Diagnostic Labs and Tests

A urinalysis is important to detect proteinuria and hematuria. Hypoalbuminemia and an elevated cholesterol level confirm the diagnosis. The proteinuria can be quantified via a urine protein/urine creatinine ratio (>2 mg/mg indicates nephrotic range proteinuria). Measures of electrolytes, blood urea nitrogen, and creatinine are useful to detect acute renal failure and hyponatremia, which can occur as a consequence of intravascular volume depletion.

Complement levels (C3 and C4) help differentiate patients with MCD from other causes of NS. A decreased C3 is seen in PSGN, lupus nephritis, and MPGN. A decreased C4 occurs in patients with lupus and in some patients with MPGN. An antinuclear antibody (ANA) test is an appropriate screening tool for lupus, especially in older children and adolescents or patients with clinical features of lupus. Patients with lupus can present with isolated NS or the combination of nephrotic and nephritic syndromes (e.g., hematuria, hypertension, renal insufficiency). PSGN causes nephritic syndrome, although some patients also have NS.

Visible hematuria or red blood cell casts on urinalysis is unusual in MCD or FSGS. Such findings should prompt a kidney biopsy except in children with a presentation consistent with PSGN (mild renal insufficiency, hypertension, decreased C3, and spontaneous resolution). A kidney biopsy is also appropriate in children with decreased complement levels, chronic renal insufficiency, a positive ANA, or age >12 years or <1 year.

Children with possible spontaneous bacterial peritonitis should have a blood culture and a peritoneal tap for cell count and culture. Blood cultures are also indicated if sepsis is suspected.

Imaging

Imaging is not central to the diagnosis of NS but can be helpful in managing complications of the disease. Children with respiratory symptoms or signs should have a chest x-ray to assess for effusions or pneumonia. Imaging studies are necessary in patients with possible thrombotic complications. In children who present with NS and renal insufficiency, a renal ultrasound can help you determine whether the renal insufficiency is chronic (small echogenic kidneys) or acute (large echogenic kidneys); ultrasound can also help you to detect renal vein thrombosis.

Treatment

The child in the present case was diagnosed with MCD and treated with oral corticosteroids. Most children with MCD respond to oral prednisone

(60 mg/m^2 or 2 mg/kg/day, given daily or divided bid; maximum dose: 60 mg/day). Proteinuria generally resolves within 2 weeks and is associated with diuresis and resolution of the edema. The initial course of daily prednisone is 4 to 6 weeks and is followed by alternate-day corticosteroids for an additional 6 to 10 weeks (e.g., 40 mg/m^2 every other day for 4 to 6 weeks, followed by a tapering dose over the next 4 weeks). Most patients with steroid-sensitive disease have relapses of NS. Treatment is similar to that for the initial episode except that the daily prednisone is continued only until proteinuria is absent for 3 days.

Patients who do not respond to corticosteroids within 4 to 6 weeks have steroid-resistant disease, which is an indication for a kidney biopsy. Treatment options for patients who have steroid-resistant FSGS or MCD include cyclosporine A, tacrolimus, high-dose corticosteroids, mycophenolate mofetil, and cyclophosphamide.

A low-sodium diet decreases edema formation. In children with severe anasarca, the combination of intravenous 25% albumin (0.4 to 1 g/kg) followed by intravenous furosemide (0.5 mg/kg) mobilizes interstitial edema and causes a diuresis. This treatment may be given 2 to 3 times per day. Diuretic therapy requires monitoring for hypokalemia. The isolated use of a diuretic can lead to intravascular volume depletion. Infectious and thrombotic complications are treated with antibiotics and anticoagulation, respectively.

Admission Criteria and Level-of-Care Criteria

Indications for admission include sepsis, acute renal failure, thromboembolism, respiratory distress, and peritonitis. Admission may also be considered for patients who have severe anasarca. Patients admitted for anasarca are managed on a general pediatric floor, while those with hemodynamic instability (i.e., from sepsis or respiratory distress) are admitted to the intensive care unit.

EXTENDED IN-HOSPITAL MANAGEMENT

Complications such as acute renal failure, spontaneous bacterial peritonitis, or thrombosis will prolong hospitalization. *Streptococcus pneumoniae* is the most common cause of spontaneous bacterial peritonitis, although gram-negative rods must also be considered. Hence patients receive empiric therapy with an intravenous third-generation cephalosporin, with adjustment based on bacterial sensitivities. Intravenous antibiotics are generally given for 10 to 14 days.

DISPOSITION

Discharge Goals

For patients admitted for anasarca, consider discharge when the patient has had a significant diuresis documented by decreased edema and weight loss.

Children admitted for peritonitis should have a normal abdominal examination and complete a course of intravenous antibiotics. Patients with positive blood cultures should have negative follow-up cultures. Children with respiratory distress due to pleural effusions are ready for discharge when they have resolution of symptoms, an improved examination, and normal pulse oximetry on room air.

Outpatient Care

A low-sodium diet should be prescribed to reduce edema formation. Instruct caregivers to check the urine for proteinuria daily, using Albustix. Caregivers should be told that 80% of children with MCD have at least one relapse, and urine monitoring at home allows detection of relapses prior to the development of edema. Early treatment of relapses with corticosteroids is critical for decreasing complications and preventing future hospitalizations. Inform caregivers about the signs and symptoms of spontaneous bacterial peritonitis and respiratory distress due to pleural effusions, both of which require immediate medical care. Children who are susceptible to varicella and who are exposed to chickenpox while on high-dose corticosteroids should receive prophylactic varicella zoster immune globulin, which decreases the risk of life-threatening disseminated varicella infection. A follow-up appointment with a nephrologist or pediatrician comfortable with managing NS should be made within 1 week of discharge.

 WHAT YOU NEED TO REMEMBER

- The four classic features of NS are proteinuria, hypoalbuminemia, edema, and hyperlipidemia.
- MCD is the most common cause of NS during childhood, and patients usually respond to treatment with corticosteroids.
- Most children with MCD have multiple relapses of NS, but home monitoring for proteinuria allows early detection and treatment.
- Complications of NS include acute renal failure, infections (spontaneous bacterial peritonitis, cellulitis, pneumonia, and sepsis), and thromboembolic events.

SUGGESTED READINGS

Eddy AA, Symons JM. Nephrotic syndrome in childhood. *Lancet* 2003;362(9384): 629–639.

Ehrich JH, Brodehl J. Long versus standard prednisone therapy for initial treatment of idiopathic nephrotic syndrome in children. Arbeitsgemeinschaft fur Padiatrische Nephrologie. *Eur J Pediatr* 1993;152(4):357–361.

International Study of Kidney Disease in Children. Nephrotic syndrome in children: prediction of histopathology from clinical and laboratory characteristics at time of diagnosis. A report of the International Study of Kidney Disease in Children. *Kidney Int* 1978;13:159–165.

Niaudet P. Genetic forms of nephrotic syndrome. *Pediatr Nephrol* 2004;19:1313–1318.

Nonaccidental Trauma

LAURA K. BRENNAN

👪 THE PATIENT ENCOUNTER

A 4-month-old boy presented to the emergency department with a several-day history of mild rhinorrhea, congestion, and cough followed by the onset of lethargy and vomiting several hours prior to presentation. On examination, his pulse was 160 beats per minute, his respiratory rate was 60 breaths per minute, and his percutaneous oxygen saturation was 98% in room air. He was afebrile with a rectal temperature of 37.4°C (99.3°F). He had a tense anterior fontanel and seemed irritable with examination, particularly when being moved or picked up. A chest radiograph revealed multiple acute rib fractures, and computed tomography (CT) of the head showed acute bilateral frontoparietal and interhemispheric subdural hemorrhage.

OVERVIEW

Definition

Child abuse can be defined as the intentional physical, sexual, or emotional maltreatment or neglect of a child <18 years of age by a parent, legal guardian, or caregiver that results in injury or emotional detriment to the child. This chapter focuses on physical abuse, also called nonaccidental trauma (NAT). NAT may take many forms, involve various organ systems, and range in severity from asymptomatic to fatal.

Epidemiology

The exact incidence and prevalence of NAT is difficult to ascertain, given the unreported nature of many cases. However, the Administration for Children and Families of the U.S. Department of Health and Human Services reports that in 2006, there were an estimated 905,000 children nationwide who were the victims of reported maltreatment, corresponding to a rate of victimization of 12.1 per 1,000 children. More than 142,000 (approximately 16%) of all maltreated children were specifically the victims of physical abuse or NAT.

Etiology

The etiology of NAT defies a simple, common-to-all-families explanation. Instead, NAT occurs within a potentially complex interaction of child, parent, family, and community factors. Child factors associated with higher rates of NAT include a difficult or fussy temperament, colic, prematurity, chronic illness, behavioral or emotional difficulties, and physical or developmental disabilities. Parent factors include alcohol or substance addiction, mental illness, poor impulse control or anger management difficulties, lack of appropriate parenting skills, unrealistic expectations of the child's behavior, and a history of having been abused as a child. Family factors include domestic violence and stressors such as homelessness and a lack of money. Community factors include poverty, unemployment, and social isolation.

ACUTE MANAGEMENT AND WORKUP

The acute management and workup help identify the extent and severity of injuries. This information can then be used to evaluate the possibility of NAT and helps to differentiate NAT from both accidental trauma and underlying organic disease.

The First 15 Minutes

The initial assessment helps determine whether to make an immediate intervention or to proceed with the history and physical examination. **First, assess vital sign stability.** Patients with severe brain injury, for example, may have Cushing's triad of bradycardia, hypertension, and irregular respirations, which signals increased intracranial pressure and impending cerebral herniation. **Second, determine whether there are obvious injuries present.** Assess the skin for burns, bruises, lacerations, or abrasions. Examine the scalp for cephalohematomas or lacerations. Examine all extremities for deformities, swelling, or pain on palpation that may indicate underlying fractures. Perform a quick neurologic assessment to evaluate for brain injury.

The First Few Hours

A detailed history, thorough physical examination, and appropriate use of labs and imaging are integral to the evaluation of possible NAT. The diagnosis of NAT is generally a diagnosis of exclusion, so a thorough evaluation is crucial to rule out accidental trauma as well as underlying organic disease.

History

Children with NAT often present for evaluation of a symptom of an injury (e.g., vomiting or seizure) or for evaluation of an injury itself (e.g., scalp cephalohematoma or a painful, swollen leg), although occasionally injuries are found incidentally, such as healing rib fractures in a child being evaluated for an acute pneumonia. The history is crucial in evaluating childhood NAT. In general, "red flags" or concern for NAT should be raised when the history is inconsistent with the injuries, the history is inconsistent with a child's developmental abilities, there are conflicting or inconsistent histories about how the injury was sustained, or there has been a significant delay in presenting for medical care in a situation where a reasonable person likely would have sought prompt medical attention.

Physical Examination

Since the history may be limited or inaccurate in cases of NAT, a thorough physical examination is especially important. The physical exam can vary from normal to finding the patient severely comatose with obvious external injuries. Ophthalmologic examination should be performed routinely to identify retinal hemorrhages. Obtain formal ophthalmology consultation in cases of intracranial hemorrhage or head injury. The skin should be examined for bruises, abrasions, burns, and scars. The extremities should be examined for deformities, tenderness, swelling, and decreased movement. A thorough neurologic exam should be performed. The abdomen should be examined carefully to assess for possible abdominal trauma, keeping in mind that a lack of external abdominal wall bruising does not rule out occult visceral injury. The frenula of the upper and lower lips as well as under the tongue should be inspected as they can tear in cases of blunt oral trauma. A child can have occult injury to the brain, abdomen, or skeletal system; therefore a normal physical examination does not exclude the possibility of serious injury. Also, the pattern of injury often suggests the mechanism of abuse. For example, vigorous shaking may lead to retinal hemorrhages, subdural hemorrhages, and posterior rib fractures.

> ### CLINICAL PEARL
>
> *Children often bruise accidentally but not usually until they begin walking (i.e., if you don't cruise, you rarely bruise). Therefore, be suspicious of abuse when you notice bruising in a nonambulating infant, especially if the bruising is located on the face.*

Labs and Tests to Consider

The proper use of labs and imaging studies helps to evaluate the nature and extent of the child's injuries and therefore can either support an accidental mechanism or lead to concern for NAT. Also, because NAT is almost always a diagnosis of exclusion in the absence of witnessed abuse or a confession, lab testing and imaging can help to support or rule out an underlying organic etiology of the child's findings.

Key Diagnostic Labs and Tests

Liver function tests, amylase, lipase, and urinalysis will facilitate the detection of abdominal trauma. If any bruising or bleeding is present, prothrombin time (PT) and partial thromboplastin time (PTT) as well as a complete blood count (CBC) are indicated to screen for the presence of an underlying coagulopathy. In any child with fractures, serum calcium, phosphorus, alkaline phosphatase, 25-OH vitamin D, and parathyroid hormone (PTH) levels are important screening tests in assessing bone health and ruling out an underlying bone disease.

The patient in the case above had completely normal abdominal trauma labs, showing no evidence of abdominal injury. His PT was 12.0 seconds, PTT was 24 seconds, and platelet count on the CBC was 256,000/μL. His serum calcium was 10.2 mg/dL; phosphorus, 5.0 mg/dL; alkaline phosphatase, 210 IU/L; 25-OH vitamin D, 38 ng/mL; and serum PTH, 36 pg/mL. All of these studies were in the normal range, which helps to rule out an underlying coagulopathy as the cause of the acute subdural hemorrhage as well as rickets or other metabolic bone disease as the cause of the rib fractures.

Imaging

A skeletal survey, which is a series of radiographs of the child's entire skeletal system, is mandatory in all cases of suspected NAT in children <2 years of age. This study may pick up metaphyseal fractures of the long bones or healing rib fractures that are often occult on exam. Brain imaging is recommended in all cases of suspected NAT in patients <1 year of age, especially in the high-risk infants <6 months of age. CT of the head can be quick and is useful if the child has mental status changes or neurologic symptoms or if there is high concern for an acute neurologic injury. Magnetic resonance imaging (MRI) of the brain is preferred, however, if the child is asymptomatic or neurologically stable because it exposes the child to no radiation and is a more detailed study. This patient's chest radiograph is shown in Figure 29-1; his CT scan is shown in Figure 29-2.

If a child has visible injuries such as bruises or scars that are concerning for NAT, photographs should be taken of the injuries and placed in the child's medical record. Always obtain appropriate consent for photos as dictated by individual institutional guidelines and label the photos with the name, medical record number, and date of birth of the child as well as with the photographer's name and the date the photos are taken.

Treatment

Treatment is aimed at managing the patient's physical injuries as well as ensuring a safe environment.

Admission Criteria and Level-of-Care Criteria

Absolute criteria for admission include the need for inpatient medical or surgical management of specific injuries. Additionally, a report should be made to the local Child Protective Services (CPS) agency regarding any child in whom NAT is suspected. If a report is made and the safety of the

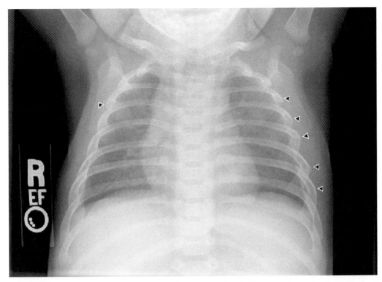

FIGURE 29-1: Chest radiograph of a 4-month-old boy with multiple bilateral acute rib fractures. The arrows point at the laterally located fractures.

child's home environment has not yet been ascertained and approved by the CPS agency, admission is indicated while the CPS investigation is ongoing.

Patients can often be managed on a general pediatric or pediatric surgical floor. However, consider admission to an intensive care unit for patients with severe neurologic injury or abdominal trauma, significant burns, or evidence of cardiovascular or respiratory instability.

EXTENDED IN-HOSPITAL MANAGEMENT

As in the illustrative case, the presence of significant intracranial bleeding can lead to prolonged hospitalization. Significant injuries, particularly neurologic or abdominal trauma, are risk factors for prolonged hospitalization and often require the services of many consultants, such as neurosurgery, general surgery, neurology, orthopedic surgery, and physical and occupational therapy. Social workers are key members of the team caring for children with suspected NAT and can facilitate communication between the hospital and the local CPS agency while also providing family support.

Because the diagnosis of NAT is often a diagnosis of exclusion that is made after a thorough evaluation and ruling out of underlying disease, it is important to keep the local CPS agency informed of the results of testing and of the current level of suspicion for NAT. It is also important to keep

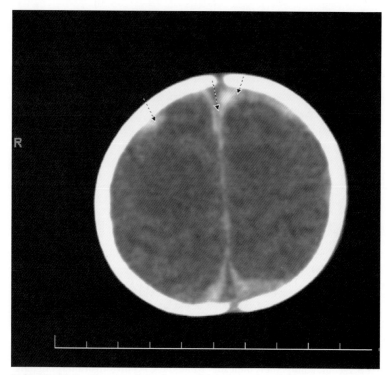

FIGURE 29-2: CT scan of the brain of the same 4-month-old boy showing bilateral and interhemispheric acute subdural hemorrhage.

CPS informed of the child's medical progress and projected discharge date and needs so that, should the child require discharge to a place other than home, CPS has adequate time to ensure alternative placement.

DISPOSITION

Discharge Goals

Consider discharge when the patient is medically stable with regard to all injuries. Additionally, once a report has been made on the hospitalized child, the child should not be discharged until "socially cleared," meaning that a discharge plan has been approved by the CPS agency.

Outpatient Care

After discharge from the hospital, patients should generally follow up with the pediatrician within 1 week. Depending on the exact nature of the injuries, follow-up may be required with specialists such as trauma surgery, general surgery, orthopedic surgery, neurology, neurosurgery, or ophthalmology. If the child is being discharged under the care and supervision of the local CPS agency, it is crucial to make CPS aware of the child's necessary medical follow-up.

WHAT YOU NEED TO REMEMBER

- NAT is generally a diagnosis of exclusion, so evaluation must be thorough to rule out accidental trauma and underlying organic disease.
- Concerns for NAT should be raised when the injuries are inconsistent with the history provided or with the child's developmental age, when there are conflicting or inconsistent histories to explain the injuries, or when there is a significant delay in presenting for medical care.
- Management is directed at specific injuries.
- Admission is indicated for medical or surgical management of injuries if needed as well as for safety while a CPS investigation is under way.

SUGGESTED READINGS

Centers for Disease Control and Prevention (CDC). Nonfatal maltreatment of infants—United States, October 2005–September 2006. MMWR—Morbidity & Mortality Weekly Report 2008;57:336–339.

Fenton SJ, Bouquot JE, Unkel JH. Orofacial considerations for pediatric, adult, and elderly victims of abuse. *Emerg Med Clin North Am* 2000;18:601–617.

Kleinman PK. Diagnostic imaging in infant abuse. *Am J Roentgenol* 1990;155: 703–712.

Martin HA, Woodson A, Christian CW, et al. Shaken baby syndrome. *Crit Care Nurs Clin North Am* 2006;18:279–286.

Rubin DM, Christian CW, Bilaniuk LT, et al. Occult head injury in high-risk abused children. *Pediatrics* 2003;111:1382–1386.

Thombs BD. Patient and injury characteristics, mortality risk, and length of stay related to child abuse by burning: evidence from a national sample of 15,802 pediatric admissions. *Ann Surg* 2008;247:519–523.

Wood J, Rubin DM, Nance ML, et al. Distinguishing inflicted versus accidental abdominal injuries in young children. *J Trauma Inj Infect Crit Care* 2005;59: 1203–1208.

Periorbital and Orbital Cellulitis

LISA HUMPHREY

THE PATIENT ENCOUNTER

An 8-year-old boy presents to the pediatrician's office with an erythematous, edematous right eyelid and fever up to 38.9°C (102°F) of 2 days' duration. His mother also notes that he has been having cough and rhinorrhea for the past 10 days. On examination, the patient complains of pain with eye movement and diplopia. The patient's past medical history is unremarkable.

OVERVIEW

Definition

Periorbital and orbital cellulitis are both infections of the tissues that surround the orbit. They are differentiated primarily by their anatomy: periorbital cellulitis is a soft tissue infection anterior to the orbital septum, while an orbital cellulitis is posterior to the septum and infects fat, muscle, and other soft tissue. However, as outlined in this chapter, they typically are also distinct in their etiology, clinical significance, and management.

Pathophysiology

Periorbital cellulitis refers to inflammation of the eyelid and surrounding soft tissues and can extend to but not past the orbital septum. Typically, it occurs as a consequence of traumatic injury to the overlying skin from a bite, laceration, or microtrauma. It can also be due to a spreading infection that began as a hordeolum, chalazion, or dacryocystitis.

Orbital cellulitis may occur by direct extension or hematogenous spread. Rarely, periorbital cellulitis can lead to a concomitant orbital cellulitis owing to a dehiscence of the orbital septum. More commonly, orbital cellulitis is due to antecedent sinusitis with subsequent extension into the muscles, fat, and other soft tissue lying posterior to the orbital septum. The bony orbit is surrounded by three sinuses: the ethmoid, frontal, and maxillary sinuses. Thus, an infection of one of these sinuses places the posterior orbit at risk for infection. The frontal and maxillary sinuses of children <7 years of age are typically underdeveloped. Therefore, orbital cellulitis in young children is often the result of an ethmoid sinusitis. The lamina papyracea, a very thin bone that constitutes the medial aspect of the bony orbit and is immediately lateral to the ethmoid sinuses, is at risk for dehiscence when the ethmoid sinuses are infected. Adolescents possess a full complement of sinuses and therefore are more likely to have an orbital cellulitis as the result of a frontal sinusitis; however, an ethmoid sinusitis is still the most common initial source of orbital cellulitis in this population. Other less common mechanisms of direct extension include trauma, surgery, dental infections, and dacryocystitis.

Bacteremia is another source of orbital cellulitis. The superior and inferior ophthalmic veins are valveless and therefore allow for easy communication between the nose, ethmoid sinuses, orbit, face, and cavernous sinuses. During an infection of the nose, face, or sinuses, there can be a resultant thrombophlebitis of these veins, with consequent spread of inflammation to the orbit as well as an orbital cellulitis.

Epidemiology

Both periorbital and orbital cellulitis are more common in children than in adults. This is because of the increased incidence of the risk factors in children, such as increased upper respiratory infections and sinusitis. Of the two, periorbital cellulitis occurs more frequently than orbital cellulitis (84% versus 16%; Weiss et al.).

Staphylococcus aureus, *Streptococcus pneumoniae*, and group A *Streptococcus* are common causes of both periorbital and orbital cellulitis. Other organisms that cause orbital cellulitis include *Streptococcus milleri* group bacteria and anaerobes such as *Prevotella* spp., *Veillonella* spp. and *Fusobacterium* spp. *Haemophilus influenzae* type b may cause periorbital cellulitis in unimmunized children. Orbital cellulitis is frequently polymicrobial because extension of infection from the sinuses is a common route of spread.

Etiology

ACUTE MANAGEMENT AND WORKUP

The initial assessment should focus on distinguishing periorbital from orbital cellulitis, as the latter warrants rapid assessment and medical intervention because of its potential complications.

The First 15 Minutes

In the first 15 minutes, take these steps:

- **First, ascertain if the patient is experiencing diplopia.** Impingement of the extraocular muscles can result from the inflammation of orbital cellulitis or a space-occupying abscess.
- **Second, examine the patient for proptosis.** Significant swelling and inflammation of the posterior orbit will cause the orbit to be displaced anteriorly and results in proptosis on examination.

- **Third, evaluate the patient for decreased visual acuity.** This finding suggests impingement of the optic nerve and presents a risk for blindness.
- **Finally, examine the patient for ophthalmoplegia.** This finding constitutes a medical emergency, as it suggests intracranial involvement.

If any of these are present, the patient needs the following:

- Urgent computed tomographic (CT) imaging of the sinuses and orbits
- Consultation with ophthalmology and otorhinolaryngology
- Establishment of intravenous access
- A complete blood count (CBC) and blood culture
- Lumbar puncture if there are signs of intracranial involvement
- Empiric intravenous antibiotic treatment

The First Few Hours
History

It can be difficult to differentiate periorbital from orbital cellulitis, as both may present with fever, eye pain, and unilateral eyelid edema and erythema. However, a thorough history can elucidate some of their subtle differences. First, ask for the fever history. With periorbital cellulitis, there can be intermittent low-grade fevers. An orbital cellulitis often presents with a sudden onset of a high fever. Second, ask about what exacerbates the pain. Periorbital cellulitis tends to cause a static pain. In contrast, the pain associated with an orbital cellulitis worsens with eye movement owing to inflammation of the extraocular muscles. Third, determine whether there is concomitant sinusitis.

CLINICAL PEARL

While a periorbital cellulitis can present with an upper respiratory infection, orbital cellulitis will more likely present with a sinusitis, as suggested by the presence of sinus tenderness, headache, halitosis, and prolonged or worsening symptoms of an upper respiratory infection.

Finally, seek a history of trauma or surgery; superficial traumas (e.g., a bug bite or abrasion) are more frequently associated with a periorbital cellulitis, whereas significant traumas with resultant orbital fractures or surgical manipulations of the eye or the patient's dentition can result in an orbital cellulitis.

In addition to using the history to differentiate a periorbital from orbital cellulitis, it is also important to use it to assess visual acuity. You should ascertain the presence of diplopia, proptosis, a limitation in extraocular movements, frank ophthalmoplegia, or a decrease in visual acuity. Determine whether the erythema and edema was initially unilateral and now is bilateral; this is seen with intracranial extension of an orbital cellulitis. Ask the parents if there has been any change in the patient's mental status, which is also seen in patients with intracranial extension. The presence of any of these findings mandates prompt evaluation and assessment.

The presence of diplopia and pain with eye movement in the case patient suggested the diagnosis of orbital cellulitis.

Physical Examination

The exam to evaluate for periorbital or orbital cellulitis can be divided into the following categories, with possible findings noted:

- *General exam:* fever, malaise, systemic symptoms of sepsis (low blood pressure, tachycardia, poor capillary refill)
- *Skin exam:* abrasions, eyelid edema, eyelid erythema, hordeolum, chalazion, dacryocystitis, eyelid abscess
- *Eye exam:* conjunctivitis, chemosis, purulent eye discharge, afferent papillary defect, decreased extraocular movement or ophthalmoplegia, decreased visual acuity, optic disc edema
- *Neurologic exam:* decreased mental status, meningeal signs, contralateral cranial nerve palsies

Table 30-1 notes how these physical examination findings correlate with periorbital and orbital cellulitis and their complications.

Labs and Tests to Consider

Lumbar puncture is not required unless the patient has signs and symptoms that raise the suspicion for meningitis.

Key Diagnostic Labs and Tests

A blood culture should usually be obtained. The likelihood of bacteremia is greater with orbital cellulitis than with periorbital cellulitis, with the prevalence of bacteremia ranging from 0% to 33% in various studies. In an afebrile, well-appearing child with periorbital cellulitis, a blood culture may not be necessary.

If a wound culture is obtained, it can provide good information. Typically, this sample is either from a sinus drainage procedure or an abscess. The abscess specimen has the best yield and purest results. Of note, there is no role for a sputum or nasal swab culture because these sites are often colonized with bacteria and isolated bacteria do not necessarily correlate with the causative species.

Clinicians frequently obtain a complete blood count (CBC). This test will often show an elevated white blood cell count ranging from the midteens to the low twenties with a left shift in the cell differential. However, because

TABLE 30-1
The Chandler Classification of Orbit Complications

Term	Definition	Presentation
Periorbital cellulitis	Infection anterior to orbital septum involving the soft tissue surrounding the orbit	Eyelid edema and erythema and pain, conjunctivitis
Orbital cellulitis	Infection posterior to orbital septum involving muscle, fat, and other soft tissues in the posterior orbit	Pain with eye movement; limited EOM; eyelid edema and erythema; chemosis
Subperiosteal abcess	Phlegmon or collection of pus located either along the superior orbital wall, adjacent to frontal sinuses, or along the medial wall, between the lamina papyracea and the periorbita	Limited EOM; proptosis; chemosis
Orbital abscess	A discrete abscess located posterior to the orbital septum and within the muscle, fat, and other soft tissues of the posterior orbit	Ophthalmoplegia, chemosis, proptosis, decreased visual acuity
Cavernous Sinus Thrombophlebitis (or other intracranial extension)	Inflammation/infection of the cavernous sinus (or intracranial inflammation)	Bilateral chemosis, ophthalmoplegia, decreased visual acuity, and proptosis, ± meningeal and/or systemic signs of sepsis

EOM, extraocular movements.

there is no clear distinction between the white blood cell count of a periorbital cellulitis and that of an orbital cellulitis, a CBC has limited diagnostic utility.

A lumbar puncture is appropriate to obtain if there are exam or radiographic concerns for intracranial extension. The lumbar puncture is ideally obtained after a CT scan and prior to the administration of antibiotics. However, it should not delay therapy and can be obtained after the start of antibiotics. The spinal fluid should be evaluated for cell count, protein, glucose, and culture.

Imaging

In most cases of periorbital cellulitis, no imaging is necessary for diagnosis; however, a CT scan of the orbits and sinuses is often necessary.

A CT scan with intravenous contrast is considered the gold standard of imaging, as it gives good information about the extent of inflammation and sinus disease and often can be done without sedation. CT scanning also permits better detection of bony defects resulting from the extension of infection. Magnetic resonance imaging (MRI) is superior in its resolution of soft tissue disease but typically requires sedation, which adds some risk and preparatory time.

Not all clinicians obtain a CT scan immediately as it involves a significant amount of radiation exposure. Some will empirically begin intravenous antibiotics and observe for clinical improvements for 24 to 48 hours. If no improvement is seen, a CT scan is then ordered.

If ordering a CT scan, obtain a contrast CT scan with thin axial and coronal cuts of the orbit and sinuses. The axial cuts allow for visualization of portions of the frontal lobes to evaluate for intracranial extension or peridural disease. Coronal views can reveal the presence and extent of a subperiosteal abscess.

Treatment

Empiric treatment for periorbital cellulitis depends on the severity of infection and the suspected mechanism. Many cases of periorbital cellulitis can be treated in the outpatient setting if follow-up within 24 hours can be assured. For infections that occur by hematogenous spread or in conjunction with sinusitis, amoxicillin–clavulanate or ampicillin–sulbactam is appropriate; clindamycin or second- or third-generation cephalosporins are appropriate alternate choices. For infections that occur after external trauma (e.g., lid abrasion), clindamycin is appropriate, given the increased prevalence of methicillin resistance among *S. aureus* isolates in the community setting. Specific predisposing conditions (e.g., a cat scratch to the eyelid) may warrant alternate antibiotic regimens. In such cases, consultation with a pediatric infectious diseases specialist is warranted.

Orbital cellulitis should initially be treated in the hospital. Appropriate empiric therapy includes ampicillin–sulbactam, with alternate regimens including piperacillin–tazobactam with or without clindamycin. Upon discharge, first-line oral antibiotic options include amoxicillin–clavulanate or clindamycin; levofloxacin is a reasonable alternative.

Admission Criteria and Level-of-Care Criteria

Orbital cellulitis mandates hospitalization as it requires an initial course of intravenous antibiotics. Conversely, periorbital abscesses can be treated in the outpatient setting with oral antibiotics. However, exceptions to this are patients <1 year of age, immunocompromised patients, and patients who have failed outpatient therapy. In any of these cases, those with a presumed periorbital cellulitis should be admitted for observation and probable intravenous antibiotics.

Most patients can be managed on a general inpatient pediatrics ward. However, if there is cavernous sinus or other intracranial involvement or the patient has significant mental status changes, he or she should be managed in an intensive care unit. Additionally, almost all inpatients merit early consultation with an otorhinolaryngologist and/or an ophthalmologist.

EXTENDED IN-HOSPITAL MANAGEMENT

Table 30-1 delineated the Chandler classification of orbital complications (see "Physical Examination," earlier in the chapter). They are listed in order of severity; however, complications can coexist. The presence of a subperiosteal abscess, an orbital abscess, or a cavernous sinus thrombophlebitis or other intracranial extension will complicate and extend a patient's course.

The presence of a subperiosteal abscess and orbital abscess may require surgical intervention, and both require consultation with an otorhinolaryngologist and/or an ophthalmologist. Indications for surgical intervention include the following:

- Proptosis >2 mm
- Decreased visual acuity
- Diminished extraocular movements
- Failure of clinical improvement after 24 to 48 hours of intravenous antibiotics
- Radiographic evidence of increased abscess formation despite intravenous antibiotics

The presence of a cavernous sinus thrombophlebitis or other intracranial extension is a surgical emergency and requires consultation with an otorhinolaryngologist and a neurosurgeon for surgical correction. This would also mandate care within an intensive care unit.

The 8-year-old presented at the beginning of the chapter merited emergent evaluation and hospitalization as he had symptoms suggestive of an orbital cellulitis. A CT scan was obtained that showed inflammation of the medial rectus muscle and surrounding fat stranding. He was admitted to the general pediatrics service after consultation with an otorhinolaryngologist and an ophthalmologist and was placed on ampicillin–sulbactam. No surgical intervention was needed, as his symptoms improved after 36 hours. He was transitioned to oral antibiotics and discharged home on amoxicillin/clavulanate for 14 days after being afebrile in the hospital for 36 hours.

DISPOSITION

Discharge Goals

Patients are maintained on intravenous antibiotics until there are clinical signs of improvement; however, there have been no studies to determine optimal length of intravenous treatment. Specifically, clinicians look for the resolution of fever, improvement in the erythema and edema, improvement in extraocular movements and visual acuity if initially impaired, and increased energy. Improvement typically occurs over 3 to 5 days. Patients can then be discharged with oral antibiotics to complete total antibiotic therapy of 10 days for periorbital cellulitis or 14 days for orbital cellulitis. Children with large undrained abscesses or extensive orbital involvement may require a longer course of therapy.

Outpatient Care

The patient is discharged home on oral antibiotics for 2 to 3 weeks. He or she should be seen by a clinician—typically, the family's pediatrician or family practitioner—within 2 to 3 days. If there was an abscess or intracranial extension initially, the consulting subspecialist will typically follow up with the patient in 2 to 3 weeks. Throughout, the patient should be monitored for fever, recurrence of erythema and/or edema, visual acuity, and extraocular muscle mobility.

 WHAT YOU NEED TO REMEMBER

- Pain with eye movement often differentiates orbital cellulitis from periorbital cellulitis.
- Decreased visual acuity implies posterior orbit involvement and mandates a CT scan.
- Proptosis also implies posterior orbit involvement, which requires a CT scan.
- Ophthalmoplegia and bilateral spread of orbital involvement imply intracranial extension and, therefore, a medical emergency.

SUGGESTED READINGS

Chandler JR, Langenbrunner DJ, Stevens ER. The pathogenesis of orbital complications in acute sinusitis. *Laryngoscope* 1970;80:1414–1428.

Dudin A, Othman A. Acute periorbital swelling: evaluation of management protocol. *Paediatr Emerg Care* 1996;12:16–20.

How L, Jones NS. Guidelines for the management of periorbital cellulitis/abscess. *Clin Otolaryngol Allied Sci* 2004;29:725.

Uzcategui N, Warman R, Smith A, et al. Clinical practice guidelines for the management of orbital cellulitis. *J Pediatr Ophthalmol Strabismus* 1998;35:73.

Osteomyelitis

SUSAN K. GOLDBERG

THE PATIENT ENCOUNTER

A 12-year-old girl presented to the emergency department with a 1-week history of progressive left leg pain. She is a gymnast and initially attributed her pain to a hard fall during practice several days earlier. She was afebrile prior to arriving at the emergency department, but on examination, her temperature was 38.9°C (102°F). She appeared nontoxic but refused to bear weight on her left leg. On examination, she was tender to palpation over her left lateral malleolus and there was mild surrounding edema, but she had full range of motion of her ankle.

OVERVIEW

Definition

Osteomyelitis is an infection of bone diagnosed on the basis of clinical, laboratory, and radiographic features in addition to response to antimicrobial therapy. Osteomyelitis is commonly described based on either the route of infection or the duration of symptoms. In children, infection usually occurs by hematogenous spread, following an episode of bacteremia; rarely, it is due to direct inoculation of pathogens (e.g., from surgery, open fractures, or puncture wounds) or to local spread of a contiguous infection (e.g., dental infections, sinusitis, or soft tissue infection). Acute osteomyelitis is defined as symptoms of infection that are present for <7 days, whereas subacute osteomyelitis has a more indolent course. Chronic osteomyelitis is defined as symptoms that are present >3 weeks or by the finding of nonviable, necrotic bone within the infection.

Pathophysiology

Acute hematogenous osteomyelitis begins during an episode of bacteremia during which organisms deposit in the slow-flowing metaphyseal capillaries and multiply. Local cellulitis develops and progressing inflammation stimulates osteoclasts to resorb nearby bone. As the infection progresses, pressure builds and accumulating exudate pushes outward toward the cortex of the bone. The subsequent course of this purulent accumulation varies based on age-related differences in bone development. During infancy, the cortex is relatively thin and the periosteum is a poor barrier, so there is frequent eruption through both into local soft tissues. In toddlers, the dense periosteum is difficult to penetrate and poorly anchored to the cortex; therefore, subperiosteal abscesses may develop. In children ≥4 years of age, the metaphyseal cortex is thick and the periosteum is more adherent, so there is rarely spread beyond the bony cortex or rupture into soft tissues.

If the acute infection progresses without diagnosis or appropriate therapy, subacute osteomyelitis develops, with continued intraosseous suppuration and granulation, creating a Brodie abscess. The overlying periosteum is displaced outward from the purulent accumulations and produces new bone, called *involucrum*, over the site of infection. Progressing infection becomes chronic osteomyelitis when necrotic areas of nonviable bone, or sequestra, develop within the poorly perfused central infection.

Infants have unique anatomy that may predispose them to a more complicated infection. From birth until 18 months, the metaphyseal nutrient capillaries cross the epiphyseal growth plate into the joint space; thus a concomitant septic arthritis may be found. Atrophy of these vessels begins at 8 months and is complete by 18 months; after this age, concomitant septic arthritis can occur in joints where the metaphysis is intracapsular (i.e., the proximal femur, proximal humerus, proximal radius, and distal tibia).

Epidemiology

Osteomyelitis occurs more frequently in younger children, with one-fourth of cases occurring in children <2 years of age and more than half of the cases occurring in children <5. Males are more commonly affected than females, and approximately one-third of patients will have a preceding history of minor trauma to the affected area. In children, osteomyelitis is usually unifocal, with the majority of such infections occurring in the metaphyses of long bones. Although any bone can be affected, up to two thirds of cases involve the long bones of the lower extremities. Another common site of infection is the humerus. Pelvic osteomyelitis and osteomyelitis of the vertebrae are also well described in children. Most children with osteomyelitis are immunocompetent, but those with immunodeficiencies, hemoglobinopathies, or indwelling vascular catheters are at increased risk of infection and may have infection with a more diverse group of pathogens.

Etiology

Staphylococcus aureus accounts for the majority of the cases in which a pathogen is found regardless of age. Neonates are also susceptible to group B *Streptococcus* and gram-negative enteric pathogens. *Haemophilus influenzae* type B historically accounted for 10% to 15% of cases in children <3 years of age but now, after vaccine institution, is exceedingly rare. Group A *Streptococcus* is the next most common pathogen after *S. aureus* but accounts for <10% of all cases. *Streptococcus pneumoniae* is a relatively uncommon cause of osteomyelitis. *Kingella kingae* is being increasingly recognized as a causative agent in musculoskeletal infections in children, perhaps partially because of improved techniques for isolation. This organism, which normally colonizes the oropharynx of young children, has been implicated in several day care–associated outbreaks of musculoskeletal infections.

Specific circumstances favor other less common pathogens. Penetrating sneaker injuries may lead to inoculation of *Pseudomonas aeruginosa* into a foot, causing osteochondritis. Hemoglobinopathies predispose to infection with *Salmonella* or gram-negative bacilli, presumably owing to decreased splenic function in clearing transient bacteremia. Other immunodeficiencies, such as chronic granulomatous disease and human immunodeficiency virus (HIV), favor infection with atypical pathogens. *Brucella*, *Bartonella*, tuberculous, and fungal infections are also reported but less common. Sick neonates with indwelling lines are more commonly infected with nosocomial pathogens such as coagulase-negative staphylococci and *Candida* species.

ACUTE MANAGEMENT AND WORKUP

The First 15 Minutes

As with any potential invasive bacterial infection, the initial encounter should be used to assess hemodynamic stability to determine if more aggressive resuscitation or immediate antibiotics are required. Most children with osteomyelitis are nontoxic at presentation. If there is suspicion for septic arthritis, orthopedic surgery should be involved to expedite early operative drainage of the joint space.

The First Few Hours

Osteomyelitis can have an indolent presentation; its diagnosis in the early stages may require a high index of suspicion. Features from a careful history and physical combined with laboratory and radiographic investigations combine to help support or refute the diagnosis. In a stable patient, any diagnostic attempts at obtaining a causative organism should be pursued prior to starting antibiotics, because isolation of a pathogen is often difficult.

History

Pain is the most common reason for seeking medical care and can manifest as a limp, refusal to use the affected area, or decreased mobility. Fever is often present but may be absent in more than half of these cases, particularly in neonates. In patients with a history of preceding trauma, the distinction of worsening pain and progressing symptoms as opposed to a static musculoskeletal injury is more suggestive of osteomyelitis. Patients with subacute pain symptoms with acute worsening may have osteomyelitis with extension into the joint space. Recent antibiotic use may attenuate symptoms and requires a lower threshold for further investigation.

Physical Examination

Bony tenderness to palpation, particularly over the metaphysis of a long bone, is the most suggestive finding of osteomyelitis. You should perform gentle systematic palpation while a child is in the least threatening position possible (usually in a parent's lap). If the evaluation of a child remains limited by fear or crying, a parent's help can be used in assessing range of motion or tenderness to palpation with the physician out of the room. A febrile child with localized bone pain has osteomyelitis until proven otherwise. Swelling and warmth may also be present, although these may be later findings, as they suggest that the infection has spread from the metaphysis into the subperiosteal space.

The surrounding joints should be carefully assessed for range of motion, warmth, erythema, or the presence of an obvious effusion, which could suggest a concurrent septic arthritis. Pain with passive joint movement, often associated with a decreased range of motion, is highly suggestive of a septic arthritis. Neonates with a concomitant septic arthritis can present with a marked immobility called *pseudoparalysis.*

Labs and Tests to Consider

Nonspecific elevation of inflammatory markers supports the diagnosis but may be absent early in the course of osteomyelitis. Radiographs may also initially be normal but can rule out other etiologies of musculoskeletal pain. Other radiographic modalities, such as plain radiographs, magnetic resonance imaging (MRI), technetium-99m (^{99m}Tc) triple-phase bone scanning, and computed tomography (CT), can demonstrate earlier signs of infection if the diagnosis is unclear.

Key Diagnostic Labs and Tests

General markers for infection are not diagnostic for osteomyelitis but can monitor response to therapy or indicate the need for surgical intervention. Usual initial investigations include a complete blood count with differential, erythrocyte sedimentation rate (ESR), C-reactive protein (CRP), blood culture, and metaphyseal aspirate for wound culture. An elevated white blood cell count is inconsistent and may be present 25% to 75% of the time. The ESR is elevated in more than 90% of cases, although it is slow to rise and may remain normal for the first 2 to 3 days. It generally peaks in 5 to 7 days despite appropriate therapy and normalizes within several weeks. The most sensitive test is the CRP, which is elevated in 98% of cases and begins to rise within hours of the start of an infection.

> ### CLINICAL PEARL
>
> *The CRP has a half-life of approximately 2 days and is expected to peak on the second day despite appropriate therapy. It then has a marked decline and should normalize within 7 to 9 days.*

Laboratory testing to isolate a pathogen should be performed before starting antibiotic therapy. Blood cultures are positive in 30% to 50% of cases, but a pathogen can be found in 50% to 80% of children who have both blood cultures and a bone aspirate. Metaphyseal aspirates should be sent for standard investigations as well as inoculated into blood culture vials to increase the likelihood of isolating *K. kingae*.

Imaging

As early as the third day of the infection, subtle soft-tissue swelling over the metaphysis and some changes in the tissue planes around the bone may be visible on plain radiographs. Views of the contralateral extremity may help delineate asymmetries. Bony changes are usually not seen until symptoms have been present for at least a week and initially manifest as periosteal elevation. Osteopenia and osteolytic lesions are later findings and become visible by plain radiographs only after >50% of the bony matrix is destroyed. If the infection progresses, significant new bone deposition and sclerotic bone on plain films usually indicates a long-standing infection that may warrant surgical intervention. Radiographs of the pelvis, vertebrae, and other nontubular bones are often normal despite several weeks of symptoms and progressing infection; thus other modalities are often required to diagnose osteomyelitis in these areas.

MRI has become the imaging modality of choice for facilitating the diagnosis of osteomyelitis. It is particularly useful to identify osteomyelitis in sites such as the vertebrae and pelvis, where osteomyelitis may present with more diffuse rather than focal symptoms and signs. MRI shows marrow edema and inflammation early in the course of osteomyelitis and, in more established disease, helps with localization of soft tissue and subperiosteal abscesses or sinus tracts for possible surgical intervention. It can also be used to differentiate osteomyelitis from soft-tissue infections, neoplastic processes, and bone marrow infarction.

^{99m}Tc triple-phase bone scanning can be used if multiple areas of infection are suspected or if the site of infection cannot be localized. A bone scan is extremely sensitive and is usually positive within 48 hours of symptoms; however, it provides little anatomic information and may yield false positives because bone remodeling as a consequence of osteomyelitis cannot readily be differentiated from other causes, such as trauma.

CT can also be used to evaluate bone and soft tissue infections of the extremities and is most sensitive at detecting gas in soft tissues; however, it has essentially been replaced by MRI owing to improved visualization and decreased concerns for radiation. Ultrasound can be used in later osteomyelitis to help guide aspiration of subperiosteal abscesses, but it is not routinely used for diagnosis. Our case patient underwent an MRI, which revealed osteomyelitis of her distal fibula (Fig. 31-1).

Treatment

The child in the case presentation was treated empirically with intravenous clindamycin. Her pain lessened substantially over the next 4 days. Over this time, her CRP decreased from a peak of 14.1 mg/dL on the second day of

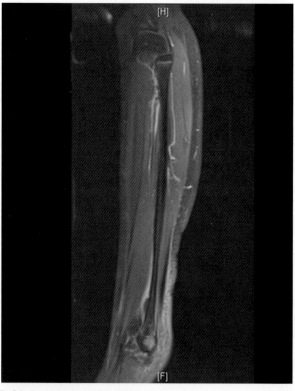

FIGURE 31-1: T1-weighted MRI image with gadolinium enhancement reveals an abnormal bone marrow signal involving the distal fibula with adjacent subperiosteal fluid collection suggestive of osteomyelitis with subperiosteal abscess.

hospitalization to 3.7 on the fourth day. In light of the clinical improvement and the declining CRP, she was switched to oral clindamycin and discharged to complete 4 weeks of total antibiotic therapy. She had a follow-up appointment scheduled 2 weeks later with a pediatric infectious diseases physician.

In a child with suspected or confirmed early osteomyelitis with no evidence of septic arthritis or obvious bony necrosis, empiric antibiotic therapy that is based on presumed pathogens with close monitoring for improvement should be instituted. All children being treated for osteomyelitis should have empiric coverage for *S. aureus* based on local rates and sensitivity patterns of community-acquired methicillin-resistant *S. aureus* (MRSA). First-generation cephalosporins and antistaphylococcal penicillins should be replaced by clindamycin and vancomycin as first-line therapies for presumed staphylococcal infections in areas where MRSA rates account for >10% of the community-acquired *S. aureus* infections.

Certain clinical scenarios require further antimicrobial therapy in addition to coverage for *S. aureus*. Infants should be evaluated and managed appropriately for a potential septic arthritis; appropriate antimicrobial therapy includes coverage for *S. aureus* plus a cephalosporin to treat group B *Streptococcus* and enteric gram-negative rods such as *Escherichia coli*. Additionally, a third-generation cephalosporin is used in combination with appropriate staphylococcal therapy in other clinical settings: (i) culture-negative osteomyelitis in children <3 years of age because of the increased prevalence of *K. kingae* (for which clindamycin and vancomycin are ineffective), which will also provide appropriate coverage for children <3 years of age with absent or partial immunization against *H. influenzae* type b; and (ii) children with sickle cell disease to cover for gram-negative pathogens, particularly *Salmonella*.

Immediate surgical therapy is indicated for osteomyelitis associated with a septic arthritis to try to preserve normal joint architecture and decrease the long-term sequelae. Surgical therapy is indicated for isolated osteomyelitis if there are large or multiple bony abscesses or a region of bone necrosis is found at presentation (e.g., if the initial diagnostic aspiration of the metaphysis demonstrates frank pus in the periosteal space or if there is radiographic evidence of chronic osteomyelitis) or if there is no improvement despite 2 to 3 days of appropriate antimicrobials. Children with penetrating sneaker injuries may require operative debridement in addition to appropriate therapy for *Pseudomonas aeruginosa* with an extended-spectrum antimicrobial such as ceftazidime, cefepime, or piperacillin–tazobactam.

Therapy can be a combination of intravenous and oral therapy once there has been a good clinical response. The total duration of antimicrobial therapy should be a minimum of 21 days to decrease the chance of recurrence; commonly, courses of 4 to 6 weeks are given. Consider sequential intravenous–oral therapy for children with uncomplicated osteomyelitis who are likely to be compliant (e.g., >2 or 3 years of age). Commonly, patients are switched from intravenous to oral antibiotics if they have demonstrated unequivocal clinical improvement, resolution of fever, and a substantive decrease in the CRP. This transition usually occurs after the fourth or fifth day of hospitalization.

Admission Criteria and Level-of-Care Criteria

Children with suspected or presumed osteomyelitis warrant admission for further investigation, initiation of parenteral antimicrobial therapy, and monitoring. Septic-appearing children with hemodynamic instability, evidence of an overwhelming systemic inflammatory response, rapidly progressing infection, or suspicion of complications such as a deep venous thrombosis may require intensive care monitoring. The majority of children can be admitted to a general pediatrics floor. An orthopedic surgeon should be available for possible operative intervention should the infection not respond appropriately to therapy.

EXTENDED IN-HOSPITAL MANAGEMENT

Most uncomplicated cases of acute hematogenous osteomyelitis are diagnosed early and respond well to antimicrobial therapy. Clinical improvement should be seen within 2 days of initiation of appropriate therapy, and serial labs can be obtained to monitor the patient's response. Surgical intervention may cause an expected transient rise in these inflammatory markers and may delay their resolution. If a child does not improve or has persistent bacteremia despite 48 to 72 hours of appropriate antimicrobial therapy, anatomic imaging with MRI and surgical debridement for a possible retained abscess should be considered. If initial cultures were negative in a child with a poor response to empiric therapy, a bone biopsy specimen should be obtained for histology and for bacterial, mycobacterial, and fungal cultures.

DISPOSITION

Discharge Goals

You can consider discharge when a patient is afebrile and showing marked clinical and laboratory evidence of improvement. Patients can be considered for transition from parenteral to oral therapy provided there is an equivalent oral antibiotic, close follow-up, anticipated good compliance, and no suspected issues with the absorption of oral antimicrobials. If there is not an appropriate oral antimicrobial regimen, it may be possible to arrange for a central line and home health administration of parenteral antimicrobials to complete the course of therapy. One exception to this general rule is that neonates require a full course of parenteral therapy and often remain in an inpatient setting because of the increased likelihood of complications of indwelling lines at this age.

The case patient was admitted to the hospital and started on empiric therapy with intravenous clindamycin. Her blood culture remained negative, but her bone aspirate from admission grew MRSA sensitive to clindamycin. She defervesced shortly after admission, was clinically improving by hospital day 4, and had marked improvement of her inflammatory markers by hospital day 5. She was discharged home with close follow-up on oral clindamycin to complete 1 month of therapy.

Outpatient Care

Patients should be followed up within several days of discharge by their primary care physician. Weekly monitoring of CRP and ESR should continue until the CRP is normal and the ESR has decreased. The patient should also be monitored to detect recrudescence of symptoms and complications of antibiotic therapy. Any fever or recurrence of pain during or in the months following therapy should be reported and evaluated by the primary care doctor with possible repeat labs and possible imaging, as approximately 5% of patients will have a recurrence of the original infection. Children with a delayed diagnosis >1 week or with septic arthritis have an increased risk of long-term sequelae on their bone growth and joint function and should have particular attention paid to their musculoskeletal exam at annual physicals.

 WHAT YOU NEED TO REMEMBER

- Acute hematogenous osteomyelitis often presents in a young child with progressive pain of an extremity.
- Concomitant septic arthritis can occur in neonates and in certain joints (hip, elbow) and require immediate diagnosis and drainage to prevent long-term damage to the joint and growth plates.
- Blood cultures and bone aspirates should be performed prior to initiation of antimicrobial therapy whenever possible.
- The majority of cases are due to *S. aureus*, but children <5 years of age or with chronic medical conditions also require empiric therapy for other pathogens.
- The treatment duration should be ≥3 weeks to minimize recurrence. If there is close follow-up, treatment can be given orally in an outpatient setting once the child is clinically improved.

SUGGESTED READINGS

Kaplan SL. Implications of methicillin-resistant *Staphylococcus aureus* as a community-acquired pathogen in pediatric patients. *Infect Dis Clin North Am* 2005;19:747–757.

Kiang KM, Ogunmodede F, Juni BA. Outbreak of osteomyelitis/septic arthritis caused by *Kingella kingae* among child care center attendees. *Pediatrics* 2005;116:e206.

Moumile K, Merckx J, Glorion C, et al. Bacterial aetiology of acute osteoarticular infections in children. *Acta Paediatr* 2005;94:419.

Stans AA. Osteomyelitis and septic arthritis. In Morrissy RT, Weinstein SL, eds. *Lovell and Winters Pediatric Orthopedics*, 6th ed. Philadelphia: Lippincott Williams & Wilkins, 2006.

Unkila-Kallio L, Kallio MJ, Eskola J, et al. Serum C-reactive protein, erythrocyte sedimentation rate, and white blood cell count in acute hematogenous osteomyelitis of children. *Pediatrics* 1994;93:59.

Yagupsky P. *Kingella kingae:* from medical rarity to an emerging paediatric pathogen. *Lancet Infect Dis* 2004;4:358–367.

Zaoutis T, Localio AR, Leckerman K, et al. Prolonged intravenous therapy versus early transition to oral antimicrobial therapy for acute osteomyelitis in children. *Pediatrics.* 2009;123(2):636–642.

CHAPTER

Pelvic Inflammatory Disease

32

DAFINA M. GOOD AND TONY COOLEY

THE PATIENT ENCOUNTER

A 17-year-old girl presents to the emergency department with complaints of lower abdominal pain, vaginal discharge, dysuria, and dyspareunia for 2 days. She presents with the following vital signs: a temperature of 38.5°C (101.3°F), a heart rate of 90 beats per minute, a respiratory rate of 12 breaths per minute, and a blood pressure (BP) of 117/70 mm Hg. On examination she is talkative and looks mildly uncomfortable; she has diffuse lower abdominal tenderness to palpation but no rebound tenderness. During pelvic examination, thick yellow discharge is seen; she has cervical motion tenderness but no adnexal tenderness with a bimanual exam. Your diagnosis is pelvic inflammatory disease (PID). She receives appropriate outpatient therapy for PID. However, 24 hours later, she returns to the emergency department with persistent vomiting and an inability to take her medications. Repeat vital signs are as follows: a temperature of 39.1°C (102.4°F), a heart rate of 110 beats per minute, a respiratory rate of 20 breaths per minutes, and a BP of 128/76 mm Hg. This time she is ill-appearing and looks moderately dehydrated. The remainder of her exam is unchanged.

OVERVIEW

Definition

PID can be defined as an infection of the upper female genital tract characterized by the presence of one of the following on examination: cervical motion tenderness, uterine tenderness, or adnexal tenderness.

Pathophysiology

PID is an ascending infection usually caused by a sexually transmitted infection (STI) that starts in the cervicovaginal area and then spreads to the upper genital tract. The uterus, fallopian tubes, and/or ovaries may be affected, leading to any combination of diseases—specifically, endometritis, salpingitis, tubo-ovarian abscess, and pelvic peritonitis.

Epidemiology

PID affects more than 1 million women each year in the United States. It is responsible for nearly 250,000 hospitalizations and 150 deaths per year. The infertility rate is estimated to be 10% per case. PID and its consequences, including chronic pelvic pain, ectopic pregnancy, and infertility, generate annual health care costs of approximately $4.2 billion (1).

PID can affect any sexually active woman that has acquired an STI. However, the peak age group for PID occurs during adolescence (ages 15 to 19 years). It is estimated that 1 in 8 sexually active adolescent girls develops PID before reaching age 20. Immaturity of the epithelial lining of the cervix and lack of local immunity have been suggested as biological factors that put adolescents at increased risk for STIs.

Etiology

Although *Chlamydia trachomatis* and *Neisseria gonorrhoeae* are the most commonly identified causes of PID, other microorganisms may be involved; these include anaerobes, *Gardnerella vaginalis*, *Haemophilus influenzae*, enteric gram-negative rods, *Streptococcus agalactiae*, cytomegalovirus, *Mycoplasma hominis*, *Urea Urealyticum*, and *Mycoplasma genitalium*.

ACUTE MANAGEMENT AND WORKUP

The acute management and workup should identify high-risk patients who have severe disease and require inpatient management as opposed to patients who may be discharged home on an outpatient antibiotic regimen.

The First 15 Minutes

You should use the first 15 minutes of any patient encounter to assess the patient's stability by rapidly assessing vital signs and ABCs (airway, breathing, and circulation). This assessment should identify critically ill patients with severe disease. In complicated cases of PID, patients may present with signs of shock (e.g., hypotension, poor perfusion, and altered mental status). In addition, patients with PID may have a significant amount of pain, possibly appearing as an acute abdomen, which must be addressed. It is our duty to assuage the patient's pain. Furthermore, the patient's discomfort may interfere with your ability to obtain a thorough history and physical exam.

The First Few Hours

The first few hours of your patient encounter will be integral in ensuring the proper diagnosis, the appropriate therapy, and the disposition of your patient.

History

Patients with PID often present with vaginal discharge and lower abdominal pain. Fever, vomiting, dysuria, abnormal bleeding, back or flank pain, and dyspareunia may be present as well.

Physical Examination

During the physical examination of a patient with PID, she typically will have lower abdominal tenderness with palpation. Mucopurulent cervicovaginal discharge is usually seen during pelvic examination. With bimanual examination, uterine tenderness, cervical motion tenderness (the "chandelier sign"), or adnexal tenderness may be elicited.

CLINICAL PEARL

Fitz-Hugh–Curtis syndrome results from ascending pelvic infection and inflammation of the liver capsule or diaphragm (i.e., acute perihepatitis). It is typically associated with acute salpingitis and manifests itself as right-upper-quadrant abdominal pain. Serum transaminases are normal because the liver parenchyma is not involved.

Labs and Test to Consider

PID is a clinical diagnosis. However, blood work and cervical cultures may help confirm and support the diagnosis of PID. Given the implications of a delayed or missed diagnosis of PID, you should have a high index of suspicion and a low threshold for treatment of any sexually active young woman at risk for PID. Minimal but adequate criteria for the diagnosis of PID are cervical motion tenderness, uterine tenderness, or adnexal tenderness. If any one of these three minimal criteria is present on physical examination, the diagnosis of PID should be made. See Table 32-1.

Key Diagnostic Labs and Tests

An elevated C-reactive protein (CRP) or erythrocyte sedimentation rate (ESR) increases the specificity of the diagnosis of PID when found in conjunction with one of the minimal physical exam criteria. Likewise, white blood cells on vaginal wet prep or evidence of *C. trachomatis or N. gonorrhoeae* on cervical Gram stain or culture also supports the diagnosis of PID.

All female patients of childbearing age with lower abdominal pain need a pregnancy test to exclude complications associated with intrauterine or ectopic pregnancy. Urinalysis may identify a urinary tract infection. Additional serologies, such as those for human immunodeficiency virus (HIV), syphilis, and hepatitis, are recommended. Although rarely performed, an endometrial biopsy with histopathologic evidence of endometritis is one of the most specific criteria for the diagnosis of PID.

The patient in the case illustrated above has a CRP of 14 mg/dL and numerous white blood cells on vaginal wet prep. Her lab findings corroborate her physical exam findings of PID.

TABLE 32-1
Criteria for the Diagnosis of Pelvic Inflammatory Disease

Minimal but Adequate Criteria for Diagnosis	Supporting Criteria	Definitive Criteria—Rarely Done
Cervical motion tenderness *or* Uterine tenderness *or* Adnexal tenderness	Fever Cervical or vaginal discharge Wet prep with WBCs Elevated ESR Elevated CRP Laboratory documentation of *N. gonorrhoeae* or *C. trachomatis*	Endometrial biopsy • Histopathologic evidence of endometritis Transvaginal sonography or MRI • Thickened, fluid-filled tubes • Free fluid in pelvis • Tubo-ovarian complex Laparoscopy

CRP, C-reactive protein; ESR, erythrocyte sedimentation rate; MRI, magnetic resonance imaging; WBCs, white blood cells.

Imaging

Although imaging studies are not routinely used in uncomplicated PID, ultrasound is the radiologic study of choice to confirm the diagnosis of PID and exclude other diagnoses that may present as female abdominal pain. Magnetic resonance imaging (MRI) has been shown to be more accurate than ultrasound, but the greater availability of ultrasound, in combination with its being easy to perform and low in cost, still make it the preferred imaging modality. On ultrasound and MRI of patients with PID, the presence of thickened fluid-filled ovarian tubes, free fluid in the pelvis, or a tuboovarian complex will confirm the diagnosis of PID.

Treatment

Parenteral and oral therapy in the treatment of PID has been shown to have similar efficacy in women with mild to moderate PID. All regimens should provide coverage of *C. trachomatis* and *N gonorrhoeae*. The recommended inpatient parenteral regimen is cefotetan 2g IV every 12 hours *or* cefoxitin 2 g IV every 6 hours *plus* doxycycline 100 mg orally or IV every 12 hours. When a tuboovarian abscess is present, metronidazole 500 mg PO every 12 hours for 14 days is often added for additional anaerobic coverage.

The outpatient oral regimen recommended by the Centers for Disease Control and Prevention (CDC)—the one that is used most commonly—is ceftriaxone 250 mg IM in a single dose *plus* doxycycline 100 mg orally twice a day for 14 days with or without metronidazole 500 mg orally twice a day for 14 days. Levofloxacin is no longer recommended as therapy because of the developing resistance of *N. gonorrhoeae.*

Admission Criteria and Level-of-Care Criteria

Admitted PID patients are generally managed on a general pediatric floor. Criteria for admission include severe disease characterized by ill-appearance, dehydration, vomiting, or high fevers. Admit patients who fail outpatient therapy either because of intolerance of the regimen, failure to improve, or noncompliance. Admit patients with concerning abdominal exams (such as those with peritoneal signs), particularly if a surgical emergency cannot be excluded. Pregnant patients or patients with a tuboovarian abscess should always be admitted.

EXTENDED IN-HOSPITAL MANAGEMENT

Once admitted, treatment with cefotaxime IV and doxycycline IV or PO is continued. If tolerated, doxycycline may be administered orally rather than parenterally because of the discomfort associated with its infusion.

Abdominal and back pain may be managed with an anti-inflammatory agent, such as ketorolac IV. Occasionally, narcotics, such as morphine, are needed. Dehydration should be managed with IV fluids in patients who cannot take enough by mouth. Antiemetics can alleviate nausea and vomiting.

If the diagnosis seems uncertain, it may be confirmed and other pathology excluded by ultrasound or MRI. Surgical consultation should be considered in patients with concerning peritonitis and when a pelvic abscess or appendicitis is suspected.

The patient in this case was admitted for parenteral antibiotic therapy. Her dehydration was corrected with IV fluids and she received ketorolac and antiemetics as needed.

DISPOSITION

Discharge Goals

Prior to discharge, patients should have clinical improvement in symptoms and be able to tolerate oral antibiotics. Lab work and radiologic imaging are not routinely used as discharge criteria. These are not routinely repeated unless they are used to follow a complication of PID, such as a tubo-ovarian abscess. When lab tests are used, CRP should decrease with treatment.

Within 48 hours, this patient was feeling much better, with minimal abdominal pain. She was tolerating a regular diet without any nausea or vomiting. A repeat CRP was 6. She was discharged home to complete a 14-day course of doxycycline.

Outpatient Care

After discharge, patients should follow up with their physician within 2 days to assess for tolerance of therapy and continued clinical improvement. Patients are discharged home to complete a total of 14 days of therapy.

WHAT YOU NEED TO REMEMBER

- PID is a clinical diagnosis made by the presence of cervical motion tenderness, uterine tenderness, or adnexal tenderness on examination.
- *C. trachomatis* and *N. gonorrhoeae* are the most common causes.
- Adolescents with PID can be treated with outpatient therapy with close follow-up.
- Patients should be admitted to the hospital for any of the following: severe illness, tubo-ovarian abscess, failed outpatient regimen, pregnancy, or suspected surgical emergencies.

REFERENCES

1. Rein DB, Kassler WJ, Irwin KL, Rabiee L. Direct medical cost of pelvic inflammatory disease and its sequelae: decreasing, but still substantial. *Obstet Gynecol* 2000;95:397–402.

SUGGESTED READINGS

American Academy of Pediatrics. Pelvic inflammatory disease. In Pickering LK, Baker CJ, Long SS, McMillan JA, eds. *Red Book: 2006 Report of the Committee on Infectious Diseases.* 27th ed. Elk Grove Village, IL: American Academy of Pediatrics; 2006: 493–498.

Benaim J, Pulaski M, Coupey SM. Adolescent girls and pelvic inflammatory disease. *Arch Pediatr Adolesc Med* 1997;151:449–454.

CDC: 2006 Sexually transmitted diseases treatment guidelines. Centers for Disease Control and Prevention. *MMWR* 2006;55(RR11):1–94.

Peritonsillar and Retropharyngeal Abscesses

NICHOLAS TSAROUHAS

THE PATIENT ENCOUNTER

A 3-year-old boy presents to the emergency department with complaints of fever, sore throat, drooling, and difficulty swallowing. His mother states that he has been sick for a few days but looks worse today. On examination, he has erythema of his posterior pharynx, but his tonsils are not enlarged. You also appreciate some mild stridor and notice that he prefers not to move his neck.

A few minutes later, you are called to see a 13-year-old girl complaining of fever, sore throat, and neck pain that has worsened over the past 3 days. On examination, she has a hard time opening her mouth fully, but you notice an erythematous pharynx with enlarged and exudative tonsils. You also appreciate fullness of the left peritonsillar area as well as deviation of the uvula to the opposite side.

OVERVIEW

Definition

Peritonsillar abscess, an infectious complication of tonsillitis or pharyngitis, results in an accumulation of purulence in the tonsillar fossa. It is also sometimes referred to as *quinsy*. A retropharyngeal abscess is an infectious complication of the lymph nodes found in the potential space between the posterior pharyngeal wall and the prevertebral fascia.

Pathophysiology

Peritonsillar Abscess

Infectious tonsillopharyngitis may progress from cellulitis to abscess. The infection starts in the intratonsillar fossa, which is situated between the upper pole and the body of the tonsil. The infection eventually extends around the tonsil. The actual abscess is a suppuration outside the tonsillar capsule, in proximity to the upper pole of the tonsil, and involves the soft palate. Purulence usually collects within one tonsillar fossa, but in some cases, it may be bilateral. Tonsillar and peritonsillar edema may lead to compromise of the airway.

Retropharyngeal Abscess

Purulent infections of the nasopharynx, posterior paranasal sinuses, and adenoids drain through their lymphatics into the retropharyngeal nodes.

Suppuration of these lymph nodes leads ultimately to abscess formation, often after passing through early stages of cellulitis, then phlegmon. Rarely, infection may be introduced by penetrating neck wounds or by extension of vertebral osteomyelitis.

Epidemiology

Although tonsillitis and pharyngitis are common in young children, peritonsillar *abscesses* are seen most commonly in adolescents and adults. In contrast, retropharyngeal abscesses are nearly always seen in children <5 years of age, as these nodes atrophy and disappear later in childhood. More than half of the cases occur in infants and children <2 years of age.

Etiology

Although the most commonly implicated microorganisms that cause peritonsillar and retropharyngeal abscesses include group A β-hemolytic streptococci (GABHS) and *Staphylococcus aureus*, it is important to remember that most of these true abscesses are polymicrobial. Furthermore, anaerobic bacteria (*Prevotella, Porphyromonas, Fusobacterium, Peptostreptococcus*) play an important role. Many describe a possible synergy between anaerobes and GABHS. Other bacteria include α-hemolytic streptococci and *Haemophilus influenzae.*

ACUTE MANAGEMENT AND WORKUP

Although the majority of children with peritonsillar and retropharyngeal abscesses are relatively stable at presentation, respiratory distress from airway obstruction is a real possibility. Your initial management must therefore identify those patients who require immediate surgical intervention and intubation.

The First 15 Minutes

Upper airway obstruction is the most feared complication, so the first priority is always to assess the adequacy of the patient's airway. Any evidence of respiratory distress should prompt immediate consultation with otolaryngology and/or critical care. Unfortunately, drooling and dysphonia, two signs commonly associated with upper airway obstruction, are commonly seen even with peritonsillar abscesses that do not obstruct the airway. However, any increased work of breathing can herald upper airway obstruction and should be considered an ominous finding.

As with a peritonsillar abscess, upper airway obstruction is the most feared complication of retropharyngeal abscess. Consequently, the first priority is to assess the adequacy of the patient's airway. Any evidence of airway compromise or respiratory distress should prompt immediate consultation with critical care and otolaryngology specialists.

The most important disease in the differential diagnosis is epiglottitis; this life-threatening airway emergency presents abruptly with fever, stridor, increased work of breathing, and drooling. Although epiglottitis is rare since the advent of the *H. influenzae* type B vaccination, the similarities in their presentations necessitate a high degree of vigilance. Patients with retropharyngeal abscess usually have a less fulminant presentation and appear slightly less toxic; but if there is still high suspicion of epiglottitis initially, they should be managed similarly. This would include blow-by oxygen delivered gently by the parent, avoidance of invasive or disturbing studies or procedures (e.g., traumatic throat exams, intravenous line placement, x-rays, etc.), and emergent anesthesia/critical care consultation.

The First Few Hours

The treatment of a true abscess without incision and drainage is often inadequate and can have airway-threatening implications. Additionally, abscesses left untreated can rupture spontaneously into the pharynx, leading to aspiration. Otolaryngology consultation is imperative when the strong possibility of an abscess exists.

The patient's state of hydration should also be quickly assessed. Many of these patients have been sick for several days. Consequently, owing to dysphagia and odynophagia, they will often have curtailed or stopped eating and drinking. Dehydration from decreased oral intake is the most common complication. Intravenous fluids may be necessary for those patients with severe disease or prolonged courses of illness. Lateral radiographs of the neck should be obtained immediately if a retropharyngeal abscess is suspected.

Antibiotics (as described below) should be initiated as soon as possible. Although it is ideal to obtain an abscess culture prior to antibiotics, this is not always practical. In general, antibiotics should be administered without delay. Also, abscess formation can often be prevented if appropriate antimicrobial therapy is initiated while the infection is still at the cellulitis stage.

History

Most patients with peritonsillar abscess will initially complain of sore throat and difficulty swallowing. Patients may also complain of unilateral neck or ear pain. Malaise and fever are also common.

Patients with retropharyngeal abscesses usually present with fever, sore throat, refusal to eat, trouble swallowing, drooling, and malaise. Most commonly they've had "cold" symptoms that include fever, runny nose, and cough. The parents usually relate that they've been sick for several days and now appear to be getting worse.

Physical Examination

Simple inspection of the throat confirms the diagnosis of peritonsillar abscess. The classic finding is unilateral peritonsillar fullness, or bulging of the posterosuperior soft palate. This is associated with uvular deviation to the contralateral side. Palpation of fluctuance of the palatal swelling supports the diagnosis. These findings are usually found in concert with an erythematous, edematous pharynx, with enlarged and exudative tonsils. Patients also commonly complain of pain with opening of the mouth (trismus). Painful swallowing also leads to drooling. When asked to speak, a muffled ("hot potato") voice is usually apparent. Neck palpation nearly always reveals cervical adenopathy. Torticollis is sometimes present.

Patients with retropharyngeal abscess always appear ill. While often showing signs of respiratory distress, usually they do not have evidence of impending airway obstruction. Stridor, however, may sometimes be present. Some children will have a neck mass, and a few will have a visible asymmetric pharyngeal bulge. Meningismus is not uncommon, sometimes confusing the diagnosis with meningitis.

CLINICAL PEARL

Children with retropharyngeal abscesses will often complain of pain with neck extension. This contrast with meningitis, where pain occurs with neck flexion.

Labs and Tests to Consider

Whereas a peritonsillar abscess can generally be diagnosed by history and physical examination alone, a lateral neck film is often necessary to confirm the diagnosis of a retropharyngeal abscess. Other diagnostic labs and tests are discussed below.

Key Diagnostic Labs and Tests

Although it is not mandatory for the diagnosis, a leukocytosis with prominent left shift is common. Similarly, the C-reactive protein is also commonly elevated. Rapid streptococcal throat antigen studies are helpful to diagnose GABHS infection. Because peritonsillar cellulitis is often associated with infectious mononucleosis, the finding of antibodies or a Monospot test to detect Epstein–Barr virus is sometimes indicated, especially in the presence of negative streptococcal studies. Of course, as with all abscesses, a Gram stain and culture of the aspirate specimen is most important to confirm the causative bacteria.

Imaging

The 13-year-old girl in the case study did not require radiologic imaging, as the physical exam was consistent with the diagnosis of peritonsillar abscess. A lateral neck x-ray was performed in the 3-year-old boy. It revealed prevertebral soft tissue swelling consistent with retropharyngeal inflammation. Computed tomography (CT) of the neck confirmed the diagnosis of retropharyngeal abscess.

Because the physical examination is nearly always diagnostic of peritonsillar abscess, radiographic studies are rarely necessary. A CT scan or intraoral ultrasound is sometimes employed to differentiate peritonsillar cellulitis from a peritonsillar abscess. The CT scan is most useful in cases where the patient cannot open his or her mouth secondary to trismus.

The initial test to diagnose a retropharyngeal abscess is a lateral neck x-ray. A retropharyngeal abscess should be suspected if, at the level of C2/C3, the prevertebral soft-tissue space is more than *half* the adjacent vertebral body diameter. In infants <1 year of age, some experts "allow" a full vertebral body diameter before calling an x-ray abnormal. Importantly, to obtain an optimal view, the neck should be positioned in mild extension, as neck flexion may lead to a "false positive" x-ray.

A CT scan is mandatory in patients suspected to have a retropharyngeal abscess by lateral neck x-ray. Done with intravenous contrast, it almost always confirms the diagnosis while also delineating the extent of disease involvement. Importantly, a distinction is made between a true retropharyngeal *abscess* and a retropharyngeal "cellulitis." Finally, the CT scan is diagnostic for a lateral pharyngeal abscess. This is very similar to retropharyngeal abscess in clinical presentation but is more difficult to diagnose because the lateral neck x-ray is often normal. These usually present in slightly older children.

Treatment

Peritonsillar abscesses should be urgently/emergently drained. In older, cooperative patients, bedside needle aspiration (usually performed by otolaryngology) is commonly employed. This is usually done after the patient's abscess has been sprayed with a topical anesthetic agent. In some cases, an anxiolytic, such as midazolam, is also used. Uncooperative patients are sometimes taken to the operative suite for surgical incision and drainage.

Retropharyngeal abscesses should be surgically drained by an otolaryngology specialist. Failure to diagnosis and drain a retropharyngeal abscess can have dire consequences, including upper airway obstruction, rupture of the abscess into the pharynx, aspiration, and mediastinitis.

Antibiotic therapy with clindamycin or ampicillin–sulbactam should not be delayed while awaiting operative intervention. Of course, fluid resuscitation and hydration maintenance are also crucial. Some experts recommend steroids (i.e., methylprednisolone, dexamethasone, or prednisone) to decrease swelling, pain, and trismus associated with peritonsillar abscesses.

Admission Criteria and Level-of-Care Criteria

Most pediatric patients with peritonsillar abscesses are admitted after needle aspiration. This is done to ensure appropriate antibiotic delivery, adequate hydration, and analgesia; it also allows for careful observation of a potential re-formation of the abscess.

Adult patients with peritonsillar abscess, however, often undergo needle aspiration in the emergency department and subsequent discharge. Selected adolescent patients may sometimes be managed in this fashion. As long as they are able to drink and have adequate pain control, some of these adolescents are discharged on antibiotics such as clindamycin, amoxillin–clavulanate (Augmentin), or penicillin.

All patients with known or suspected retropharyngeal abscesses are admitted. The only initial disposition question is whether the patient needs to be rushed to the operative suite for emergent surgical intervention.

EXTENDED IN-HOSPITAL MANAGEMENT

After undergoing needle aspiration, children with peritonsillar abscess admitted for parenteral antibiotics should show improvement (defervescence, no abscess reaccumulation) within 24 to 48 hours. If no improvement is apparent, surgical drainage with tonsillectomy should be considered. Some children will respond to antibiotic therapy but still require several days of hospitalization secondary to pain control and hydration issues.

Children admitted for retropharyngeal "cellulitis" are treated with parenteral antibiotics and observed closely for clinical improvement (defervescence, improvement in airway and respiratory symptoms.) If clinical improvement is not apparent within 24 to 48 hours, surgical intervention is mandatory. Patients who have undergone surgical drainage, similarly, should improve clinically within 24 to 48 hours. Once again, some children have protracted stays for hydration issues secondary to refusal to drink.

DISPOSITION

Discharge Goals

Patients may be discharged when they are afebrile, comfortable swallowing, and drinking well and when peritonsillar swelling has subsided.

Outpatient Care

Patients are discharged on oral antibiotics to complete a 10- to 14-day course. Patients with peritonsillar abscesses should follow up with their primary care provider within 48 hours of discharge in order to ensure that the abscess has not reformed. Children with severe or recurrent peritonsillar abscesses should follow up with otolaryngology for discussion of the possible need for tonsillectomy. Patients with a retropharyngeal abscess usually require follow-up with otolaryngology within 1 week of discharge from the hospital.

WHAT YOU NEED TO REMEMBER

- Peritonsillar *abscesses* are seen most commonly in adolescents and adults. In contrast, retropharyngeal abscesses are nearly always seen in children <5 years of age.
- The physical examination is diagnostic for peritonsillar abscess; inspect for a unilateral peritonsillar bulge of the posterosuperior soft palate.
- Radiographic imaging is not necessary to make the diagnosis of peritonsillar abscess but is required to make the diagnosis of retropharyngeal abscess.
- Needle aspiration is a crucial part of the adequate management of peritonsillar abscess, while many cases of retropharyngeal abscess require intraoperative drainage.
- Children >5 years of age rarely develop retropharyngeal abscesses because these nodes atrophy and disappear later in childhood.

SUGGESTED READINGS

Abdel-Haq NM, Harahsheh A, Asmar BI. Retropharyngeal abscess in children: the emerging role of group a beta hemolytic *Streptococcus*. *South Med J* 2006;99(9): 927–931.

Blotter JW, Yin L, Glynn M, et al. Otolaryngology consultation for peritonsillar abscess in the pediatric population. *Laryngoscope* 2000;110:1698–1701.

Brook I. Microbiology and management of peritonsillar, retropharyngeal, and parapharyngeal abscesses. *J Oral Maxillofac Surg* 2004;62(12):1545–1550.

Cherukuri S, Benninger MS. Use of bacteriologic studies in the outpatient management of peritonsillar abscess. *Laryngoscope* 2002;112:18–20.

Etchevarren V, Bello O. Retropharyngeal abscess secondary to traumatic injury. *Pediatr Emerg Care* 2002;18(3):189–191.

Galioto NJ. Peritonsillar abscess. *Am Fam Physician* 2008;7(2):199–202.

Johnson RF, Stewart MG, Wright CC. An evidence-based review of the treatment of peritonsillar abscess. *Otolaryngol Head Neck Surg* 2003;128:332–343.

Kirse DJ, Roberson DW. Surgical management of retropharyngeal space infections in children. *Laryngoscope* 2001;111(8):1413–1422.

Lee SS, Schwartz RH, Bahadori RS. Retropharyngeal abscess: epiglottitis of the new millennium. *J Pediatr* 2001;138(3):435–437.

Toback Seth, Herr S. Retropharyngeal abscess in a toxic-appearing infant. *Pediatr Emerg Care* 2001;17(4):255–257.

Pneumonia

GARY FRANK AND SAMIR S. SHAH

THE PATIENT ENCOUNTER

A 3-year old girl was taken to her pediatrician with a 3-day history of fever and worsening cough. On examination, her respiratory rate was 50 breaths per minute and her percutaneous oxygen saturation was 98% in room air. A chest radiograph revealed a left-lower-lobe infiltrate and she was prescribed oral amoxicillin for community-acquired pneumonia. Over the next 3 days, she continued to spike high fevers, became increasingly short of breath, and complained of left-sided chest pain. She presented to the emergency department with a temperature of 39.7°C (103.5°F) and a respiratory rate of 55 breaths per minute. On examination, she was noted to be ill-appearing and tachypneic. Her breath sounds were diminished over her left lower and midlung fields.

OVERVIEW

Definition

Pneumonia can be defined as the presence of fever or acute respiratory symptoms accompanied by new parenchymal infiltrates on chest radiography. This chapter will focus on community-acquired pneumonia (CAP). CAP may be complicated by significant necrosis, abscess, pleural effusion, empyema, or pneumatocele formation.

Pathophysiology

Pneumonia occurs by three primary mechanisms. First, inhalation of aerosolized droplets can spread among *infected* close contacts. This mode of infection is commonly seen with viruses and atypical bacteria, such as *Mycoplasma pneumoniae* and *Chlamydophila* (formerly *Chlamydia*) *pneumoniae*. Second, colonization of the nasopharynx may lead to subsequent aspiration or inhalation into the lung, often in the context of transient or chronic impairment of normal host defenses. The bacteria then lodge in bronchioles and proliferate, initiating an inflammatory process that begins in alveolar spaces with an outpouring of protein-rich fluid. Finally, transient bacteremia may lead to hematogenous seeding of the lung. *Staphylococcus aureus* most commonly causes CAP by this mechanism.

While CAP most commonly presents in normal hosts, certain risk factors predispose to the development of bacterial pneumonia. For example, anatomic abnormalities such as cleft palate predispose to aspiration of gastric contacts. Other predisposing factors include physiologic abnormalities (e.g., swallowing dysfunction, gastroesophageal reflux), primary immune deficiency (e.g., hyper-IgE syndrome, IgA deficiency), and acquired immune deficiency (e.g., human immunodeficiency virus [HIV] infection).

Epidemiology

More than 4 million children are diagnosed with CAP each year in the United States. The annual incidence of CAP of 34 to 56 per 1,000 in children <5 years of age is higher than at any other time of life except perhaps in adults >75 years of age. This incidence decreases to approximately 16 cases per 1,000 children ≥5 years of age. Approximately 1 in 7 children with CAP require hospitalization, although mortality occurs in <1% of hospitalized children.

Etiology

Common causes of CAP are summarized in Table 34-1. *Mycobacterium tuberculosis* is a less common cause of pneumonia in the industrialized world, although the presence of a pleural effusion should raise suspicion for this condition.

TABLE 34-1
Common Etiologies of Community-Acquired Pneumonia

Neonates	1–3 months	>3 months–5 years	>5 years
Group B *Streptococcus*	Lower respiratory viruses[a]	Lower respiratory viruses[a]	*Mycoplasma pneumoniae*
Gram-negative enteric bacilli	*Streptococcus pneumoniae*	*Streptococcus pneumoniae*	*Chlamydophila pneumoniae*
Cytomegalovirus	*Chlamydia trachomatis*	*Mycoplasma pneumoniae*	*Streptococcus pneumoniae*
Listeria monocytogenes	*Bordetella pertussis*	*Staphylococcus aureus*	Influenza A or B
Herpes simplex virus			*Staphylococcus aureus*

[a]Includes respiratory syncytial virus, adenovirus, parainfluenza viruses (types 1, 2, and 3), influenza viruses (A and B), human metapneumovirus, and human bocavirus.

ACUTE MANAGEMENT AND WORKUP

The acute management and workup help to identify those patients with severe or life-threatening illness who require more intensive inpatient management as compared with the majority of patients, who can be safely and successfully treated with oral antibiotics in an outpatient setting.

The First 15 Minutes

In an ill-appearing child, the initial assessment helps determine whether to make an immediate intervention or to proceed with the history and physical examination. **First, ask the patient to recite the alphabet.** Uncooperative or extremely anxious patients may have life-threatening hypoxia. Those who can recite only the first few letters of the alphabet are in severe distress and could have impending respiratory failure. **Second, determine whether supraclavicular retractions are present.** Children have compliant chest walls, so suprasternal, subcostal, and intercostal retractions are common in the setting of mild or moderate respiratory distress. In contrast, supraclavicular retractions suggest severely diminished air entry.

The First Few Hours

A good history, thorough physical exam, and appropriate use of labs and imaging are integral to developing an appropriate plan of action. Adult literature strongly emphasizes the importance of early antibiotics, but this has not been duplicated in children.

History

Children with CAP typically have fever, cough, and labored breathing. Chest pain, vomiting, and decreased activity are often noted. Abdominal pain is a common complaint in children with basilar pneumonia because the T9 dermatome is shared by the lung and the abdomen. Children with atypical pneumonia often develop fever, cough, and malaise, as well as other constitutional symptoms. In such cases, wheezing or diffuse rales develop during the second week of illness as the primary complaints resolve; thus, the designation of "walking pneumonia."

Physical Examination

Tachypnea is the most reliable predictor of pneumonia in children, with a sensitivity of 50% to 85% and a specificity of 70% to 90%. The child may exhibit grunting, flaring of the alae nasi, splinting, and subcostal or intercostal retractions. Dullness to percussion over the affected lung field has a low sensitivity but high specificity for the diagnosis of CAP. On auscultation, rales, tubular breath sounds, egophony, bronchophony, and whispered pectoriloquy may be appreciated, although these findings are uncommon in children <5 years of age. The presence of wheezing suggests a viral or atypical bacterial cause.

Labs and Tests to Consider

The judicious use of labs and imaging studies help confirm the diagnosis of pneumonia and allows for the evaluation of complicating factors, such as pleural effusions or empyemas. However, given a convincing history and exam, you should consider pneumonia even in the absence of an identifiable infiltrate on chest x-ray, because imaging findings tend to lag behind clinical findings.

Key Diagnostic Labs and Tests

Blood cultures are positive in <2% of patients with pneumonia who are well enough to be managed in the outpatient setting. However, blood cultures are positive in 7% to 10% of patients requiring hospitalization for pneumonia and in up to 25% of patients with pneumonia complicated by pleural effusion.

Additional laboratory studies may include an arterial blood gas (to detect hypoxemia and metabolic acidosis), a complete blood count, and electrolytes (to detect hyponatremia, renal insufficiency, metabolic acidosis, etc.). An elevated C-reactive protein (CRP) does not reliably differentiate viral from bacterial causes of CAP; however, a decrease in an initially elevated CRP can serve as an objective laboratory marker of patient improvement.

In young infants, *C. trachomatis* can be detected by direct fluorescent antibody testing or culture of a nasopharyngeal (NP) or conjunctival swab. Polymerase chain reaction (PCR) testing of an NP aspirate is very sensitive for *B. pertussis*, whereas a culture is time-consuming and direct fluorescent antibody testing has poor sensitivity. In a patient with diffuse wheezing, *M. pneumoniae* and *C. pneumoniae* can be detected by PCR testing of an NP aspirate; if PCR is not available, acute and convalescent serum antibody titers are appropriate. Viruses can be detected in NP aspirates by PCR or immunofluorescence, but identification of a virus does not rule out bacterial superinfection. Tuberculin skin testing should be performed if tuberculosis is suspected.

The patient in the case illustrated earlier had a peripheral white blood cell count of 27,000/μL with 14% bands and 70% segmented neutrophils. Her CRP level was 17 mg/dL and her sodium level was 130 mmol/L. The leukocytosis and elevated CRP suggested an inflammatory process and were consistent with the initial diagnosis of CAP.

Imaging

A chest radiograph is required for an accurate diagnosis. A bacterial cause is likely in the presence of lobar or segmental consolidation or a unilateral pleural effusion. If the diaphragm is obscured, a lower lobe pneumonia is likely. If the right heart border is indistinct, a right middle lobe pneumonia is likely. Pneumatoceles (air-filled cavities resulting from alveolar rupture) are detected in approximately two-thirds of patients with pneumonia caused by *S. aureus*. Viral and atypical bacterial pneumonias commonly manifest as diffuse interstitial infiltrates. Nodular infiltrates are commonly caused by endemic fungi (e.g., *Histoplasma capsulatum* and *Pneumocystis jiroveci* [formerly *P. carinii*]) and less commonly by viruses and atypical bacteria.

CLINICAL PEARL

Mycoplasma pneumoniae *infections, although typically multifocal, may cause unilateral lobar consolidation (<10% of cases) or small bilateral pleural effusions (approximately 20% of cases).*

Computed tomography (CT) of the chest should be performed to more clearly define specific abnormalities such as nodular infiltrates, lung abscesses, necrotizing pneumonia, and pleural effusions. The patient's CT scan is presented in Figure 34-1.

Treatment

Table 34-2 summarizes empiric therapy for children with CAP. The typical duration of therapy is 10 to 14 days except for azithromycin, which is used for 5 days.

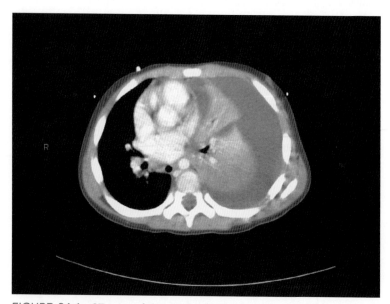

FIGURE 34-1: CT scan of the chest of a 3-year-old girl with complicated pneumonia. The scan shows a large left pleural effusion causing rightward shift of the mediastinum.

TABLE 34-2
Summary of Empiric Treatment of Community-Acquired Pneumonia

Patient Age Group	Inpatient	Outpatient
Neonate	First-line: ampicillin + aminoglycoside Alternate: ampicillin + cefotaxime; piperacillin–tazobactam ± vancomycin[a]	**Outpatient therapy not recommended**
1–3 months	First-line: ampicillin or cefotaxime Alternate: add erythromycin if *Chlamydia trachomatis* or *Bordetella pertussis* suspected	**Outpatient therapy not recommended**
>3 months to 5 years	First-line: ampicillin or clindamycin Alternate: cefotaxime or ceftriaxone; add azithromycin or clarithromycin for diffuse wheezing to cover for atypical bacteria	First-line: amoxicillin or clindamycin
>5 years	First-line: ampicillin or clindamycin Alternate: levofloxacin; cefotaxime; for extremely ill patients, use azithromycin plus cefotaxime; also consider adding vancomycin	First-line: amoxicillin or clindamycin Alternate: levofloxacin[b]; switch to levofloxacin or add azithromycin or clarithromycin for diffuse wheezing to cover for atypical bacteria

[a]If hospital-acquired rather than perinatally or community-acquired.
[b]Not currently approved by the U.S. Food and Drug Administration for children <18 years of age, although there is published evidence to support its use in younger children.

Admission Criteria and Level-of-Care Criteria

Absolute criteria for admission include evidence of sepsis, hypoxia, respiratory distress, and a patient age <3 months. Admission should be considered for patients with underlying medical conditions (e.g., prematurity, congenital heart disease, cystic fibrosis), mild to moderate dehydration, failed outpatient therapy, an inability to tolerate oral fluids, or an unreliable social situation. Patients with extensive consolidation, a low white blood cell count, or a high white blood cell count with immature neutrophils (i.e., a "left shift") may also merit admission.

Patients can often be managed on a general pediatric floor. However, consider admission to an intensive care unit for patients with severe respiratory distress or failure, evidence of sepsis, or an oxygen requirement >50% to 60% FiO_2.

EXTENDED IN-HOSPITAL MANAGEMENT

As in the illustrative case, the presence of significant pleural effusions will lead to prolonged hospitalization. A pleural effusion should be suspected in the following cases: (i) pleuritic chest pain, (ii) fever more than 48 hours after starting antimicrobial treatment, (iii) clinical deterioration during the treatment of CAP, (iv) isolation of S. aureus from blood cultures, and (v) development of hemolytic–uremic syndrome in a patient with CAP. Examination reveals dullness to percussion and diminished breath sounds over the affected lung. In contrast to adults, a pleural effusion in a child with CAP is almost always caused by infection. Common pathogens include *Streptococcus pneumoniae*, *S. aureus*, group A beta-hemolytic *Streptococcus*, and *M. tuberculosis*.

Early pleural fluid drainage appears to decrease the length of hospital stays in children with pneumonia complicated by pleural effusion. The optimal method of initial drainage (i.e., chest tube versus video-assisted thoracoscopic surgery [VATS]) remains controversial, although several retrospective studies suggest that children undergoing VATS have a shorter length of stay and require fewer repeat drainage procedures.

The following tests are often sent from the pleural fluid: cell count, bacterial culture, mycobacterial culture, Gram stain, glucose, pH, lactate dehydrogenase, and acid-fast stain. In general, low pH (<7.1), low glucose (<40 mg/dL), high pleural fluid LDH (>1,000 IU/L), and an elevated pleural fluid:serum LDH ratio (>0.6) suggest empyema. The presence of mononuclear white blood cells in the pleural fluid suggests tuberculosis. The presence of eosinophils in the pleural fluid suggests tuberculosis, fungi, parasites, and hypersensitivity reactions.

Empiric therapy for a child with a pleural effusion may include clindamycin alone, clindamycin plus a third-generation cephalosporin (i.e., cefotaxime or ceftriaxone), or vancomycin plus a third-generation cephalosporin. The duration of therapy depends on the clinical course. In general, most patients require antibiotics for 7 to 10 days after the resolution of fever; the typical treatment course is 17 to 21 days, although patients with discrete abscesses often require longer therapy. The patient in this case underwent early VATS with placement of a chest tube and was treated empirically with intravenous ceftriaxone and vancomycin because of her ill appearance in the context of a complicated pneumonia.

DISPOSITION

Discharge Goals

Consider discharge when patients are clinically improved and are able to take adequate oral intake. Patients should be able to maintain an oxygen saturation of at least 93% on room air and should be afebrile for a minimum of 12 to 24 hours. If labs are followed, look for a downward trend in the C-reactive protein and normalization of the white blood cell count. If blood cultures were initially positive, repeat blood cultures should document clearance of bacteremia. Follow-up chest radiographs are not necessary in a clinically improving patient as resolution of radiographic abnormalities lags behind clinical improvement by days to weeks. The case patient's chest tube was removed on the fourth day after VATS and her last fever occurred on the seventh day after VATS. She received 10 days of intravenous antibiotics and was discharged on another week of oral antibiotics.

Outpatient Care

After discharge from the hospital, patients should have a follow-up visit with their pediatrician within 2 to 3 days. Patients with complicated pneumonia may be discharged on intravenous or oral antibiotics. Repeat chest radiographs are not routinely necessary but should be considered 4 to 6 weeks later for patients with pneumatoceles, extensive lung necrosis, and protracted symptoms. Patients with significant necrosis or pneumatocele formation require regular follow-up with a pulmonologist. Patients who develop increased respiratory distress or fever within a week after discharge have likely failed oral therapy and require a repeat chest radiograph and reevaluation of the antibiotic regimen.

 WHAT YOU NEED TO REMEMBER

- Tachypnea is the most sensitive sign/symptom of pneumonia.
- Abdominal pain is a common complaint in children with basilar pneumonia.
- *Mycoplasma pneumoniae* infections are typically multifocal but may cause unilateral lobar consolidation or small bilateral pleural effusions.
- Early pleural fluid drainage appears to decrease the length of hospital stay in children with pneumonia complicated by pleural effusion or empyema.

SUGGESTED READINGS

Avansino JR, Goldman B, Sawin RS, et al. Primary operative versus nonoperative therapy for pediatric empyema: a meta-analysis. *Pediatrics* 2005;115:1652–1659.

Black SB, Shinefield HR, Ling S, et al. Effectiveness of heptavalent pneumococcal conjugate vaccine in children younger than five years of age for prevention of pneumonia. *Pediatr Infect Dis J* 2002;21:810–815.

British Thoracic Society Guidelines for the Management of Community Acquired Pneumonia in Childhood. *Thorax* 2002;57:s1–24.

Dowell SF, Jupronis BA, Zell ER, et al. Mortality from pneumonia in children in the United States, 1939 through 1996. *N Engl J Med* 2000;342:1399–1407.

Grijalva CG, Nuorti JP, Arbogast PG, et al. Decline in pneumonia admissions after routine childhood immunization with pneumococcal conjugate vaccine in the USA: a time-series analysis. *Lancet* 2007;369:1179–1186.

Raty R, Ronkko E, Kleemola M. Sample type is crucial to the diagnosis of *Mycoplasma pneumoniae* pneumonia by PCR. *J Med Microbiol* 2005;54:287–291.

Seizures

DARRYL R. MORRIS AND DAVID A. HSU

THE PATIENT ENCOUNTER

Last night you admitted a 9-month-old previously healthy baby girl with fever, vomiting, and dehydration. During morning rounds, you are paged by the baby's nurse, who says that the baby is seizing. You arrive to the room and notice that the baby is having a generalized tonic–clonic seizure. The nurse informs you that she had a fever of 39.4°C (103°F) 15 minutes before the seizure began, and that the baby has been seizing nonstop for the past 5 minutes.

OVERVIEW

Seizures are common phenomena of childhood and are a frequent cause of visits to the pediatric emergency department and hospitalizations. This chapter focuses on the acute management of seizures in the hospital setting: status epilepticus, seizures with fever, febrile seizures, neonatal seizures, and infantile spasms.

Definition

Febrile seizures are those in which the child has a fever, usually ≤39°C (102.2°F), before or at the time of the seizure but without evidence of central nervous system (CNS) infection or underlying epilepsy. The usual age range for febrile seizures is 6 months to 5 years. Seizure with fever that begins >5 years of age is likely to be a manifestation of epilepsy and not a febrile seizure. **Simple febrile seizures** are generalized tonic–clonic seizures, lasting ≤15 minutes, and occur only once in a 24-hour period. A **complex febrile seizure** is a seizure with fever that is focal, lasts >15 minutes, or is associated with one or more additional seizures within 24 hours after the initial seizure.

Status epilepticus describes either a single prolonged seizure or multiple consecutive seizures without return of normal consciousness with a total duration of ≤30 minutes. Status epilepticus is associated with significant morbidity and mortality and is a medical emergency.

Younger children are more likely to suffer long-term sequelae of status epilepticus, such as epilepsy, brain injury, and developmental delay. The prognosis depends upon the etiology of status epilepticus.

Neonatal seizures occur in infants ≤28 days of age. Seizures in neonates should raise the suspicion of underlying brain pathology. Because of their immature CNS myelination, neonates who seize do not typically develop generalized tonic–clonic activity.

Infantile spasm, also known as **West syndrome,** is the most common of the catastrophic epilepsy syndromes. The age of onset is between 3 and 8 months of age. The spasms consist of brief, repetitive flexor or extensor contractions of the extremities, head, or trunk that are usually bilateral. These contractions can occur in clusters often throughout the day and are most frequent with drowsiness or on awakening from sleep. They can resemble but are distinct from myoclonic or tonic seizures. West syndrome consists of a triad of infantile spasms, psychomotor retardation, and hypsarrhythmia, which is a characteristic finding on electroencephalography (EEG) and consists of a chaotic pattern of high-amplitude slow-wave activity with multifocal spikes.

Symptomatic infantile spasms are those with an identified etiology. The great majority of children with symptomatic infantile spasms do not develop normally. Sequelae include mental retardation, developmental disorders, epilepsy (especially Lennox–Gastaut syndrome), and death. Cryptogenic infantile spasms are associated with a better prognosis, although about half or more of these children eventually show some neurocognitive impairment.

Nonfebrile seizures in children are most commonly idiopathic but can be due to a wide variety of conditions. Important causes to consider include intracranial hemorrhage (which can be a sign of nonaccidental trauma), brain tumor, brain malformation (especially cortical dysplasias), hypoglycemia, hypocalcemia, hyponatremia, drug or toxin ingestion, ventriculoperitoneal shunt malfunction, or an inborn error of metabolism.

Pathophysiology

The pathophysiology of seizures is complex and multifactorial. Essentially, seizures result from an imbalance of the excitatory and inhibitory forces that act on cortical principal neurons in favor of excitation. Contributory factors include abnormalities in ion channels, extracellular ion homeostasis, energy metabolism, receptor function, transmitter uptake, and neural connectivity.

Epidemiology

Seizures in children can occur at any age but are more common in those <3 years of age. The lifetime risk of epilepsy is approximately 1%. However, 4% to 10% of children will have at least one seizure during childhood, with febrile seizures being the most common type.

After a first febrile seizure, the risk of recurrence of febrile seizures is 30%; the rate of recurrence is highest when the first febrile seizure occurs <12 months of age, with relatively low fevers, or in the context of a family history of febrile seizures. The recurrence risk of febrile seizures is 70% if all four risk factors are present. There is a slightly increased risk of epilepsy in children with febrile seizures (2% to 4%), with an additional increased risk in those with a history of complex febrile seizures, a developmental delay, or a family history of epilepsy. The risk of epilepsy rises to 20% to 50% if all risk factors are present.

Etiology

Febrile seizures are most often associated with routine childhood illnesses, such as otitis media, viral syndromes, and viral or bacterial gastroenteritis. *Shigella* enteritis is classically associated with febrile seizure. Viruses commonly associated with febrile seizures include influenza, parainfluenza, respiratory syncytial virus (RSV), rotavirus, adenovirus, and human herpesvirus 6 (HHV-6).

In children, status epilepticus is most often precipitated by fever or infection, but it can also be caused by traumatic or hypoxic brain injury, brain malformations and tumors, electrolyte abnormalities, metabolic disorders, or underlying epilepsy. A child with a seizure lasting ≥10 minutes or who has three or more tonic–clonic seizures within a 24-hour period is at risk of developing status epilepticus.

The most common cause of neonatal seizures is hypoxic–ischemic encephalopathy, which can occur as early as the first 24 hours of life. Other etiologies include intracranial hemorrhage; CNS infection, including herpes simplex virus encephalitis; brain malformations; inborn errors of metabolism; hypoglycemia; and electrolyte abnormalities. A rare cause of early-onset neonatal seizures is pyridoxine deficiency, which should be considered if the seizures do not respond to conventional anticonvulsant treatment.

Most infantile spasms are symptomatic (85% to 90%), with etiologies such as a prior history of hypoxic–ischemic encephalopathy, CNS infection, intracerebral hemorrhage, or brain malformations. Any genetic or metabolic disorder that affects the brain can also cause infantile spasms.

ACUTE MANAGEMENT AND WORKUP

If the patient is having a seizure, begin emergency management immediately.

The First 15 Minutes

For an actively seizing child, as for any critically ill child, the ABCs (airway, breathing, and circulation) are the most important first steps in management. Prolonged seizures are associated with hypoxia, which can lead to significant complications if not addressed promptly. In addition, many of the antiepileptic drugs are respiratory depressants, and apnea or respiratory failure can occur after repeated doses. Children should be placed on supplemental oxygen, and the physician should be ready to perform endotracheal intubation if the child develops respiratory insufficiency. For an ongoing seizure, intravenous access should be rapidly obtained.

TABLE 35-1

Antiepileptic Drugs Commonly Used in the Initial Management of Seizures

Medication	Dose	Maximum Cumulative Dose	Notes
Lorazepam (Ativan)	0.05–0.1 mg/kg IV	4 mg/dose	May repeat once in 10 min
Diazepam (Valium)	0.2–0.5 mg/kg IV (1 mo–12 yr) 5–10 mg IV (>12 yr)	5 mg (1 mo–5 yr) 10 mg (5–12 yr) 30 mg (>12 yr)	May repeat once in 10 min; avoid use in neonates; short antiepileptic effect (20–30 min)
Diazepam (Diastat)	0.5 mg/kg PR (2–5 yr) 0.3 mg/kg PR (6–11 yr) 0.2 mg/kg PR (>11 yr)		Can be used if IV access cannot be rapidly obtained

The next goal is to stop the seizure. The preferred initial antiepileptic drug is a benzodiazepine—in particular, lorazepam (Table 35-1). If intravenous (IV) access cannot be immediately obtained, diazepam can also be administered rectally. If the seizure does not stop after two doses of a benzodiazepine, the child should be loaded with an anticonvulsant intravenously. Table 35-2 describes these anticonvulsant drugs, including fosphenytoin (which is preferred over phenytoin because it can be administered more rapidly), phenobarbital, valproic acid, and levetiracetam.

The First Few Hours

If the seizure does not stop after an IV benzodiazepine plus one or two subsequent IV anticonvulsant drugs, you should consider intubation and putting the child into a pharmacologically induced coma. The usual agents are continuous pentobarbital, midazolam, or propofol. Propofol is used with care in pediatrics because of the risk of metabolic acidosis, particularly with prolonged use.

TABLE 35-2

Anticonvulsant Drugs Available in Intravenous Form

Medication	Loading Dose	Maintenance Dose	Notes
Phenytoin (Dilantin)	20 mg/kg IV	5 mg/kg/day PO/IV divided bid	Adjust dose based on levels
Fosphenytoin (Cerebyx)	20 mg PE/kg IV	5 mg PE/kg/day IV divided bid–tid; Max: 3 mg PE/kg/min to 150 mg PE/min IV	Begin maintenance dose 12 hr after loading dose
Phenobarbital (Luminal)	20 mg/kg IV	5 mg/kg qd–bid	May give load 10 mg/kg at a time; watch for respiratory depression; begin maintenance dose 12 hr after loading dose; adjust dose based on levels
Valproic acid (Depakene)	20 mg/kg IV bid–tid	Max 60 mg/kg/day	Use with caution in children <2 yr of age owing to risk of hepatotoxicity
Levetiracetam (Keppra)	20 mg/kg IV	Max 20–60 mg/kg loading dose, then divided bid	May give 20 mg/kg boluses as needed

PE, phenytoin sodium equivalents.

After the seizure has stopped and the child is stable from a respiratory standpoint, you should seek an etiology for the seizure. For a simple febrile seizure with a clear focus of infection, such as otitis media or gastroenteritis, and if the mental status is appropriate for the patient's age (i.e., the baby is alert, interactive, and shows appropriate interest in parents and feeding), no additional workup is necessary.

History

The history provided by the parents is an essential guide to the evaluation of any seizure. A history of persistent poor feeding and growth associated with vomiting, lethargy, an altered level of consciousness, and apnea is suggestive of an inborn error of metabolism. Severe headache with vomiting or focal neurologic signs, such as ataxia or changes in behavior, raises concern for a CNS process such as a brain tumor or an intracranial hemorrhage. A history of accidental or intentional medication or drug ingestion is suggestive of a toxigenic seizure.

Physical Examination

A seizure with fever can be a sign of a CNS infection. The child may have findings on examination supportive of CNS infection, such as an altered mental status, meningismus, or a telltale rash; however, exam findings are less reliable in infants, especially those <3 months of age. In addition to a thorough neurologic exam, patients should be examined for stigmata of the underlying syndromes or disorders that may be associated with seizures.

Labs and Tests to Consider

Children with simple febrile seizures may not require any laboratory tests. Children <18 months of age are more difficult to assess for the presence or absence of signs of meningitis and, therefore, may warrant lumbar puncture even in the absence of specific signs of meningitis. For a first nonfebrile seizure, laboratory tests should be ordered based on individual clinical circumstances such as vomiting, diarrhea, dehydration, or failure to return to baseline alertness. A toxicology screen should be considered for those children with a question of drug exposure or abuse.

Key Diagnostic Labs and Tests

Children with complex febrile seizures, status epilepticus, or neonatal seizures should receive a more extensive workup. Initial labs should include a basic metabolic panel, a measure of calcium and magnesium levels, a complete blood cell count, and a blood culture. Other labs to consider include antiepileptic drug levels for children who have epilepsy, urinalysis and urine culture for young children with fever, blood and urine toxicology screens if ingestion is suspected, and ammonia and liver function tests. If the history, physical examination, or initial laboratory studies are suggestive of an inborn error of metabolism, your workup should also include serum lactate and pyruvate, plasma amino acids, urine organic acids, free and total carnitines, plasma acylcarnitine profile, and a blood gas. Children with infantile spasms should receive these metabolic screens as well as high-resolution chromosome analysis.

If CNS infection is suspected on the basis of the physical exam or history, or in a young infant when the physical examination is not felt to be reliable, a lumbar puncture for cerebrospinal fluid (CSF) analysis should be performed.

An EEG is recommended after a first nonfebrile seizure and for all infants with new-onset neonatal seizures or infantile spasms. It should be considered for children with status epilepticus and for patients with complex febrile seizures. An EEG is generally not necessary in the acute setting for children with a simple febrile seizure, bacterial meningitis, or patients with a known history of epilepsy. For children admitted to the hospital, the EEG ideally should be obtained within the first 24 to 48 hours after the seizure to improve the yield of diagnostic findings.

Imaging

For a brief nonfebrile or simple febrile seizure in a child with a normal prior history and a normal current physical examination, neuroimaging is not indicated in the acute setting. Neuroimaging is indicated for suspected CNS infection, unexplained status epilepticus, persistent focal neurologic signs, or a persistently altered mental status. A computed tomography (CT) scan of the head is acceptable in this setting. Magnetic resonance imaging (MRI) of the brain is recommended for the workup of infantile spasms and for focal seizures or focal EEG findings; this study can be deferred to the subacute setting if the child is otherwise stable.

CLINICAL PEARL

Children with sickle cell anemia and those undergoing treatment for cancer should always receive a brain MRI with a first seizure because of the high risk of stroke in sickle cell disease and the risk of CNS complications in children undergoing chemotherapy.

The infant in the case presentation had spontaneous resolution of her seizure after 10 minutes. A lumbar puncture was performed because her young age and irritability in the context of fever made it difficult to exclude the possibility of meningitis solely based on physician examination. Her CSF had only one white blood cell per cubic millimeter; the CSF culture was subsequently negative.

Treatment

Patients who have been stabilized and admitted to an inpatient unit should be placed on seizure precautions (padded side rails, bag-mask apparatus at bedside, and frequent neurologic checks). Children who have had a cluster of seizures or a single prolonged seizure and those who had cyanosis or respiratory depression and who are still postictal need cardiorespiratory monitoring and IV access.

The decision about whether to continue antiepileptic drugs after the initial seizure has ended depends on the estimated risk of seizure recurrence. A rough rule of thumb is that children who have had two or more unprovoked seizures need to start maintenance antiepileptic drugs.

Admission Criteria and Level-of-Care Criteria

Children with a first nonfebrile seizure or simple febrile seizure generally do not need to be admitted to the hospital if there is no evidence of CNS infection and the child is clinically well after the seizure, with no focal neurologic signs or altered mental status. All infants <1 month of age and young infants (<3 months) with seizure and fever generally require admission to the hospital. Children with complex febrile seizures, new-onset neonatal seizures, focal deficits or altered mental status, CNS infection, or those in status epilepticus generally require admission to the hospital. Patients who need management in an intensive care unit include those who develop significant respiratory compromise or those with refractory status epilepticus.

EXTENDED IN-HOSPITAL MANAGEMENT

Consultation with a pediatric neurologist is recommended for children with infantile spasms, neonatal seizures, status epilepticus, and atypical febrile seizures. If an inborn error of metabolism or a genetic disorder is suspected, consultation with a geneticist may also be considered. The management of CNS infection often necessitates consultation with an infectious disease specialist.

DISPOSITION

Discharge Goals

The patient may be discharged once seizures are under control, the patient is able to tolerate oral antiepileptic drugs (if required) without difficulty, and relevant cultures and tests for infectious agents are known.

Outpatient Care

Follow-up with the child's pediatrician or family practitioner within 72 hours after discharge is recommended. Depending on the clinical scenario, follow-up with a pediatric neurologist and a geneticist may also be indicated. Communication between the hospital team and the primary care physician is essential to ensure continuity of care after discharge.

WHAT YOU NEED TO REMEMBER

- Seizures are common in childhood. Most are brief and self-limited with no long-term sequelae.
- Important etiologies to consider in the acute setting include bacterial meningitis, herpes simplex virus (HSV) encephalitis, trauma (including nonaccidental trauma), structural intracranial abnormalities, and metabolic disorders. The early recognition and management of children with these findings as well as children in status epilepticus is essential to prevent significant morbidity or mortality.

SUGGESTED READINGS

Beghi E. Management of a first seizure. General conclusions and recommendations. *Epilepsia* 2008;49(Suppl):58–61.

Blumstein MD, Friedman MJ. Childhood seizures. *Emerg Med Clin North Am* 2007; 25:1061–1086.

Major P, Thiele EA. Seizures in children: determining the variation. *Pediatr Rev* 2007;28:363–370.

Riviello JJ Jr, Ashwal S, Hirtz D, et al. Practice parameter: diagnostic assessment of the child with status epilepticus (an evidence-based review): Report of the Quality Standards Subcommittee of the American Academy of Neurology and the Practice Committee of the Child Neurology Society. *Neurology* 2006;67:1542–1550.

Sadleir LG, Scheffer IE. Febrile seizures. *BMJ* 2007;334:307–311.

Septic Arthritis

WENDALYN K. LITTLE AND JESSE J. STURM

THE PATIENT ENCOUNTER

A 15-month-old previously ambulatory infant presents with a 2-day history of a fever and an increasing refusal to bear weight on his right leg. The child is ill-appearing, with a temperature of 39.7°C (103.5°F), and is lying on the bed with his right hip externally rotated and slightly flexed. This is slightly warm and tender on palpation and exquisitely tender on attempts to rotate it.

OVERVIEW

Definition

Septic or suppurative arthritis is a serious bacterial infection within the articular capsule of the joint and presents a true surgical emergency. It must be differentiated from postinfectious joint effusions, which are sterile and attributable to antigen–antibody complex deposition. This chapter focuses on the important physical exam, history, and laboratory findings to differentiate these two processes.

Pathophysiology

Septic arthritis occurs by three primary mechanisms: (1) hematogenous dissemination of bacteria to the highly vascular synovium of the joint space, (2) contiguous spread from surrounding infected soft tissues, and (3) direct extension from osteomyelitis at the epiphysis into the neighboring joint space.

Pyogenic infection within the joint space causes increased pressure within the minimally distensible joint capsule, resulting in derangements in the vascular and lymphatic supply. These changes can compromise vascular flow and result in ischemic injury to the bone. Bacterial and leukocyte proliferation also occur, causing the release of proteolytic enzymes, which directly damage the intra-articular cartilage. Significant articular damage can occur within as little as 8 hours.

Eighty to ninety percent of septic joints occur in the lower extremities. The knee and the hip are the two most commonly affected joints. The hip is one of the few joints in the body in which the physis is intracapsular, allowing ready inoculation of the joint space from infection in the proximal femoral metaphysis. In >90% of cases, infections involve only a single joint. Infections at multiple joints are more common in neonates or in sexually active adolescents with disseminated *Neisseria gonorrhoeae* infection.

Epidemiology

The epidemiology of septic arthritis of the hip is not well defined, but an early peak appears to occur in the first months of infancy, with an overall average age of 3 to 6 years. Males and females seem to be at approximately equivalent risk. The annual incidence in children ranges from 5 to 37 cases per 100,000.

Etiology

The organisms responsible for septic arthritis are typically those that also cause osteomyelitis. *Staphylococcus aureus* is the most commonly involved organism. *Haemophilus influenzae* type b, once a leading cause of septic arthritis, rarely occurs in immunized children. Group A *Streptococcus* and *Streptococcus pneumoniae* are now increasingly common causes of septic arthritis in children. Other bacterial causes include group B *Streptococcus* and gram-negative enteric bacteria in neonates, *N. gonorrhoeae* in sexually active adolescents, and *Salmonella* in patients with sickle cell disease. *Kingella kingae*, a gram-negative rod, has been isolated as a cause of pediatric bone and joint infections.

Community-acquired methicillin-resistant *S. aureus* (Ca-MRSA) has increasingly been documented as a cause of septic arthritis, with some recent evidence that it now accounts for ≥40% of all bone and joint infections in children.

ACUTE MANAGEMENT AND WORKUP

The acute management and workup should attempt to differentiate septic arthritis from other causes of acute joint inflammation, such as trauma or transient synovitis of the hip. Transient synovitis is a self-limited process that typically occurs after a viral illness. It may be difficult to differentiate from septic arthritis but it is important to do so because untreated septic arthritis may progress rapidly and cause permanent joint damage.

The First 15 Minutes

For a child who appears septic or "toxic," perform a quick, focused history and physical evaluation with special attention to matters of airway, breathing, and circulation. Patients with septic arthritis may present with signs and symptoms of septic shock, necessitating immediate stabilization. In a less ill-appearing child, consider providing appropriate analgesia, which may ensure a more cooperative patient and therefore a more revealing physical examination.

The First Few Hours

A thorough history and physical examination and judicious use of laboratory and imaging studies are crucial for arriving at an appropriate diagnosis and treatment plan. Early consultation with an orthopedic surgeon should be considered in cases of suspected septic arthritis.

History

Children with septic arthritis generally present with a history of fever and joint pain. If the affected joint is in the lower extremity, the patient may have a limp or may refuse to bear weight. Young infants may present with only fever and increased irritability, especially during routine handling for diaper changes or bathing. The presence or absence of trauma may be misleading; young children frequently fall during running or play; seemingly minor trauma may also predispose to the development of joint infections.

Physical Examination

Patients with septic arthritis are often febrile and ill-appearing. Pain and muscle spasm often lead to a "pseudoparalysis" of the affected joint; the patient will tend to hold the joint in the position that maximizes the intra-articular space and therefore decreases the pressure within it. A red, hot, swollen, and tender joint is the hallmark finding in septic arthritis. For smaller joints such as the knee, elbow, wrist, or ankle, these findings should arouse a strong suspicion for an intra-articular infection. The most common site of septic arthritis in children, however, is the hip, and these telltale signs of infection may be difficult or impossible to detect in that location. A child with septic arthritis of the hip will typically lie with the leg flexed and externally rotated at the hip. He or she will generally refuse active movement or weight bearing on the affected extremity and may resist attempts at passive movement of the joint.

Labs and Tests to Consider

Laboratory tests and imaging studies may help differentiate septic arthritis from other causes of joint inflammation, such as transient synovitis of the hip.

Key Diagnostic Labs and Tests

Blood cultures should be obtained in all patients suspected of having septic arthritis. Although blood cultures are positive in <50% of patients with septic arthritis, a positive result may help guide antibiotic therapy. Sexually active patients should be evaluated for possible gonococcal infection by culture or polymerase chain reaction (PCR). Laboratory studies in children with hip pain and normal radiographs may help differentiate septic arthritis from self-limited causes of inflammation, such as transient synovitis. An elevated peripheral white blood cell (WBC) count may suggest septic arthritis but is generally a poor test for differentiating septic arthritis from other causes of joint inflammation. Several studies have examined the utility of C-reactive protein (CRP) and the erythrocyte sedimentation rate (ESR) in differentiating infectious from noninfectious causes of joint pain. Although no single laboratory test or value has been found to definitively diagnose septic arthritis, abnormalities of WBC, CRP, and ESR values may identify those patients who warrant more aggressive evaluation for suspected joint infection.

If a high suspicion for septic arthritis exists based on clinical and/or laboratory and imaging data, diagnostic aspiration of the joint should be performed. This may be accomplished in the ER or clinic setting for smaller joints such as the knee. Children with septic arthritis of the hip may require ultrasound-guided joint aspiration. The synovial fluid should be inspected for general appearance and sent for laboratory evaluation. Cloudy, purulent-appearing fluid suggests bacterial infection. An elevated joint fluid WBC count, low glucose content (compared with serum), and the presence of bacteria on the Gram stain all suggest septic arthritis. Joint fluid should also be cultured; pretreatment with antibiotics or the presence of a fastidious organism may lead to negative cultures, but a positive culture will be very useful in guiding antibiotic therapy. Early consultation with an orthopedic specialist is needed in suspected cases of septic arthritis to assist with diagnosis and treatment.

CLINICAL PEARL

Inoculating joint fluid into a blood culture bottle (rather than culturing on conventional blood agar plates) will increase the likelihood of detecting fastidious pathogens such as K. kingae.

Imaging

Patients presenting with joint pain or a limp should have plain radiographs of the affected joint, and consideration should be given to imaging the contralateral joint for comparison. Plain radiographs may initially be normal in septic arthritis or may show only an effusion. Later in the course of the illness, radiographic evidence of bone and joint destruction may become apparent. In patients with hip pain and normal radiographs, ultrasound may be useful for detecting joint effusions, although it cannot differentiate infectious from noninfectious causes. Computed tomography (CT) and magnetic resonance imaging (MRI) are more sensitive than plain radiographs for demonstrating bone and joint abnormalities, but definitive management of septic arthritis should not be significantly delayed in order to obtain imaging.

Treatment

The flexed and externally rotated position of the hip of the child in the case presentation suggested the presence of a moderate amount of joint fluid. Ultrasound-guided needle aspiration of joint fluid was performed. The white blood cells were at $95,000/mm^3$, a value consistent with bacterial arthritis. The child was taken to the operating room for open drainage several hours later.

The treatment of septic arthritis involves surgical drainage and/or debridement as well as appropriate antibiotic therapy. Surgical drainage may be accomplished through closed-needle aspiration in smaller joints, but arthroscopy or open drainage may be necessary for larger joints such as the knee or hip.

Initial antibiotic therapy should be broad-spectrum and should be chosen to cover the most likely pathogens. Historically, antistaphylococcal penicillins (such as oxacillin or nafcillin) or cephalosporins were used to treat staphylococcal infection. The emergence of Ca-MRSA as a leading cause of septic arthritis warrants using clindamycin or vancomycin as first-line treatment for septic arthritis pending culture results. Linezolid also has good activity against MRSA and may be considered for MRSA joint infections. All patients with septic arthritis should receive antibiotic therapy effective against staphylococcal infections. Additional therapy such as cefotaxime or ceftriaxone should be considered in neonates against gram-negative enteric organisms, in adolescents against *N. gonorrhea*, and in patients with sickle cell disease against *Salmonella* spp. Results of blood and/or synovial fluid cultures may help in guiding antibiotic therapy.

ADMISSION CRITERIA AND LEVEL-OF-CARE CRITERIA

Extended In-Hospital Management

Children with septic arthritis often require operative drainage of the affected joint as well as close monitoring of their clinical status and laboratory values. Appropriate analgesia should be provided. Patients with involvement of smaller joints, including the knee, may be treated with sequential intravenous–oral therapy. Patients with septic arthritis of the hip will require intravenous antibiotic therapy. These patients will require a week or more of parenteral antibiotics and may require placement of a peripherally inserted central catheter or other semipermanent intravenous access for parenteral antibiotics both in the hospital and after discharge home.

DISPOSITION

Discharge Goals

Consider discharge when the patient is clinically improved and has regained a nearly normal degree of joint mobility. Look for a downward trend in the white blood cell count, the CRP, and the ESR, as well as a negative blood culture to document clearance of bacteremia.

Current recommendations and consensus guidelines recommend ≤3 weeks of antibiotics, with at least the first week's treatment delivered parenterally. Consideration may then be given to transitioning to an appropriate oral antibiotic (for patients who do not have septic arthritis of the hip); however, therapy should be continued until ESR/CRP levels and clinical symptoms normalize.

Outpatient Care

After discharge from the hospital, patients should have a follow-up visit with their pediatrician within 2 to 3 days. Any episodes of fever or recurrent joint symptoms should be evaluated promptly with a repeat physical exam and laboratory studies, including ESR, CRP, and WBC.

WHAT YOU NEED TO REMEMBER

- Patients with septic arthritis of the hip will maintain the joint in a flexed, externally rotated position to maximize the joint space volume and minimize pain.
- The CRP and ESR are elevated at presentation in most patients with septic arthritis.
- Patients with involvement of small joints, such as the ankle or knee, may be switched from an intravenous to an oral antibiotic regimen for completion of therapy.

SUGGESTED READINGS

Arnold SR, Elias D, Buckingham SC, et al. Changing patterns of acute hematogenous osteomyelitis and septic arthritis: emergence of community-associated methicillin-resistant *Staphylococcus aureus*. *J Pediatr Orthop* 2006;26:703–708.

Chen CJ, Chiu CH, Lin TY, et al. Experience with linezolid therapy in children with osteoarticular infections. *Pediatr Infect Dis J* 2007;26:985–988.

Fleischer G, Ludwig S, Henretig FM. *Pediatric Emergency Medicine*, 5th ed. Philadelphia: Lippincott Williams & Wilkins, 2006:828–829.

Garcia-De La Torre I. Advances in the management of septic arthritis. *Infect Dis Clin North Am* 2006;20:773–788.

Kocher MS, Zurakowski D, Kasser JR. differentiating between septic arthritis and transient synovitis of the hip in children: an evidence-based clinical prediction algorithm. *J Bone Joint Surg* 1999;81:1662–1670.

37

Sickle Cell Disease

SHER LYNN GARDNER

THE PATIENT ENCOUNTER

A 6-year-old girl with known sickle cell disease presented to the pediatric emergency department with a 2-day history of runny nose, cough, and chest pain. She was given pain relievers at home without improvement of her chest pain. She had developed a fever at home earlier that day and was found to have a temperature of 38.9°C (102°F) in the emergency department. On examination, she appeared ill but not toxic. She had a respiratory rate of 35 breaths per minute and was taking shallow breaths secondary to the chest pain. Her breath sounds were decreased on the right in the middle and lower segments.

OVERVIEW

Definition

Sickle cell disease (SCD) is an autosomal recessive group of hemoglobin disorders in which sickle hemoglobin chains predominate. Normal hemoglobin is termed Hgb A (adult). Homozygous sickle cell disease (Hgb SS) is the most common; other common genotypes include Hgb SC and Hgb Sβ thalassemia. The complications of SCD are numerous, but this chapter focuses on the following: (i) anemia, (ii) pain crises, (iii) bacteremia and sepsis, (iv) acute chest syndrome, and (v) splenic sequestration. Priapism and cerebrovascular accidents are also potential complications of SCD but are beyond the scope of this chapter.

Pathophysiology

The abnormal hemoglobin leaves the erythrocyte vulnerable to destruction. Consequently, in SCD, the erythrocytes are destroyed prematurely, resulting in a chronic anemia.

Low oxygen tension results in polymerization of the abnormal hemoglobin chains. This polymerization distorts the shape of the red blood cells into a "sickle" shape. These sickle-shaped red cells do not move smoothly through the body's microvasculature and can be lodged in these spaces. The red cells also become adherent to the endothelial lining of these blood vessels, resulting in microvascular occlusions. The occlusive events result in significant pain. These events are called "pain crises." Such a crisis is the most frequent manifestation of SCD and can occur in any part of the body (1).

Young children with SCD have altered splenic function. The spleens of these patients have markedly reduced phagocytic and reticuloendothelial functions. This makes them more susceptible to infections with encapsulated organisms, most specifically pneumococci.

Acute chest syndrome (ACS) describes acute pulmonary disease in SCD. ACS occurs when any inciting agent (atelectasis, infection, inflammation, bronchospasm, etc.) causes deoxygenation and polymerization of the abnormal hemoglobin in the microvasculature of the lungs; it leads to a new pulmonary infiltrate on chest x-ray plus one or more of the following: hypoxia, changes on pulmonary auscultation, chest pain, increased work of breathing, or fever. It is the second most common cause of hospitalization in this population (behind vaso-occlusive crisis) and also the most common cause of death (2).

Splenic sequestration occurs as a result of vaso-occlusion in the spleen. This leads to pooling of blood in the spleen with resultant splenic enlargement. When severe, it can lead to severe anemia and hypovolemic shock. Splenic sequestration is more common in younger children whose spleens have not yet undergone the autoinfarction and fibrosis that typically occurs over time in older children with SCD.

Epidemiology

SCD affects millions of people worldwide. It most commonly occurs in people of sub-Saharan African descent as well as others of South American, Central American, Saudi Arabian, Indian, and Mediterranean descent. In the United States, it affects about 72,000 people, most of them African American. It occurs in about 1 in 500 African American births and in 1 in 1,000 to 1,400 Hispanic American births. About 1 in 12 African Americans carry the sickle cell trait (3).

Etiology

SCD is a genetic disorder affecting chromosome 11 and is due to substitution of a single amino acid (valine for glutamic acid) in the sixth position of the beta chain of hemoglobin (3).

ACUTE MANAGEMENT AND WORKUP

The acute management and workup of children with clinical manifestations of SCD can help differentiate those children who can be managed as outpatients and those who require hospitalization for prolonged treatment.

The First 15 Minutes

First, assess the overall appearance of the patient. In patients with fever or ACS, lab specimens should be drawn quickly and antibiotics administered urgently. For children with ACS, immediately assess for the work of breathing and hypoxia. Supplemental oxygen should be administered to a hypoxic patient. A child with significant splenic enlargement should initially be assessed for evidence of shock, including hypotension, cool extremities, prolonged capillary refill, tachycardia, and a history of decreased urine output.

The First Few Hours

A full history and physical examination are important in the first few hours to better assess the degree of illness and develop a more comprehensive medical plan.

History

Children with severe anemia may complain only of being tired or weak. The parents may state that the child is sleeping more or just has a decreased activity level.

Patients who present with vaso-occlusive crisis will simply complain of pain, which can be located anywhere. In some, the pain will have a predilection for one or two areas of the body. These children may have taken some pain medications at home prior to presentation with little or no improvement in symptoms. Many children are admitted multiple times for pain crises and others will have very few admissions.

The source of fever in a patient with SCD is not necessarily different from that in other children. Those with possible pneumonia will have increased work of breathing, cough, fatigue, and, at times, abdominal pain. Osteomyelitis and cellulitis can present with pain in the affected area. Patients will occasionally report edema or erythema in such cases. Children with urinary tract infections typically have abdominal or flank pain accompanying their fever. Some patients also complain of dysuria. Children with SCD and a general viral illness will have constitutional symptoms (fever, malaise, aches, chills).

Children with SCD who present with ACS typically have fever, cough, increased work of breathing, and occasionally abdominal complaints secondary to referred pain from a basilar pulmonary process. These children may also complain of chest pain either at baseline or pain increases with respirations.

Patients who present with an enlarged spleen due to splenic sequestration usually complain of abdominal pain.

Physical Examination

A child with severe anemia may appear pale. Pallor can be difficult to assess in darker-skinned individuals, but patients' palms and soles as well as oral mucosa and conjunctiva can be used in its evaluation. Severe anemia also leads to tachycardia with a hyperdynamic precordium secondary to cardiac compensatory mechanisms.

Patients with SCD who have fever may appear uncomfortable. They may be tachycardic and or tachypneic. Other physical manifestations will depend on the actual cause of the fever.

A child with a significant vaso-occlusive crisis generally appears quite uncomfortable. With severe pain, he or she may be lying perfectly still in order to minimize pain associated with movement. Such a child can, however, look relatively comfortable but be in significant pain. A patient with a vaso-occlusive crisis may have tenderness to touch in the affected area(s), but this is not always the case.

Patients who exhibit the clinical manifestation of ACS also appear generally ill. These patients are usually febrile can have labored breathing; they may have intercostal and subcostal as well as supraclavicular retractions. They may also have nasal flaring and grunting. Upon auscultation, decreased breath sounds over the affected lung field(s) can be heard. Tubular breath sounds may also be heard and indicate an increased severity of consolidation.

Patients with splenic sequestration may be well- or ill-appearing. They may have pallor if the degree of sequestration is severe, with resultant increased anemia. The spleen will be palpable on exam. A careful technique should be used in palpating the spleen. It is important to begin palpation at the right iliac crest and work upward until the edge of the spleen is felt. Many patients with splenic sequestration may also have an enlarged liver.

CLINICAL PEARL

A markedly enlarged spleen (with extension into the pelvis) may go undetected if you begin palpation in the left upper quadrant rather than the right iliac crest.

Dactylitis, a common manifestation of vaso-occlusive crises in young children with homozygous sickle cell disease, manifests with painful swelling of the hands or feet.

Labs and Tests to Consider

Careful selection and diligent follow-up on labs and x-rays are essential in the comprehensive assessment of patients with clinical manifestations of SCD. Along with a careful history and physical, labs are helpful in determining the degree of illness and the need for additional or more intensive intervention.

Key Diagnostic Labs and Tests

A complete blood count with differential help determine the degree of anemia (relative to baseline) for symptomatic children with SCD. The hemoglobin and hematocrit levels can be low during any manifestation of illness in these children. The cell counts of patients with splenic sequestration can fall rapidly and should be followed carefully. Reticulocyte counts are used to evaluate whether the patient's bone marrow is producing an appropriate number of red cell precursors in response to the degree of anemia. If the reticulocyte count is inappropriately low (i.e., <1%), suspect an aplastic crisis and draw parvovirus B19 titers.

Obtain blood cultures from any febrile child with SCD. Repeat cultures may be necessary in a persistently febrile patient. When osteomyelitis is suspected, a baseline C-reactive protein can be helpful in objectively tracking resolution of the infection. A bone biopsy may sometimes be necessary when there is no clinical response to treatment. *Salmonella* is a common cause of osteomyelitis in this patient population.

Imaging

A chest x-ray is used to diagnose ACS. Lobar patterns suggest bacterial causes such as *Streptococcus pneumoniae* or *Staphylococcus aureus*. A more diffuse pattern is consistent with viral pneumonia. Infection with *Mycoplasma pneumoniae* may be lobar or more diffuse.

Plain radiographs can be helpful in diagnosing avascular necrosis of the femoral and/or humeral head, which can occur in patients with SCD. However, magnetic resonance imaging (MRI) is more sensitive than plain films, especially in the early stages of avascular necrosis. MRI can also be helpful in confirming a diagnosis of osteomyelitis. Bone scans are not helpful in this setting as they will "light up" secondary to the pain crisis itself.

Treatment

The child in the case presentation had fever, tachypnea, and an abnormal lung examination. Chest x-ray revealed right-middle- and right-lower-lobe infiltrates, suggesting ACS precipitated by pneumonia. She was treated with azithromycin and ampicillin. A summary of common treatment options for children with clinical manifestations of SCD is given in Table 37-1. Pain control is also a critical element of managing the complications associated with sickle cell disease. A continuous narcotic infusion with additional patient-administered "bolus" medications (i.e., patient-controlled analgesia) as needed is the preferred management strategy for most school-age children with pain associated with sickle cell disease.

Admission Criteria and Level-of-Care Criteria

Patients with SCD with vasoocclusive crises should be admitted if their pain is not adequately controlled after outpatient and emergency department management. All younger children (those ≤5 years of age) with fever,

TABLE 37-1

Summary of Treatment Options for Children with Clinical Manifestations of Sickle Cell Disease

Clinical Manifestation	Treatment Options
Severe anemia	Blood transfusion
Vasoocclusive crisis	Opioid (morphine, fentanyl, nalbuphine) and NSAIDs (ketorolac, ibuprofen) work synergistically. Use a stool softener and an H2 blocker to counteract side effects. Administer IVFs at 1¼ times the maintenance rate.
Bacteremia	Third-generation cephalosporin and vancomycin. Be prepared to respond to shock (IVFs and pressors).
Acute chest syndrome	Ampicillin or third-generation cephalosporin in combination with azithromycin. Supplemental oxygen if needed, with added positive-pressure device. Use caution when giving IVFs, which can cause pulmonary edema and worsen the clinical picture. Start with three quarters of the maintenance fluid rate.
Splenic sequestration	IVFs at 1¼ times the maintenance rate to attempt to liberate some red cells from the spleen. With persistently falling red cell counts, clinical symptoms, and continued enlargement of the spleen, transfuse with packed RBCs (give slowly).

IVFs, intravenous fluids

severely anemic patients, and children with ACS should be admitted to the inpatient service. Patients who have rapidly enlarging spleens and falling blood counts should also be admitted for inpatient management. These patients can usually be managed safely on a general pediatric or hematology service. Any acute decompensation (e.g., respiratory distress, hypoxia not responding to supplemental oxygen, falling blood pressure) warrants immediate transfer to an intensive care unit.

EXTENDED INHOSPITAL MANAGEMENT

Patients with refractory vaso-occlusive crises often warrant longer hospital stays. At times, patient-controlled analgesia is needed when scheduled pain medications do not adequately control and improve the pain crisis. Child-life specialists can play a vital role in helping these patients cope with their pain. Child psychiatry is also instrumental in offering the patients adjunct therapies when dealing with chronic pain.

Patients with ACS who have complications may warrant longer stays as well, especially if they develop an effusion and/or empyema. Most bacteremic and all septic children should complete a full course of antibiotics as inpatients.

DISPOSITION

Discharge Goals

Children with severe anemia are ready for discharge after transfusion if their hemoglobin has returned to the desired level and they are no longer symptomatic (e.g., tachycardia has resolved). Patients with vaso-occlusive crises are ready for discharge once their pain has resolved or is adequately treated with oral medications. A patient with fever is ready for discharge once blood cultures are negative at 48 hours, the patient is afebrile for 24 hours, and the patient is eating and/or drinking well. Children with ACS are ready for discharge once they are no longer hypoxic, have an easy work of breathing, breath sounds have improved, and chest pain has resolved. A follow-up chest x-ray is unnecessary if the clinical picture is reassuring. A patient with splenic sequestration is ready for discharge once spleen size has decreased, cell counts have normalized, and clinical symptoms have improved.

Outpatient Care

Upon discharge from the hospital, follow-up with the patient's primary care physician should be scheduled within a week. Patients with fever and negative blood cultures require no medications other than their routine penicillin and folic acid. Those with pneumonia or other bacterial infections will require antibiotic therapy to complete the prescribed course. Children with vaso-occlusive crises will require home pain mediation management (usually acetaminophen with codeine and ibuprofen). Patients with ACS will require oral antibiotics to complete a prescribed course (usually 10 days except for azithromycin, which is 5 days). Children with splenic sequestration need only their routine penicillin and folic acid.

WHAT YOU NEED TO REMEMBER

- Fever, ACS, and severe anemia in children with SCD should be considered medical emergencies.
- Children with vaso-occlusive crises may appear to be healthy but may be in significant pain.
- Rapid but careful interventions for sickle cell complications can significantly reduce the rate of progression.

REFERENCES

1. Vichinsky E, Schrier S, Landaw S. Overview of the clinical manifestations of sickle cell disease February 4, 2008. Available at: www.uptodateonline.com/online/content/topic.
2. Heeney M, Mahoney D, Acute chest syndrome in children and adolescents with sickle cell disease. February 7, 2008. Available at: www.uptodateonline.com
3. National Institutes of Health. *Genetic Disease Profile: Sickle Cell Anemia*. NIH publication No. 96-4057. Available at: www.ornl.gov?sci/techresources/Human_Genome/posters/chromosome/sca.shtml.

SUGGESTED READINGS

Claster, S, Vichinsky EP. Managing sickle cell disease. *BMJ* 2003;327(7424):1151–1155.
Ellison AM, Shaw K. Management of vasoocclusive pain events in sickle cell disease. *Pediatr Emerg Care* 2007;23(11):832–841.

38
Skin and Skin Structure Infections

LINDSAY H. CHASE

THE PATIENT ENCOUNTER

A 2-year-old boy is taken to the emergency department (ED) by his parents for a spreading area of redness on his leg. His parents think it started with an insect bite. He was seen at his pediatrician's office 2 days prior and was started on cephalexin. Since then, the affected area has grown and has become more tender. In the ED, he is febrile to 39°C (102.2°F). Examination reveals an area of erythema and an induration on his right thigh; it is tender and warm to the touch.

OVERVIEW

Definition

Cellulitis is an acute infection of the skin. A variety of terms are used to further describe infections of the skin and skin structures. **Impetigo** is a superficial, intradermal infection that presents as vesiculopustular lesions. **Folliculitis** is inflammation and infection of the hair follicle. The term *furuncle* is also used to describe an infected hair follicle. When a group of follicles get infected and result in a painful deep mass, it is called a *carbuncle.* An **abscess** is a collection of pus in a cavity formed as a result of the body's immune response to infection or a foreign body. **Erysipelas** is an acute superficial skin infection involving the dermal lymphatics, usually caused by infection with group A streptococci. **Necrotizing fasciitis** is an infection of the deeper layers of skin and subcutaneous tissues that spreads across fascial planes within the subcutaneous tissue.

Pathophysiology

Often there is a break in the skin that serves as a portal of entry for bacteria. The bacteria trigger an immune inflammatory response that increases blood flow and white blood cell influx to the area. Inflammation of the dermis and subcutaneous tissues causes swelling, warmth, redness, and tenderness, the typical symptoms of cellulitis. The surrounding healthy tissue may wall off the infected area to keep the infection from spreading, which results in the formation of an abscess. Unfortunately, this allows the bacteria to continue to grow because antibiotic penetration into the abscess is limited. The bacteria may also produce toxins or virulence factors that lead to the rapid destruction of soft tissues, sometimes resulting in necrotizing fasciitis.

Epidemiology

Skin and soft tissue infections are a common reason for visits to pediatricians' offices, urgent care centers, and EDs. It is difficult to estimate a true incidence and prevalence because cellulitis is not a reportable condition.

Etiology

The most common causative organisms of cellulitis are *Staphylococcus aureus* and group A *Streptococcus*. Gram-negative bacteria, specifically *Aeromonas*, should be considered if there was soil or freshwater exposure. In immunocompromised individuals, rapidly progressing infection may be due to *Streptococcus pneumoniae*. Cellulitis in neonates may be due to group B streptococci. Animal bites may cause infections with *Pasteurella multocida* (cat bites) and *Capnocytophaga* spp. (dog bites). *Pseudomonas aeruginosa* may cause soft tissue infections of the foot after a puncture wound through a sneaker. Fasciitis is most commonly caused by group A *Streptococcus*. *Vibrio vulnificus*, *Clostridium perfringens*, and *Bacteroides fragilis* should also be considered as potential causes of necrotizing fasciitis.

ACUTE MANAGEMENT AND WORKUP

Most patients with skin infections can be treated with oral antibiotics in an outpatient setting; however, the acute management and workup identifies those patients with systemic signs of illness who require more aggressive and immediate treatment.

The First 15 Minutes

Assess the patient for the severity of illness and toxicity, because even a simple cellulitis can rapidly progress to toxic shock. If there are signs of toxic shock (tachycardia, low blood pressure, diffuse flushing, altered mental status), place an intravenous (IV) line, give a fluid bolus, and start antibiotics immediately.

The First Few Hours

Once you know your patient is stable, it is time for a thorough history and physical exam. Laboratory and imaging studies may be indicated. If possible, obtain specimens for culture before antibiotics administration because culture results can ultimately help guide therapy.

History

Be sure to ask about the onset, the rate of progression, inciting events (insect bite, eczema, trauma, nail through the sneaker), systemic signs of illness (fever, vomiting), associated pain, or limitations in activities (walking, moving a joint). Do a complete review of systems, as other symptoms could point to other diagnoses related to the skin condition, such as human immunodeficiency virus (HIV) infection or malignancy. Review any treatments (antihistamines, antibiotics, topicals) that have been tried and note whether they helped. Ask about past skin infections and other medical problems (e.g., sickle cell or diabetes). Take a complete exposure history, including recent travel and exposure to soil, water, animals, and tuberculosis (family members in jail, in nursing homes, with a cough, etc). Ask if there is a family history of skin infections. If there is a strong family history of recurrent skin infections, methicillin-resistant *S. aureus* (MRSA) should be considered as the causative organism until proven otherwise.

Physical Examination

Thoroughly examine overlying and underlying structures to determine the extent of infection, especially if it is on the face or over a joint. Evaluate for areas of fluctuance that could be drained for both diagnostic and therapeutic purposes. Evaluate for a foreign body. Check for lymphadenopathy in the chains draining the site of infection. Also check for secondary or other sites of infection. Do not forget to check the scalp and under clothes and diapers.

> ### CLINICAL PEARL
>
> *On your initial exam, mark the outside of the area of erythema with a pen or marker. This will be helpful in follow-up exams to determine if the infection is progressing or resolving.*

Labs and Tests to Consider

Other than a culture, labs are not routinely indicated in well-appearing patients with focal disease. However, consider a more extensive workup in patients with signs of systemic illness.

Key Diagnostic Labs and Tests

Culture, culture, culture. If there is any pus or drainage, send it for Gram stain and culture. An actual specimen is best, but if you are using swabs, be sure to send at least two. Gram stains may be done immediately and can provide useful information to guide initial therapy if organisms are seen. Cultures will take at least 1 to 2 days to yield results.

Consider a complete blood count with differential, C-reactive protein (CRP) and blood culture in patients with systemic signs of illness. CRP can be helpful in following response to treatment.

Imaging

Although imaging is not routinely indicated for cellulitis, it can be helpful to evaluate the extent of infection and check the integrity of underlying structures. Ultrasound can be helpful to check for loculations and abscesses that can be drained. Computed tomography (CT) can be helpful in evaluating a facial cellulitis to be sure that infection has not progressed to orbital cellulitis with intracranial extension. Magnetic resonance imaging (MRI) can be helpful to evaluate for spread to muscles or bones.

Treatment

If there is pus, it must be drained. Small abscesses are often drained in the ED under local or moderate sedation. More extensive infections may require surgical consultation for drainage or debridement. Drains or packing may be placed into deep or extensive infections. Although antibiotics are typically initiated in all patients, some studies indicate that incision and drainage of small abscesses is often curative, even without the addition of antibiotics.

The child in the case presentation underwent incision and drainage in the ED. Gram stain of the purulent drainage revealed many white blood cells and gram-positive cocci in clusters. The child was empirically treated with clindamycin. MRSA, which was sensitive to clindamycin, was subsequently isolated from culture.

Admission Criteria and Level-of-Care Criteria

Patients with extensive or rapidly progressing infections, systemic signs of illness, failure to respond to oral antibiotics, or an inability to tolerate oral antibiotics should be admitted to the hospital for further care. Consider admission for very young patients (especially those <2 months), patients with facial infections or infections over a joint, and patients without access to appropriate follow-up. Patients with rapidly progressing infection or signs of shock should be considered for intensive care unit admission.

EXTENDED IN-HOSPITAL MANAGEMENT

Most patients are admitted on IV antibiotics. Knowing the susceptibility/resistance patterns in the community and any special patient factors is key to instituting the appropriate therapy. For inpatient therapy, clindamycin is a good choice. Vancomycin should be considered for severe infections with systemic signs or joint involvement. It is important to obtain cultures prior to starting vancomycin; otherwise, it may be difficult to transition to oral antibiotics. For facial cellulitis, ceftriaxone or another antibiotic with good coverage for *Haemophilus* spp. and oral flora should be added. Broader coverage is also needed if there was freshwater, soil, or sneaker exposure.

DISPOSITION

Discharge Goals

The patient should be afebrile and the site of infection improving prior to discharge. If the wound is packed or a drain is in place, the parents should be taught how to do dressing changes, and appropriate follow-up should be arranged.

Outpatient Care

Patients need close follow-up after discharge (either from the hospital or the ED) in order to monitor progression/resolution of the infection. For outpatient therapy, clindamycin is often a good choice, as it covers most MRSA as well as group A *Streptococcus*. However, it is important to know the local susceptibility patterns, as sometimes methicillin-sensitive *Staphylococcus aureus* (MSSA) as well as MRSA is resistant to clindamycin. Cephalexin should not be considered first-line therapy if there are high rates of MRSA in the community. Trimethoprim–sulfamethoxazole is sometimes used, but it does not cover group A *Streptococcus* and can cause Stevens–Johnson syndrome on rare occasions.

WHAT YOU NEED TO REMEMBER

- Measure and mark the area of erythema so that you can evaluate its progression.
- Often, cellulitis is accompanied by abscess. Feel for fluctuance—if there's pus, it must be drained.
- Culture, culture, culture. If at all possible, get a Gram stain and culture of pus prior to starting antibiotics.
- Think about antibiotic resistance patterns in your area and your patient's risk factors.

SUGGESTED READINGS

Bingöl-Koloğlu M, Yildiz RV, Alper B, et al. Necrotizing fasciitis in children: diagnostic and therapeutic aspects. *J Pediatr Surg* 2007;42(11):1892–1897.

Daum RS. Skin and soft-tissue infections caused by methicillin-resistant *Staphylococcus aureus*. *N Engl J Med* 2007;357(4):380–390.

Eady EA, Cove JH. Staphylococcal resistance revisited: community-acquired methicillin resistant *Staphylococcus aureus*—an emerging problem for the management of skin and soft tissue infections. *Curr Opin Infect Dis* 2003;16(2):103–124.

Khangura S, Wallace J, Kissoon N, et al. Management of cellulitis in a pediatric emergency department. *Pediatr Emerg Care* 2007;23(11):805–811.

Purcell K, Fergie J. Epidemic of community-acquired methicillin-resistant *Staphylococcus aureus* infections: a 14-year study at Driscoll Children's Hospital. *Arch Pediatr Adolesc Med* 2005;159(10):980–985.

THE PATIENT ENCOUNTER

A 5-year-old boy with a history of asthma was taken to the emergency department (ED) for a 2-day history of wheezing and increased work of breathing, which had been worsening at home despite the administration of albuterol every 4 hours. He was seen at his pediatrician's office earlier in the day and received three nebulized albuterol treatments without significant relief. On examination in the ED, he was afebrile with a heart rate of 120 beats per minute, a respiratory rate of 48 breaths per minute, and an oxygen saturation of 88% on room air. He was in moderate to severe respiratory distress with suprasternal retractions and nasal flaring. Pulmonary auscultation revealed symmetrically decreased breath sounds with diffuse expiratory wheezing.

OVERVIEW

Definition

Status asthmaticus can be defined as an acute asthma exacerbation that is refractory to initial bronchodilator therapy in an emergency setting. The components that characterize asthma include inflammation, airflow obstruction, and airway hyperresponsiveness.

Pathophysiology

Asthma is a chronic inflammatory disease of the airways. Status asthmaticus may be triggered by either allergic or nonallergic exposures. Allergic antigens such as pollen, pets, mold, or dust mites trigger bronchoconstriction via an IgE-dependent release of inflammatory mediators from mast cells. Nonallergic stimuli such as smoke, respiratory viruses, aspirin, ibuprofen, and cold air can also cause bronchoconstriction via a non-IgE mediated pathway. Both allergic and nonallergic triggers lead to smooth muscle contraction within minutes of exposure, which narrows the airways and interferes with airflow.

Epidemiology

Asthma is the most common chronic disease of childhood, currently affecting more than 6 million children, or about 9% of the population under 18 years of age (1). It is more prevalent in males, non-Hispanic blacks, and poor families.

In children, asthma accounts for approximately 700,000 ED visits per year, 200,000 admissions, and 200 deaths (2). Most children with asthma present by 5 years of age. Risk factors for death from asthma include a previous severe exacerbation requiring intubation or intensive care unit (ICU) admission, two or more hospitalizations for asthma in the past year, three or more visits to the ED in the past year, a hospitalization or ED visit for asthma in the past month, low socioeconomic status, and the lack of a written asthma action plan.

Etiology

The etiology is unknown but likely includes a genetic component with exacerbation in the context of specific environmental triggers.

ACUTE MANAGEMENT AND WORKUP

When status asthmaticus is suspected, the goals of the acute management and workup are to stabilize the patient from a cardiorespiratory standpoint, consider other causes of respiratory distress, and begin definitive treatment with inhaled beta-agonists and systemic corticosteroids.

The First 15 Minutes

While walking to the bedside, rapidly assess the patient's mental status, color, and the degree of respiratory distress. If the patient is drowsy or confused, cyanosis is present, or accessory muscle use and retractions are severe, immediate resuscitative efforts may be indicated.

If emergent intervention is not necessary, first determine if there is a history of asthma, as this will decide the breadth of your differential diagnosis and the degree to which it is explored in the evaluation. At the bedside, obtain a set of vital signs, paying particular attention to the respiratory rate and oxygen saturation, and compare them with the age-appropriate normal values. If the oxygen saturation is <90%, supplemental oxygen should be administered. Next, ask the child some questions to determine his or her degree of dyspnea. A child who is able to speak only in single words or short phrases is experiencing severe respiratory distress. Then assess the degree of intercostal, subcostal, and supraclavicular retractions, accessory muscle use, and nasal flaring up close while auscultating the lung fields. Note the degree of air movement heard and the quality of the wheezing. Absence of wheezing may indicate severe obstruction and imminent respiratory failure. In a patient with a brief history and an exam consistent with a moderate to severe asthma exacerbation, inhaled beta-agonists and systemic corticosteroids should be initiated early in the ED course.

The First Few Hours

A thorough history and physical exam should be performed with careful consideration of the differential diagnosis. After the initial evaluation, the child should be reassessed often to determine the response to treatment and need for escalation of pharmacologic therapy and hospitalization.

> ### CLINICAL PEARL
>
> *In the first few hours, the oxygen saturation may decrease with beta-agonist therapy because of an accentuation of the V/Q mismatch that occurs in status asthmaticus. Because cardiac output rises to a greater degree than bronchodilation in response to the beta agonist, perfusion to a nonuniformly ventilated lung increases and the oxygen saturation may decrease transiently.*

History

While taking the history in children with suspected status asthmaticus, it is important to consider other possibilities, including pneumonia, bronchiolitis, foreign body aspiration, cardiac disease, pulmonary edema, anaphylaxis, anatomic anomalies (vascular ring, mass, tracheoesophageal fistula, tracheobronchomalacia, diaphragmatic hernia), vocal cord dysfunction, and gastroesophageal reflux. Chronic disease other than asthma, such as cystic fibrosis, pulmonary hemosiderosis, alpha-1 antitrypsin deficiency, and bronchopulmonary dysplasia, should also be considered in patients with recurrent episodes of wheezing.

Determine the onset, duration, and trigger of this episode. Did the patient's caretakers notice increased cough, rapid breathing, wheezing, or fever, and how did those symptoms evolve prior to presentation? Fever may suggest a viral illness as a trigger or an underlying pneumonia. Ask about the therapy that was given at home and how frequently it was given—not only the interval between doses but how many times it was given in a 24-hour period. Some families will report giving albuterol every 4 hours, but only while the child is at home and awake, which may only be twice per day.

In children with a history of asthma, determine the severity of prior exacerbations. Ask specifically about triggers, prior hospitalizations, prior ICU admissions, prior intubations, recent ED visits, and recent steroid bursts. If the family has an asthma action plan, review the asthma medications and assess whether the family knows the plan and if they followed it with this exacerbation. If they did not, what were the barriers? In the winter months, ask if the patient has received the influenza vaccine, as influenza disease causes significant morbidity in children with asthma. Finally, determine if the patient has any allergies or other medical conditions that may influence his or her care.

Physical Examination

The physical exam focuses on rapidly triaging the patient's degree of illness based on the mental status, color, and severity of respiratory distress (Table 39-1). In addition to the auscultatory findings already discussed, crackles may be present owing to atelectasis or a coexisting pneumonia. Also, pay attention to the hydration status, as these patients have increased insensible losses and may be prone to dehydration.

Labs and Tests to Consider

Most children with status asthmaticus do not need an extensive laboratory workup. The key tests to consider are peak expiratory flow (PEF) rate and arterial blood gas (ABG).

Key Diagnostic Labs and Tests

Determination of the PEF is a quick and easy measure of airflow obstruction in children ≥ 5 years of age, but it is difficult for some children to perform and cannot distinguish between poor effort, obstructive disease such as asthma, and restrictive disease such as pneumonia. Nevertheless, PEF can provide useful information about the severity of an exacerbation in a cooperative patient with proper coaching (see Table 39-1). If available, measurement of the forced expiratory volume in one second (FEV$_1$) may be more useful.

ABG measurement may be used in the evaluation of a child with severe status asthmaticus in whom projected respiratory failure is a concern. Early in the course of an exacerbation, the PaO$_2$ and PaCO$_2$ are both mildly decreased, reflecting the ventilation/perfusion mismatch. As the exacerbation worsens, the PaCO$_2$ begins to rise into and above the normal range; the pH subsequently falls. A "normal" PaCO$_2$ in a patient with status asthmaticus who also has tachypnea and an increased work of breathing indicates a high risk of respiratory failure.

Imaging

Imaging is not routinely necessary, although chest radiographs may be indicated in the following situations: wheezing unresponsive to treatment; persistent focal findings on auscultation after therapy; and signs and symptoms consistent with pneumonia, foreign body aspiration, pneumothorax, or cardiac disease. Some pediatricians prefer to obtain a chest x-ray on all first-time wheezers to rule out other causes of wheezing such as a mass compressing the airway. Chest radiography findings consistent with status asthmaticus include hyperinflation, peribronchial thickening, and atelectasis.

Treatment

The initial treatment of an asthma exacerbation includes the following:

• Supplemental oxygen if the percutaneous oxygen saturation is <90% on room air.

TABLE 39-1

Factors Helpful in the Determination of the Severity of Asthma Exacerbation[a]

Factor	Mild	Moderate	Severe	Respiratory Arrest Imminent
Mental status	Normal to agitated	Often agitated	Often agitated	Drowsy or confused
Color	Normal	Normal to pale	Pale to cyanotic	Cyanotic
Breathlessness	While walking	While at rest[c]	While at rest[d]	While at rest[d]
Position	Can lie down	Prefers sitting	Sits upright	Sits upright
Speaks in	Sentences	Phrases	Words	Words
Respiratory rate	Normal to increased	Increased	Often >30/min	Often >30/min
Oxygen saturation	>95%	90%–95%	<90%	<90%
Accessory muscle use	Usually not	Commonly	Usually	Paradoxical thoracoabdominal movement

(continued)

TABLE 39-1

Factors Helpful in the Determination of the Severity of Asthma Exacerbation[a] (Continued)

Factor	Mild	Moderate	Severe	Respiratory Arrest Imminent
Wheeze	Often only end-expiratory	Throughout exhalation	Throughout inhalation and exhalation	Absence of wheezing
PEF, % predicted or % personal best[b]	≥70%	40%–69%	<40%	<25%

PEF, peak expiratory flow rate; $PaCO_2$, arterial partial pressure of carbon dioxide.

[a]These parameters are general guidelines that may help determine the severity of an exacerbation, but many have not been systemically studied.

[b]Peak expiratory flow may be useful in children ≤5 years of age.

[c]Infants may have a softer, shorter cry and experience difficulty feeding.

[d]Infants may stop feeding.

Source: Adapted from National Asthma Education and Prevention Program Expert Panel. *Report 3: Guidelines for the Diagnosis and Management of Asthma Full Report 2007* (NIH Publication No. 07-4051). Bethesda, MD: National Institutes of Health, National Heart, Lung, and Blood Institute, August 2007.

- Albuterol given via a metered-dose inhaler (MDI) with a spacer (4 to 8 puffs inhaled every 20 minutes for three doses) or via a nebulizer (0.15 mg/kg inhaled every 20 minutes for three doses).
  - Beta-agonist given via an MDI with a spacer produces equivalent bronchodilation to a nebulizer (3), and offers quicker setup and delivery, a lower cost, and the opportunity to provide education on home MDI use.
  - Levalbuterol administered in half the milligram dose of albuterol provides comparable efficacy and safety to albuterol, although at a significantly higher cost.
- Ipratropium bromide (inhaled) via a MDI or nebulizer.
  - This is not a stand-alone therapy, but it reduces the likelihood of hospital admission when administered concomitantly with albuterol in the ED (4).
- Systemic corticosteroids (oral prednisolone or IV methylprednisolone 1 to 2 mg/kg x1 to max 60 mg/dose).
  - Corticosteroids should be administered promptly to patients presenting with moderate to severe asthma exacerbations or in patients presenting with mild exacerbations who do not respond adequately to initial beta-agonist therapy. Oral dosing is preferred over IV unless the patient is unable to tolerate medications by mouth.

Following initial treatment with an inhaled beta-agonist, ipratropium, and corticosteroids, the patient should be reassessed. Patients with a good response (i.e., no respiratory distress, a normal exam, and a PEF reading >70% predicted/personal best) may be considered for discharge. Those with a poor or incomplete response will likely require admission to the ward or ICU and may need escalation of therapy with additional medications (see later discussion). The most critically ill patients need noninvasive ventilation, such as continuous positive airway pressure (CPAP) or intubation and mechanical ventilation.

Additional medications to consider in status asthmaticus include the following:

- Continuous albuterol via a nebulizer (0.5 mg/kg/hr inhaled to a maximum of 15 mg/hr).
  - Start continuous albuterol immediately in patients presenting with severe asthma exacerbations or in those with minimal improvement after three doses of intermittent albuterol.

In patients without significant improvement despite therapy with continuous albuterol, consider adding one or more of the following:

- Magnesium sulfate (25 to 75 mg/kg IV to a maximum of 2 g).
  - This may cause hypotension, so the patient's blood pressure must be monitored.

- Epinephrine 1:1,000 (0.01 mL/kg subcutaneously to a maximum of 0.5 mL).
- Terbutaline 0.1% (0.01 mL/kg subcutaneously to a maximum of 0.25 mL every 20 minutes for three doses OR a loading dose of 10 μg/kg IV over 10 minutes followed by a continuous IV infusion of 0.4 μg/kg/min (titrate up by 0.2 μg/kg/min, usual effective range is 3 to 6 μg/kg/min).
- In critically ill patients with life-threatening exacerbations, consider adding heliox (helium/oxygen mixture administered by facemask) to the above therapies.

Admission Criteria and Level-of-Care Criteria

Children with status asthmaticus typically require admission. This encompasses children with an oxygen saturation of <90% on room air, a PEF <70% predicted/best, persistent respiratory distress, or tachypnea on reevaluation. In addition, children who have been seen in the ED <24 hours earlier and those with complicating pulmonary or cardiac disease should receive additional consideration for admission. Patients in severe respiratory distress who require >40% FiO_2, continuous albuterol, magnesium sulfate, subcutaneous epinephrine, or terbutaline should be admitted to the ICU.

EXTENDED IN-HOSPITAL MANAGEMENT

Patients admitted to the hospital should continue on inhaled beta-adrenergic therapy via a MDI with a spacer or nebulizer, twice-daily systemic corticosteroids, and their usual home medications. Once the patient has stabilized and is beginning to improve, the frequency of beta-adrenergic therapy can be decreased until the patient is able to tolerate an acceptable frequency (i.e., no more frequently than every 4 hours) and dosage for home use. The patient's asthma action plan should be reviewed and updated. The action plan should outline medications and environmental control measures for daily management as well as clues to recognizing exacerbations of asthma (symptoms as well as PEF values, if used) and the appropriate response. For a sample asthma care plan, visit the "Resources for Professionals" section of the Community Asthma Prevention Program of Philadelphia's website, http://www.chop.edu/consumer/jsp/division/generic.jsp?id=77576.

The patient illustrated in the encounter was started on oxygen via nasal cannula and was given albuterol and ipratropium via a MDI with spacer, treatment being given every 20 minutes for a total of three times, along with 2 mg/kg of prednisolone, but there was no significant improvement. He was then admitted to receive continuous albuterol with 40% FiO_2. After 1 hour on continuous albuterol, he had some improvement but still had a moderately increased work of breathing, nasal flaring, and loud expiratory wheezing. Magnesium sulfate was given intravenously and the patient was admitted to the ICU, where he continued on the albuterol and prednisolone. Within 8 hours, he was markedly improved, and the dose of his continuous albuterol was cut in half. He was weaned off the supplemental oxygen. The next morning he was changed to albuterol administered via MDI with spacer, treatments being given every 2 hours, and transferred to the general pediatric ward. His parents attended asthma education classes and the residents reviewed the patient's asthma action plan with his family. Since his mother reported that he awoke coughing or four times per month, the team added fluticasone, a twice-daily inhaled corticosteroid, to his action plan. That evening his albuterol dosing was changed to every 4 hours. The inactivated influenza vaccine was administered. He tolerated the increased interval well and the next morning was discharged home to continue the prednisolone for a total of 7 days.

DISPOSITION

Discharge Goals

As illustrated in the patient encounter, consider discharge when the patient is stable on room air with no respiratory distress, tolerating albuterol every 4 hours at the dose to be received at home (usually two puffs, as opposed to the higher dosing that may be indicated in the hospital). If available, administer the influenza vaccine. Also ensure that the patient has received and understands the family's asthma action plan prior to discharge. The team should notify the primary care physician of the admission and discuss any changes made to the asthma action plan.

Outpatient Care

After discharge from the hospital, patients should have a follow-up visit arranged with their primary care physician within 2 to 3 days. Oral corticosteroids are typically used for a total of 5 to 10 days. Treatment >10 days may require a taper.

Asthma is classified by symptom severity into the following four categories: intermittent, mild persistent, moderate persistent, and severe persistent. Important factors that affect the classification include the frequency of daytime symptoms, nighttime awakenings, activity limitations, albuterol and oral corticosteroid requirements, and FEV_1. Based upon the asthma severity, a stepwise approach to medication management is recommended. For further details, view the latest guidelines from the National Asthma Education and Prevention Program Expert Panel at http://www.nhlbi. nih.gov/guidelines/index.htm.

WHAT YOU NEED TO REMEMBER

- Patients with moderate to severe exacerbations should receive both beta-agonist therapy and systemic corticosteroids as soon as possible following a brief initial evaluation.
- The absence of wheeze on physical examination in a patient with severe respiratory distress may be a sign of diminished airflow and impending respiratory failure.
- The patient's asthma action plan should be evaluated and updated during any ED visit and inpatient hospitalization; any changes should be reviewed with the family and communicated to the primary care physician.

REFERENCES

1. Bloom B, Cohen RA. *Summary Health Statistics for U.S. Children: National Health Interview Survey, 2006.* Vital and Health Statistics 2007;10(234):4–9.
2. Moorman JE, Rudd RA, Johnson CA, et al. MMWR Surveillance for Asthma—United States, 1980–2004. *MMWR* 2007;56(SS-8):1–6.
3. Cates CJ, Crilly JA, Rowe BH. Holding chambers (spacers) versus nebulisers for beta-agonist treatment of acute asthma. *Cochrane Database Syst Rev* 2006;(2): CD000052.
4. Qureshi F, Pestian J, Davis P, Zaritsky A. Effect of nebulized ipratropium on the hospitalization rates of children with asthma. *N Engl J Med* 1998;339:1030–1035.

SUGGESTED READINGS

Busse WW, Lemanske RF Jr. Asthma. *N Engl J Med* 2001;344:350–362.
National Asthma Education and Prevention Program. *Expert Panel Report 3: Guidelines for the Diagnosis and Management of Asthma Full Report 2007* (NIH Publication No. 07-4051). Bethesda, MD: National Institutes of Health, National Heart, Lung, and Blood Institute, August 2007.
Rodriguez-Roisin R. Gas exchange abnormalities in asthma. *Lung* 1990;168:599–605.
Resources for Professionals. *Community Asthma Prevention Program of Philadelphia.* Available at: http://www.chop.edu/consumer/jsp/division/generic.jsp?id=77576. Accessed February 25, 2008.

Syncope

CARMEN M. LEBRÓN AND DEBORAH W. YOUNG

THE PATIENT ENCOUNTER

A 2-year-old boy with no past medical conditions presents to the emergency department because of episodes of loss of consciousness that have been occurring approximately twice a week for the past 4 months. The episodes are described as unexpected sudden pallor after minor trauma, which is then followed by a fall with loss of consciousness, rolling of the eyes, and clonic movements for approximately 30 seconds. Consciousness is regained spontaneously over the next 2 minutes before the patient drifts off to sleep. Results of a complete physical exam include normal vital signs, growth parameters, and cardiac and neurologic exams.

DEFINITION

Syncope, also known as fainting, passing out, or falling out, is defined as a temporary episode of loss of consciousness with loss of postural tone that resolves spontaneously.

Pathophysiology

All true syncopal episodes are caused by a decreased substrate (i.e., oxygen, glucose) supply to the brain. The most common mechanism is a momentary decrease in oxygenation and perfusion that then leads to the fainting episode. Most fainting episodes in children are benign in origin, but there are a small percentage of cases that can have a serious cause with the potential for sudden death. Nearly all life-threatening causes of syncope are cardiac in origin.

Most syncopal episodes in children are caused by benign alterations in vasomotor tone. In patients with hemodynamic alterations as an etiology to their syncope, the triggering stimulus activates the nucleus tractus solitarius of the brainstem, which results in simultaneous enhancement of the parasympathetic nervous system (vagal) tone and withdrawal of the sympathetic nervous system tone. This, in turn, can cause a continuum of responses. At one end of the continuum is the cardioinhibitory response, which is characterized by a drop in heart rate. The decreased heart rate then leads to a decrease in blood pressure significant enough to cause loss of consciousness. On the other end of the continuum is the vasodepressor response, which presents as a decrease in blood pressure without much change in the heart rate. This is due to vasodilatation secondary to withdrawal in the sympathetic nervous system tone. Most patients have a mixed response between the two ends of the spectrum. The Bezold–Jarisch reflex is thought to maintain blood pressure during orthostatic stress. In patients prone to vasomotor syncope, this reflex is thought to be exaggerated.

Epidemiology

Syncopal events account for 1% to 3% of all emergency department visits. By the time of the initial assessment by the physician, the patient has already regained consciousness. Up to 15% of children experience a syncopal episode by the end of adolescence, and up to 47% of college students report having had at least one episode of fainting.

> ## CLINICAL PEARL
>
> *Approximately 75% of pediatric patients who faint have neurocardiogenic ("vasovagal") syncope. Other causes of "fainting" include migraines (11%), seizures (8%), and cardiac causes (6%).*

Etiology

Fainting can be broadly categorized into three groups: true syncope, seizures, and psychological causes. The most common causes of syncope in children and teens are orthostatic hypotension, vasovagal etiologies, and breath-holding spells.

True syncope can be further categorized as autonomic, cardiovascular, or metabolic.

- *Autonomic syncope.* Autonomic syncope (also known as neurocardiogenic syncope, reflex or situational syncope, and common fainting) typically occurs while the patient is standing or during a rapid positional change from supine or sitting to standing. A brief prodrome or presyncopal phase progresses to sudden unconsciousness that lasts 1 to 2 minutes with a spontaneous return to the previous state of arousal within a short time. Precipitating events or triggers include prolonged standing; stress, such as pain, fear, or anxiety; confinement in enclosed or poorly ventilated spaces; and environmental heat. These increase circulating catecholamines in response to a real or perceived threat. Reflex precipitants, such as swallowing, hair grooming, and micturition, have also been described. The patient will typically have a prodrome, which can include symptoms such as light-headedness, nausea, tinnitus, dizziness, visual changes (blurred, double, or tunnel vision), pallor, diaphoresis, or shortness of breath. The patient may remain pale, nauseated, and diaphoretic for several hours after the syncopal episode. Autonomic syncope is considered to be a benign illness and carries a favorable prognosis. The full syncopal episode can be avoided if the patient is taught to identify the prodromal symptoms and assumes a supine position during their onset. Additionally, the patient can be instructed salt-enriched tablets during athletic activity or environmental stress.

Another common and usually benign variant of vasovagal syncope in the pediatric population is breath-holding spells. They typically occur from 6 to 24 months of age and are triggered by an emotional insult such as pain, anger, or fear. Breath-holding spells can be pallid or cyanotic, with the latter occurring more commonly (in 80% of cases).

• *Cardiac syncope.* Life-threatening conditions that cause syncope are generally cardiac in origin. They include structural heart disease and electrical disturbances. The common etiologies include arrhythmias, known cardiac defects, and electrolyte abnormalities such as hypokalemia and hypocalcemia. Cardiac defects commonly seen as an etiology include tetralogy of Fallot (postsurgical), hypertrophic cardiomyopathy, and aortic stenosis.

Baseline abnormalities of cardiac conduction, as seen in heart block conditions and bradycardia syndromes, also cause a decrease in cardiac output that leads to syncope. Arrhythmias responsible for recurrent syncope include supraventricular tachycardia (SVT), ventricular tachycardia, Wolff–Parkinson–White syndrome, and prolonged-QT syndrome. SVT is the most common arrhythmia seen in a normally structured heart. Decreased ventricular filling time results in a decrease in the blood flow to the lungs and the brain. Prolonged-QT syndrome is characterized by a prolongation of the corrected QT interval >0.45 seconds (Fig. 40-1). Prolonged QT syndrome can be either congenital or acquired. Acquired etiologies include electrolyte abnormalities, increased intracranial pressure, and

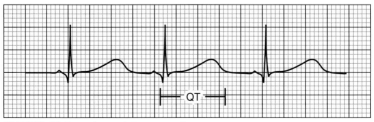

FIGURE 40-1: Prolonged QT interval.

medications such as psychotropic medications (tricyclic antidepressants), phenothiazines, and nonsedating antihistamines.

- *Metabolic and other causes of syncope*. Metabolic conditions can also cause syncope. Hypoglycemia can present with weakness, hunger, diaphoresis, dizziness, and pallor unrelated to position that then progresses to loss of consciousness. Unconsciousness may be prolonged and seizures may occur as a result of the hypoglycemia. Often glucose administration will be required for the resolution of symptoms. Hypoxia can also cause syncope, especially when it is associated with carbon monoxide poisoning. Resolution of the fainting occurs with removal of the patient from the environment where the exposure occurred.

Some conditions may resemble syncope. Seizures typically include loss of consciousness and, if unwitnessed, may be difficult to differentiate from true syncopal episodes. Migraine syndromes, particularly basilar migraines, may present with symptoms similar to syncope, such as loss of consciousness, but are usually preceded by an aura and are accompanied by a severe headache, ataxia, and/or vertigo. Hyperventilation is associated with high anxiety and emotional events. It classically occurs in adolescents, who may complain of shortness of breath, chest pain, paresthesias, dizziness or light-headedness, and visual disturbances. Hyperventilation may result in a true loss of consciousness thought to be mediated by cerebral vasoconstriction in response to self-induced hypocapnia. Hysteria or conversion disorders can be similar to syncopal episodes, occurring most commonly in adolescent patients. The "fainting" episode can be associated with hyperventilation and classically occurs in front of others. Narcolepsy may mimic syncope. An abrupt onset of sleep occurs when the patient has cataplexy, which is defined as the sudden intrusion of rapid-eye-movement sleep into the waking period.

ACUTE MANAGEMENT AND WORKUP

The purpose of the evaluation of a pediatric patient with syncope is to identify life-threatening conditions or conditions that can be associated with significant injury. A cardiac etiology for syncope is particularly important to identify.

The First 15 Minutes

Special attention should be paid to the ABCs (airway, breathing, and circulation), evaluating the vital signs and assessing for hemodynamic stability, including orthostatic blood pressure and pulse oximetry as well as mental status changes. An electrocardiogram (ECG) should be obtained and reviewed to eliminate symptomatic arrhythmias or long-QT syndrome as the cause for the syncopal event. A measurement of serum glucose should be obtained in patients who remain symptomatic.

The First Few Hours

A complete and detailed history along with a meticulous physical exam and evaluation of the ECG will direct the patient's management, appropriate imaging, and consultation.

History

Careful history taking is the most important tool in recognizing the cause of the syncopal episode and is most helpful in directing the workup. Studies have identified specific historical features associated with specific syncopal etiologies: prolonged upright posture (vasovagal), triggers identified for the event (vasovagal), exercise-related syncope (cardiac), and recurrent syncope (psychogenic or cardiac).

The precipitating events just prior to the syncopal episode should be identified. Documenting the position that the child was in when the syncope occurred is also important. Fainting that occurs after prolonged standing or after a sudden change in position (from sitting or lying down to standing) is associated with a vasovagal etiology. Syncope occurring during exercise or exertion is very concerning for a cardiac etiology. Fainting *after* exercise could be cardiac or vasovagal/orthostatic in origin.

Certain triggers have been associated with primary electrical disturbances. For example, the most common genotypes of congenital long-QT syndrome have as associated triggers being startled (acute arousal) or auditory stimuli (such as a loud alarm). Patients with familial catecholaminergic polymorphic ventricular tachycardia can develop arrhythmias in response to emotional or physical stress.

A detailed description of the event should be documented. A typical vasovagal spell will present with symptoms prior to the event that include dizziness, light-headedness, diaphoresis, nausea, and visual changes. Difficulty breathing, palpitations and/or chest pain prior to or during the event are concerning for a cardiac origin of the syncope. Orthostatic or vasovagal syncope may recur when the patient tries to sit up or stand after the event.

A medical history with a focus on cardiac and neurologic history should be obtained. Any history of congenital heart disease (corrected or uncorrected) or a history of cardiac surgery or arrhythmias should be documented. Ask about prior syncopal events or seizures. A menstrual history and access to prescribed medications or illicit drugs are also very important.

Search for a cardiac cause for the syncopal episode when there is a family history of sudden cardiac deaths prior to age 45, a sudden death that involves unexplained accidents such as drowning, and a history of known arrhythmias or familial heart disease. A family history of vasovagal syncope may be present in ≤90% of patients with this condition.

TABLE 40-1

Differentiation of Syncope From Other "Spells"

	Syncope, Vasovagal	Metabolic Syncope	Seizure	Breath-Holding Spell
Unconsciousness	Seconds	Variable	Minutes or longer	Seconds
Prodrome	Fright, pain, "Feels faint"	Confusion, AMS, ↑HR, sweating	Occasional aura	Pain or fright→vigorous cry→apnea→LOC
Incontinence	Absent	Absent	May occur	Absent
Confusion on Awakening	Absent/mild	Mild	Marked	Absent
Tonic-clonic movements	May occur if LOC is prolonged	May occur	Commonly present	Rare; may see 1 to 2 beats
EEG	Normal	Normal	May be abnormal	Normal

AMS, altered mental status; HR, heart rate; LOC, loss of consciousness; EEG, electroencephalogram.

Physical Examination

Perform a complete physical examination, including evaluating vital signs, paying particular attention to the cardiac and neurologic exams. Heart rate and blood pressure should be measured first while the patient is lying down and then while he or she is standing. Orthostatic vital signs are considered positive if there is an abnormal decrease in systolic blood pressure (>20 mm Hg) or if there is an abnormal increase (>20 beats per minute) in the heart rate. A return of the symptoms upon changing position from lying down to standing is more significant than any measurement.

During the cardiac exam, pay particular attention to any abnormal heart sounds, gallops, rubs, or outflow obstruction murmurs. Systolic ejection murmurs and ejection clicks are characteristic of aortic stenosis. An outflow murmur that decreases in intensity with increased venous return to the heart (i.e., during a Valsalva maneuver or squatting) is characteristic of hypertrophic cardiomyopathy. The finding of rales, gallops, and/or hepatomegaly is consistent with cardiac disease.

A careful neurologic evaluation should be performed to look for focal deficits. Also assess the patient's hydration status and consider the presence of any toxidromes.

Labs and Tests to Consider

The ECG is considered to be a usual part of the syncope workup. In an asymptomatic patient, extensive blood work, such as complete blood counts and a measure of serum electrolytes, and/or glucose, are rarely helpful.

Key Diagnostic Labs and Tests

An ECG should be included in all initial evaluations for syncope, and patients should be placed on a continuous cardiac monitor to assess heart rate, rhythm, and conduction intervals. ECG findings in cardiac syncope may include nonsinus rhythms, bradycardia, or a complete atrioventricular block. A corrected QT interval >0.45 seconds is suggestive of long-QT syndrome. Pseudo–right bundle branch block and persistent V1 to V3 ST-segment elevation is suggestive of Brugada syndrome. Delta waves are seen in syndromes with preexcitation, such as Wolf–Parkinson–White. Ventricular hypertrophy and strain patterns are consistent with hypertrophic cardiomyopathy. Myocardial injury signs on ECG are suggestive of congenital coronary artery anomalies. Right ventricular hypertrophy is suggestive of tetralogy of Fallot or primary pulmonary hypertension.

Other studies are dictated by careful history taking. A bedside glucose determination might be useful for patients who present immediately after the episode. A measure of hematocrit might be useful for children who are at risk for anemia. A urine pregnancy test is indicated in all postmenarchal females. A urine toxicology screen for drugs of abuse may be useful for patients with altered mental status. A serum carboxyhemoglobin determination should be obtained in those who are at risk for exposure. Holter monitoring is costly, rarely diagnostic in children, and is rarely included in the initial workup. Event recorders are similar in size and have replaced Holter monitors in many medical centers in the evaluation of a child with syncope.

Our case patient's ECG revealed normal sinus rhythm with a QTc interval of 0.40 seconds. An outpatient EEG was normal. EEG with ocular compression testing showed bradycardia with a brief 4-second episode of reversible asystole, from which he recovered spontaneously, thus confirming the diagnosis of syncope and ruling out seizures as the etiology of his episodes.

Imaging

An echocardiogram can identify hypertrophic cardiomyopathy or obstructive disease in patients who have an abnormal ECG, a pathologic murmur, a history of cardiac disease, or exercise-induced syncope. Emergent neuroimaging is indicated in patients with focal findings on their neurologic exams, a persistently altered mental status, or a significant head injury.

Treatment

For patients with a diagnosis of vasovagal syncope, reassurance and education regarding the benign nature of the process should be initiated. The patient should be taught to identify the prodromal symptoms and to adopt a sitting or lying position as soon as these signs are identified. Another simple measure is avoidance of dehydration. Salt-enriched diets may be encouraged during periods of exercise, and 1 g/day of oral salt supplementation, with or without fludrocortisone acetate (0.1 mg/kg/day), is often therapeutic. Refractory cases may need β-adrenergic blockade (with atenolol or propranolol). Disopyramide, transdermal scopolamine, and cardiac pacing are used more rarely.

Children who have cyanotic breath-holding spells may be treated with iron, even in the absence of anemia. Parents must also be reassured as to the benign nature of these episodes. Pallid breath-holding spells are also benign in nature. If they should become severe or frequent, anticholinergic therapy is available.

The treatment of arrhythmias ranges from pharmacologic intervention to ablation therapy and pacing. The parents of patients diagnosed with long-QT syndrome should be instructed to avoid macrolide antibiotics and cisapride for their child, because these may precipitate fatal arrhythmias. Beta-blockers may be lifesaving, and parents of children with long-QT syndrome need to be taught cardiopulmonary resuscitation because exercise restriction and pharmacotherapy are insufficient in some children.

Admission Criteria and Level of Care Criteria

Most patients can be followed as outpatients. Admission to the hospital should be considered for patients with evidence of cardiovascular disease, an abnormal ECG, chest pain, cyanotic spells, apnea or bradycardia that resolves only with a vigorous stimulus, focal neurologic findings, orthostasis that does not resolve with fluid therapy, or acute toxic ingestions.

EXTENDED INHOSPITAL MANAGEMENT

In patients with a cardiac etiology, inpatient evaluation with cardiac catheterization and electrophysiologic testing with invasive monitoring may be needed. Radiofrequency ablation of aberrant conduction or pacer implantation may be indicated. Patients with atrial myxomas or congenital cardiac structural defects will need surgical correction of their conditions.

DISPOSITION

Discharge Goals

Most patients presenting for an evaluation of syncope will be able to go home with reassurance and instructions for outpatient follow-up. Those who do not have a concerning history or physical findings for cardiac syncope and who have responded appropriately to medical intervention (i.e., intravenous hydration) may be discharged home.

Outpatient Care

Patients should have a follow-up visit with their primary care physician. Patients with a history and physical exam findings consistent with seizures, patients with migraines, and patients with altered mental status or focal neurologic findings will need to see a neurologist. Those patients with suspected hysteria or a psychological etiology to their fainting warrant referral to a psychiatrist.

WHAT YOU NEED TO REMEMBER

- Syncope is a sudden, brief loss of consciousness and postural tone that resolves spontaneously.
- Most syncopal episodes in the pediatric population are benign in etiology.
- Most dangerous causes of syncope are cardiac in origin.
- Conditions that imitate syncope include seizures, migraines, hyperventilation, and hysteria.

SUGGESTED READINGS

Delgado C. Syncope. In Fleisher GR, Ludwig S, Henretig FM. *Textbook of Pediatric Emergency Medicine,* 5th ed. Philadelphia:Lippincott Williams & Wilkins, 2006.

Sapin SO. Autonomic syncope in pediatrics: a practice-oriented approach to classification, pathophysiology, diagnosis, and management. *Clin Pediatr* 2004;43(1): 17–23.

McLeod KA. Syncope in Childhood. *Arch Dis Child* 2003;88(4):350–353.

Systemic Lupus Erythematosus

BRIAN MCALVIN

THE PATIENT ENCOUNTER

A 16-year-old girl presented to the emergency department with 2 weeks of fever. She was upset because she had recently developed a bright red rash involving her forehead, nose, and cheeks. She complained of a flaky rash on her scalp and behind her ears. She also reported that her ankles and the soles of her feet had become extremely tender and swollen. Her mother was worried about her daughter's persistent vomiting and 20-pound weight loss. On examination, the patient's temperature was 37.6°C (99.7°F), her blood pressure was 111/81 mm Hg, her pulse was 89 beats per minute, her respirations were 16 breaths per minute, and her SaO₂ was 99% on room air. Her face had a raised erythematous rash over the malar eminences with sparing of the nasolabial folds. Superficial scalp desquamation as well as scattered petechiae and purpuric lesions over the lower extremities were noted. Both ankles were warm, swollen, and tender.

OVERVIEW

Systemic lupus erythematosus (SLE) is a multisystem autoimmune disease of unknown etiology with symptoms that vary over time. Clinically, it is a relapsing and remitting illness that can affect almost any organ system.

Definition

SLE is diagnosed by the presence of 4 or more of the 11 diagnostic criteria (see Table 41-1). These may occur serially or simultaneously during any interval of observation.

Pathophysiology

The disease mechanism of SLE is not fully understood; however, its hallmark is the production of autoantibodies against self-antigens such as nuclear proteins, membrane phospholipids, ribosomes, platelets, erythrocytes, coagulation factors, and leukocytes. Initially these self-antigens are abnormally processed by antigen-presenting cells (APCs), which bind B-cell receptors and stimulate the production of IgG autoantibodies. APCs also activate helper T cells, which in turn stimulate the autoreactive B cells. In SLE, these B cells and helper T cells are abnormally hyperactivated and are

TABLE 41-1
Diagnostic Criteria for SLE[a]

Criterion	Definition
1. Malar rash	Fixed erythema, flat or raised, over the malar eminences, tending to spare the nasolabial folds.
2. Discoid rash	Erythematous raised patches with adherent keratotic scaling and follicular plugging; atrophic scarring may occur in older lesions.
3. Photosensitivity	Rash as a result of unusual reaction to sunlight (elicited by patient history or physician observation).
4. Oral ulcers	Oral or nasopharyngeal ulceration, usually painless, observed by a physician.
5. Arthritis	Nonerosive arthritis involving two or more peripheral joints, characterized by tenderness, swelling, or effusion.
6. Serositis	Pleuritis: convincing history of pleuritic pain or rub heard by a physician or evidence of pleural effusion. OR Pericarditis: documented by ECG or rub or evidence of pericardial effusion.
7. Renal disorder	Persistent proteinuria >0.5 g/day or >3+ if quantitation not performed. OR Cellular casts: may be red blood cell, hemoglobin, granular, tubular, or mixed.
8. Neurologic disorder	Seizures: in the absence of offending drugs or known metabolic derangements (e.g., uremia, ketoacidosis, or electrolyte imbalance). OR Psychosis: in the absence of offending drugs or known metabolic derangements (e.g., uremia, ketoacidosis, or electrolyte imbalance).

TABLE 41-1

Diagnostic Criteria for SLE[a] (Continued)

Criterion	Definition
9. Hematologic disorder	Hemolytic anemia, with reticulocytosis. OR Leukopenia: $<4,000/mm^3$ total on two or more occasions. OR Lymphopenia: $<1,500/mm^3$ on two or more occasions. OR Thrombocytopenia: $<100,000/mm^3$.
10. Immunologic disorder	Anti-DNA antibody to native DNA in abnormal titer. OR Anti-Smith: presence of antibody to Smith nuclear antigen. OR Positive finding of antiphospholipid antibodies based on (1) an abnormal serum level of IgG or IgM anticardiolipin antibodies; (2) a positive test result for lupus anticoagulant using a standard method, or (3) a false-positive serologic test for syphilis known to be positive for at least 6 months and confirmed by *Treponema pallidum* immobilization or fluorescent treponemal antibody absorption test (FTA-ABS). Standard methods should be used in testing for the presence of antiphospholipid.
11. Antinuclear antibody	An abnormal titer of antinuclear antibody by immunofluorescence or an equivalent assay at any time and in the absence of drugs known to be associated with "drug-induced lupus syndrome."

[a]The presence of 4 or more of the 11 criteria serially or simultaneously during any interval of observation is diagnostic of systemic lupus erythematosus.
Source: Updating the American College of Rheumatology revised criteria for the classification of systemic lupus erythematosus. *Arthritis Rheum* 1997;40:1725.

able to escape the normal process of immune tolerance. Normally, suppressor T cells regulate the B-cell response, but in SLE suppressor T cells may function abnormally. The autoantibodies produced by the B cells bind various self-antigens and form immune complexes that result in complement activation and tissue injury. Normally, these immune complexes bind to complement receptors on the surface of red blood cells, which carry them to the mononuclear phagocytic system for clearance. However, in SLE, the phagocytes may have diminished function, resulting in poor clearance of immune complexes.

Epidemiology

Prevalence data in the United States for SLE vary depending on the population. Among Caucasian men, the prevalence is 10/100,000; in African American men, it is 50/100,000; in Caucasian women, it is 100/100,000; and in African American women, it is 400/100,000. Hispanic, Native American, and Southeast and South Asian populations have a higher prevalence than Caucasian populations. Female predominance is observed in all populations and varies from 4:1 before puberty to 8:1 after puberty.

Etiology

The etiology of SLE is multifactorial. Multiple genetic haplotypes have been identified that predispose individuals to the development of SLE. Many environmental factors have been implicated, including ultraviolet light, sex hormones, dietary factors, infectious agents, and exposure to certain medications.

ACUTE MANAGEMENT AND WORKUP

The acute management and workup should identify patients with severe or life-threatening illness who require more intensive inpatient management as compared with those who can be treated as outpatients.

The First 15 Minutes

The manifestations of lupus are highly variable. In the ill-appearing child, your initial assessment should identify whether stabilization is necessary. This requires careful attention to identify patients with cardiopulmonary compromise, thromboembolic disease, neuropsychiatric complications, or severe infection that can result from immunosuppression.

The First Few Hours

Whether the diagnosis of lupus is established or suspected, the clinician must identify which organ systems are involved and how severely they are affected. This is accomplished by a thorough history and physical examination coupled with appropriate screening laboratory tests. These should include a complete blood count (CBC) with differential and reticulocyte count, a comprehensive metabolic panel, urinalysis, and evaluations of C3 and C4, antinuclear antibodies, erythrocyte sedimentation rate (ESR), and C-reactive protein level. A chest x-ray and electrocardiogram may be helpful when pleuritis or pericarditis is suspected.

History

The presentation of SLE can be highly variable, but patients most frequently complain of fever, fatigue, joint pain, and rash. Because the diagnosis of lupus is largely clinical, a thorough history is essential. Ask about photosensitivity, rashes, oral or nasal ulcers, joint pain, chest or abdominal pain (serosal inflammation), seizures, and behavioral changes (see Table 41-1). The symptoms may be present simultaneously or serially over time as the disease waxes and wanes. Other manifestations not listed in the table are possible. Inquire about other family members who may have SLE or autoimmune disease.

Physical Examination

A thorough physical examination is essential because of its role in the diagnosis of SLE. All joints should be evaluated for effusions, swelling, warmth, and tenderness. Carefully examine the skin for rashes and inspect the mucous membranes for ulcerations. Serosal inflammation may result in evidence of a pleural effusion (diminished breath sounds, lack of fremitus, and dullness to percussion) as well as a pleural or pericardial friction rub. Hypertension or edema can result from nephritis. Assess the patient's mental status and identify focal neurologic deficits.

Labs and Tests to Consider

Laboratory evaluation plays an important role in SLE, not only for diagnosis but also for identifying major organ involvement, monitoring disease activity, and following its progression in major organs. Furthermore, many of the clinical manifestations are associated with specific autoantibodies.

Key Diagnostic Labs and Tests

Key laboratory tests should be used to identify active disease as well as predict disease manifestations.

Diagnostic Laboratory Evaluations. Key lab tests are guided by the American College of Rheumatology diagnostic criteria (Table 41-1). The presence of 4 or more of the 11 criteria, serially or simultaneously during any interval of observation, is diagnostic. Titers for antinuclear antibodies should be obtained. Persistent proteinuria and cellular casts can be identified by urinalysis with microscopic evaluation. Proteinuria can be quantified with a 24-hour urine collection. The hematologic derangements can be identified by obtaining a CBC with differential and reticulocyte count. Immunologic abnormalities are identified by obtaining serum antibody titers for double-stranded DNA, Smith nuclear antigen, antiphospholipid, anticardiolipin, and lupus anticoagulant.

Markers of Disease Activity. High antibody titers of anti-ds-DNA, elevated ESR, and low serum complement (CH_{50}, C_3, C_4) levels are reliable markers of active disease.

Predictors of Disease Manifestations. Many of the clinical manifestations of SLE are associated with the presence of specific autoantibodies. For example, antiphospholipid antibodies are associated with the antiphospholipid antibody syndrome, Coombs antibodies with hemolytic anemia, lupus anticoagulant with hypercoagulability, and antiribosomal P antibody with cerebritis.

 CLINICAL PEARL

The kidney is the most commonly involved visceral organ in patients with SLE.

Although most patients have renal disease on biopsy, only 50% will ever have clinical manifestations, such as hypertension, edema of the lower extremities, retinal changes, clinical manifestations associated with electrolyte abnormalities, nephrosis, and acute renal failure. Renal disease is more frequently observed in children than in adults. Other associations that have been identified are not discussed here.

Imaging

Imaging studies should be guided by clinical manifestations. Chest x-rays are useful for the evaluation of interstitial lung disease, pulmonary hemorrhages, and pleural effusions. All can be further characterized by computed tomography, which is also useful for pulmonary emboli. Echocardiography is used to detect pericardial effusions and vegetations from Libman–Sacks endocarditis. Brain magnetic resonance imaging/magnetic resonance angiography (MRI/MRA) is helpful for detecting vasculitis, stroke, and cerebritis.

Treatment

Because the treatment of SLE is associated with significant side effects, you must decide whether conservative therapy is adequate or if aggressive treatment is needed. Steroids effectively treat most manifestations of SLE;

however, many symptoms can be treated with other medications. Conservative measures include analgesics, topical steroids, sunscreens, nonsteroidal anti-inflammatory drugs (NSAIDs), salicylates, and antimalarials. Aggressive therapy consists of high-dose glucocorticoids and cytotoxic/immunosuppressive drugs.

Mild arthritis, arthralgia, and myalgia can be treated with analgesics, NSAIDs, and antimalarial medication, with steroids reserved for severe symptoms. Cutaneous lupus can be treated with topical steroids, antimalarial medications, and isotretinoin, with systemic steroids reserved for refractory disease. Serositis is usually treated with salicylates, NSAIDs, antimalarials, or low-dose steroids; however, high-dose steroids are sometimes needed.

Severe, active disease requires aggressive therapy with high-dose steroids and cytotoxic agents. Important treatment decisions are largely based on major organ involvement, including nephritis, neuropsychiatric disease, and hematologic derangements. The exact steroid dose and preferred route of administration are controversial. These agents can be given orally in divided doses, intravenously, or as a combination of both. If the response and toxicity are acceptable, the steroids can be gradually tapered to the lowest effective dose, which can be given daily or every other day. Adverse effects of corticosteroids include hyperglycemia, hypertension, gastritis, osteopenia, cataracts, and cushingoid body habitus.

If the response to steroids is inadequate or if the toxicity is unacceptable, then the addition of a cytotoxic agent may be necessary. The two most commonly used cytotoxic agents are cyclophosphamide and azathioprine. These drugs in are used in conjunction with glucocorticoids to control active disease, prevent organ damage, and minimize steroid requirements. Other steroid sparing drugs used in the treatment of SLE include methotrexate, cyclosporine, and mycophenolate mofetil.

For the case patient, initial laboratory evaluation revealed leukopenia (WBCs 2,840/mm^3), lymphopenia (682/mm^3), hypocomplementemia (C3, 12 mg/dL; C4, 4 mg/dL), hematuria (10 RBCs per high-power field), proteinuria (2+ dipstick), and elevation of her hepatic and pancreatic enzymes (AST 765 U/L, ALT 230 U/L, amylase 313 U/L, lipase 1947 U/L). Serum IgG titers for ribonuclear protein, SS-A (Ro), SS-B (La), and ds-DNA were elevated. She was diagnosed with SLE with hepatitis, pancreatitis, and nephritis. She was hospitalized and intravenous methylprednisolone (1 g daily) was initiated.

Admission Criteria and Level-of-Care Criteria

Because the manifestations of lupus vary greatly, the decision to hospitalize must be done on a case-by-case basis. Admission criteria include any life- or organ-threatening manifestations. Examples are severe hematologic complications, neuropsychiatric disease, thromboembolic events, and cardiopulmonary compromise from heart or lung disease. Immuno-suppressed patients with fever who appear ill should be admitted and started on antibiotics until the appropriate culture results are known. Most patients can be managed on the pediatric floor; however, admission to the intensive care unit should be considered for patients who require higher levels of respiratory or cardiovascular support, those with signs and symptoms of sepsis, and those with life-threatening central nervous system disease.

EXTENDED INHOSPITAL MANAGEMENT

When possible, a rheumatologist should be consulted. Complications such as pericardial tamponade, thromboembolic disease, pulmonary complications, nephritis, or neuropsychiatric illness also warrant appropriate consultation.

In evaluating the patient's response to therapy, a combination of clinical and laboratory parameters should be used. For example, in patients with nephritis, serum creatinine, blood urea nitrogen, and complement levels (C3 and C4), as well as the measurement of urine protein, are used to gauge improvement. Other manifestations, such as psychosis and cognitive changes, are followed clinically. As patients improve, complement levels should increase and titers of nuclear antibodies should fall. Once the patient has begun to show both clinical and laboratory improvement, the glucocorticoid dose can be gradually tapered.

DISPOSITION

Discharge Goals

Prior to discharge, it is important for the patient and family to understand that full disease remission may not be achieved. The most important measures of improvement are clinical, such as stable renal function (with or without proteinuria), safe hematologic counts, mild arthralgias, and mild skin lesions. Consider discharge when these measures have been met and the patient is established on an immunosuppressive regimen than can be followed at home.

Outpatient Care

The goal of outpatient care is to maximize disease control while minimizing the predictable side effects of therapy. Normalization of serum levels of complement, antibodies to DNA, and ESR have been shown to reduce the number of flares; however, controversy exists over whether or not this should be the goal of therapy. Ultimately, the patient and clinician must decide together if the severity of symptoms warrants aggressive therapy or if they can be treated conservatively.

WHAT YOU NEED TO REMEMBER

- SLE is a multisystem autoimmune disease that can affect any organ system.
- SLE is more common in African Americans and women.
- The diagnosis of SLE is confirmed by the presence of any 4 of the 11 criteria listed in Table 41-1, simultaneously or over time.
- The most common initial symptoms are fever, fatigue, joint pain, and rash.
- Therapy, whether conservative or aggressive, is guided by which organ systems are affected.
- The goal of treatment is to balance mild, non–life-threatening symptoms with the toxic side effects of therapy.

SUGGESTED READINGS

Behrman R. *Nelson Textbook of Pediatrics*, 17th ed. Philadelphia: Elsevier Saunders, 2004.

Benseler SM, Silverman ED. Systemic lupus erythematosus. *Pediatr Clin North Am* 2005;52(2):443–467.

Grimaldi CM. Sex and systemic lupus erythematosus: the role of the sex hormones estrogen and prolactin on the regulation of autoreactive B cells. *Curr Opin Rheumatol* 2006;18(5):456–461.

Harris ED, Jr., Ruddy S, Firestein GS, et al. *Kelley's Textbook of Rheumatology*, 7th ed. Philadelphia: Elsevier Saunders, 2005.

Helmick CG, Felson DT, Lawrence RC, et al. National Arthritis Data Workgroup. Estimates of the prevalence of arthritis and other rheumatic conditions in the United States. Part I. *Arthritis Rheum* 2008;58(1):15–25.

Hochberg MC. Updating the American College of Rheumatology revised criteria for the classification of systemic lupus erythematosus. *Arthritis Rheum* 1997;40(9):1725.

Rojas-Serrano J, Cardiel MH. Lupus patients in an emergency unit. Causes of consultation, hospitalization and outcome. A cohort study. *Lupus* 2000;9(8):601–606.

Testicular Torsion

THAO M. NGUYEN AND NAGHMA S. KHAN

THE PATIENT ENCOUNTER

A 15-year-old sexually active male presented to the emergency department with acute left-sided scrotal swelling and pain of 4 hours' duration. He denied any provoking event, fever, or penile discharge. He felt nauseous but had not vomited. Vital signs revealed a temperature of 37.4°C (99.3°F), a heart rate of 94 beats per minute, a respiratory rate of 18 breaths per minute, and blood pressure of 132/87 mm Hg. Physical examination of the abdomen was benign and there was no inguinal hernia. His genitourinary exam showed pubescent changes with a sexual maturity rating of 4, normal right testis, and a tender, enlarged, mildly erythematous left testis with horizontal lie. Cremasteric reflex was absent on the left side.

OVERVIEW

Every male patient with the acute onset of scrotal pain and swelling requires immediate evaluation to diagnose or exclude testicular torsion. Testicular torsion is a true urologic emergency in which a delay in diagnosis and management can lead to loss of the testicle.

Definition

Testicular torsion is a surgical emergency in which torsion of the spermatic cord of the testis causes strangulation of gonadal blood supply, leading to testicular necrosis and atrophy.

Pathophysiology

Testicular torsion refers to twisting of the spermatic cord structures. Torsion obstructs venous return, leading to subsequent testicular and spermatic cord swelling and congestion, which ultimately impedes arterial flow, with resultant testicular ischemia and atrophy. The degree of ischemia and the viability of the torsed testis depend on the duration of torsion and the degree of rotation of the spermatic cord. Irreversible ischemia of the testes can occur as soon as 4 hours after torsion; testicular loss is almost certain after 24 hours. The degree of torsion may vary from 180 to 720 degrees, with greater degrees of rotation leading to a more rapid onset of ischemia.

Epidemiology

The incidence of testicular torsion is 1 in 4,000 males younger than 25 years of age. Although it can occur at any age, peak incidences are seen in the neonatal period, with a much larger peak observed during puberty. Approximately 65% of cases occur in boys between the ages of 12 and 18 years. It is the most frequent cause of testicular loss in adolescent males.

Etiology

The two types of testicular torsion are intravaginal and extravaginal torsion. Normal testicular suspension ensures fixation of the testis posteriorly and prevents twisting of the spermatic cord. Intravaginal torsion, which accounts for the majority of cases, results from a congenital malformation in which the tunica vaginalis completely surrounds the epididymis and spermatic cord. This creates the "bell-clapper deformity," in which the long axis of the testicle is oriented transversely rather than cephalocaudally, thus allowing abnormally mobile testis to rotate freely within the tunica space (Fig. 42-1). This deformity is typically bilateral, although the left testis is more frequently involved in torsion. An increase in testicular volume (often associated with puberty), trauma, and testicular tumor predispose to intravaginal torsion.

Extravaginal torsion occurs in utero in the setting of normal anatomy. The entire structure (testis, spermatic cord, and tunica vaginalis) freely rotates prior to the development of testicular fixation and the infant is born with a large, firm, nontender, and nonviable testis.

ACUTE MANAGEMENT AND WORKUP

Testicular torsion must be excluded in all cases of acute scrotum because a delay in diagnosis can lead to testicular loss. A careful history and examination along with diagnostic imaging will establish the appropriate diagnosis. The most common causes of testicular loss after torsion are delay in seeking medical attention (58%), incorrect initial diagnosis (29%), and a delay in treatment (13%).

The First 15 Minutes

The initial assessment helps to determine if the patient is clinically stable. In patients who are comfortable at rest and do not appear in pain, a thorough directed history and exam may be performed.

The First Few Hours

Time is of essence for successful testicular salvage. Consult urology immediately if clinical suspicion is high for testicular torsion. A Doppler ultrasound imaging study should be ordered for equivocal cases; however, imaging should not delay urologic consultation. Scrotal exploration is necessary

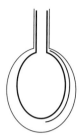

A Normal Testicle and Tunica Vaginalis

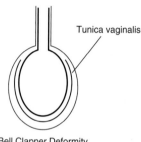

Tunica vaginalis

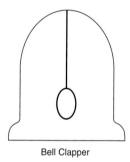

B   Bell Clapper Deformity   Bell Clapper

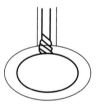

C   Testicular Torsion

FIGURE 42-1: Illustration of **(A)** normal testicle and tunica vaginalis, **(B)** bell-clapper deformity, and **(C)** testicular torsion with a transverse lie.

for definitive exclusion if the clinical examination and imaging cannot exclude testicular torsion. A negative surgical exploration is preferable to a missed diagnosis.

All patients should be provided with adequate pain control. Oral intake should be withheld until a surgical condition has been ruled out.

History

Most patients presenting with acute scrotal pain do not have testicular torsion. It is, however, the most important diagnosis to differentiate from other less emergent causes of acute scrotal pain, such as torsion of the appendix testis, epididymitis, scrotal trauma, and hydrocele. A focused history of urinary tract and gastrointestinal symptoms will provide significant clues to the specific diagnosis. Special attention should be paid to the onset and duration of the pain and swelling, the presence of nausea or vomiting, a history of previous urinary tract trauma or infection, and a history of sexual exposure.

An abrupt, sudden onset of severe pain is characteristic of testicular torsion; this pain may occur at rest or may relate to sports or physical activities. Gradual, mild to moderate pain that develops over a few days is more suggestive of epididymitis or a torsed appendix testis. Nausea and vomiting are common in testicular torsion, whereas fever and voiding problems or painful urination are more suggestive of epididymitis. A history of similar but self-limiting painful episodes may suggest intermittent testicular torsion.

Physical Examination

The evaluation of patients with acute scrotum should include a detailed examination of the abdomen, inguinal region, and genitalia. The degree of swelling, the presence and location of erythema, the lie of the testicles, and the degree of thickening of the scrotal skin should be carefully observed. The cremasteric reflex is elicited by stroking the inner aspect of the upper thigh, which should normally stimulate contraction of the cremasteric muscles and elevation of the ipsilateral testicle. The testicle is best examined by grasping it between the thumb and first two digits. The epididymis should be palpable on the posterior and superior aspects of the testicle. Tenderness over the entire testicle is consistent with testicular torsion. The presence of the "blue-dot sign," a small, bluish discoloration over the superior pole of the testicle, indicates appendiceal torsion. The physical examination is most helpful within the first 12 hours after symptom onset; with time, significant erythema and scrotal wall thickening result in the loss of the anatomic landmarks of the testis and epididymis, making it difficult to differentiate the causes of acute scrotal pain.

The physical examination of a typical prepubertal patient with testicular torsion may reveal a swollen, tender, high-riding testis with an abnormal horizontal lie. The absence of the cremasteric reflex in a patient with acute scrotal pain is the most sensitive and specific sign of testicular torsion on physical examination.

Labs and Tests to Consider

Laboratory examinations of urine and blood are seldom helpful except to confirm the absence of cord torsion in cases where surgical intervention is believed to be unnecessary. The presence of pyuria on urinalysis with or without bacteria would be unusual in testicular torsion but is suggestive of epididymitis. A complete blood count may show leukocytosis, which is a nonspecific finding in both testicular torsion and epididymitis.

The patient illustrated in the case above had a peripheral white blood cell count of 18,000/mm³, with 5% bands and 65% segmented neutrophils. The white blood cell count in the urine was increased to 10 cells per high-power field, with no bacteria present. The leukocytosis suggested an inflammatory process and the sterile pyuria could possibly indicate a urinary infection rather than torsion.

Imaging

Imaging should be done only in equivocal cases where suspicion for torsion is low or the duration of pain is >12 hours. Any patient with a history and physical examination suspicious for torsion with a duration of pain <12 hours should have immediate urologic evaluation and surgical exploration.

Color Doppler ultrasonography (US) is the imaging modality of choice. Torsion is diagnosed when intratesticular blood flow is diminished or absent within the affected testis compared with the normal testis. Occasionally, false-negative results may occur because of increased blood flow to highly inflamed scrotal tissues secondary to the devascularized testis. It is important to also visualize the coiled spermatic cord. US findings also associated with testicular torsion include the absence of scrotal wall edema, swollen testis, decreased testicular echogenicity, and normal epididymis. The case patient underwent ultrasound imaging while awaiting urology arrival. His US showed both the symptomatic and contralateral testes.

Radionuclide scanning using ⁹⁹ᵐTc-pertechnetate, once the study of choice, is more limited because it evaluates only testicular blood flow and does not provide any anatomic data. It is rarely available on a 24-hour basis and usually takes longer to perform, resulting in a significant delay in diagnosis.

Treatment

Successful testicular salvage is directly related to the duration of torsion.

CLINICAL PEARL

The testicular salvage rate is approximately 90% if detorsion occurred <6 hours from the onset of symptoms; this rate falls to 50% after 12 hours and close to zero after 24 hours.

Emergency surgical exploration with intraoperative detorsion is the definite treatment for testicular torsion to alleviate testicular ischemia and prevent subsequent atrophy. If viable, the affected testis as well as the contralateral testicle are surgically fixed in the scrotum (orchiopexy) to prevent future torsion. Orchidectomy is indicated for nonviable testes.

While awaiting surgery, preoperative manual detorsion of the spermatic cord can save a testicle by the immediate restoration of blood flow in patients presenting with early symptoms. Because testes usually twist in an inward (medial) direction with anteromedial rotation of the spermatic cord, manual detorsion should proceed with lateral (outward) rotations, like "opening a book." For example, if it is the right testicle and you are facing the patient, rotate the right testicle *outward* or *laterally* 180 degrees toward the right thigh. This may need to be repeated several times, depending on the degree of the torsion. The lack of resistance during rotation indicates the proper direction of manipulation. Relief of pain is the best indication of successful manual detorsion, which should be confirmed sonographically. Mild sedation or analgesia prior to manipulation will not impair accurate assessment of pain relief that accompanies successful detorsion. Manual detorsion is not a substitute for surgical exploration, and orchiopexy remains mandatory to prevent recurrence.

After urologic evaluation, the case patient was immediately brought to the operating room, where he underwent surgical exploration of his symptomatic testis. Torsion of the spermatic cord was confirmed by direct visualization. The patient had a bell-clapper deformity. The testis was still viable after detorsion and was subsequently fixed to the scrotum with nonabsorbable suture. He also had orchiopexy of his contralateral testis.

Admission Criteria and Level-of-Care Criteria

These criteria are at the discretion of the urologist.

EXTENDED IN-HOSPITAL MANAGEMENT

Extended in-hospital management is usually not indicated or needed.

DISPOSITION

Discharge Goals

The patient should be free of pain and able to tolerate oral fluids.

Outpatient Care

Urology will arrange for a follow-up appointment within 1 to 2 weeks for the evaluation of potential testicular atrophy.

WHAT YOU NEED TO REMEMBER

- Torsion of the spermatic cord is a surgical emergency. It must be excluded in all presentations of acute scrotal swelling.
- The classic presentation of testicular torsion is typically a prepubertal male with sudden, severe testicular pain for ≤6 hours, nausea and vomiting, high-riding or horizontal testis, and decreased or absent cremasteric reflex.
- Color Doppler ultrasound is indicated for equivocal presentation; the decrease or absence of testicular blood flow is diagnostic of testicular torsion.
- Imaging should not delay urologic evaluation and/or surgical exploration if there is a high index of suspicion for testicular torsion.
- Testicular salvage is most successful if the duration of torsion is <6 hours. After 24 hours, testicular viability approaches zero.

SUGGESTED READINGS

Arce JD. Sonographic diagnosis of acute spermatic cord torsion. *Pediatr Radiol* 2002;32:485–491.

Ciftci AO. Clinical predictors for differential diagnosis of acute scrotum. *Eur J Pediatr Surg* 2004;14:333–338.

Edelsberg JS. The acute scrotum. *Emerg Med Clin North Am* 1988;6:521–546.

Garel L. Preoperative manual detorsion of the spermatic cord with Doppler ultrasound monitoring in patients with intravaginal acute testicular torsion. *Pediatr Radiol* 2000;30:41–44.

Karmazyn B. Clinical and sonographic criteria of acute scrotum in children: a retrospective study of 172 boys. *Pediatr Radiol* 2005;35:302–310.

Kass EJ. The acute scrotum. *Pediatr Clin North Am* 1997;44:1252–1266.

Lam WW. Colour Doppler ultrasonography replacing surgical exploration for acute scrotum: myth or reality? *Pediatr Radiol* 2005;35:597–600.

Ringdahl E. Testicular torsion. *Am Fam Physician* 2006;74:1739–1743.

Schneck FX. Abnormalities of the testes and scrotum and their surgical management. In Wein AJ, ed. *Campbell-Walsh Urology*, 9th ed. Philadelphia: Elsevier Saunders, 2007.

Urinary Tract Infections

MERCEDES M. BLACKSTONE

THE PATIENT ENCOUNTER

A 6-month-old white girl presented to her pediatrician with a 2-day history of fevers. On review of systems, she had some nasal congestion and a mild cough for the previous few days. She had two loose stools on the day prior to the visit. She had normal oral intake and urine output. Her parents are unaware of any ill contacts but she does attend day care. In the office, her temperature was 39.2°C (102.6°F). Her physical exam was unremarkable with the exception of some nasal congestion and fluid behind her tympanic membranes bilaterally. She was diagnosed with a viral upper respiratory infection and sent home. The next day, the patient was not acting like herself, was vomiting, and was continuing to spike high fevers. Her parents brought her to the emergency department, where a transurethral catheterization of the bladder was performed to obtain urine for urinalysis and culture.

OVERVIEW

Definition

A urinary tract infection (UTI) is defined by the presence of microorganisms within the normally sterile urinary tract. UTIs are typically divided into lower tract disease, in which infection is localized to the bladder and urethra (cystitis and urethritis), and upper tract disease, in which it extends to the ureter and kidney (pyelonephritis). Pyelonephritis in childhood is associated with renal scarring, which has been linked to risks for subsequent hypertension, chronic renal disease, and preeclampsia. Young febrile infants with a UTI are assumed to have pyelonephritis and are treated accordingly.

Pathophysiology

The vast majority of UTIs are caused by bacterial pathogens, but viruses, fungi, and parasites can cause infection as well. This chapter focuses on bacterial UTIs. Urinary tract infection occurs when enteric stool pathogens or skin flora ascend through the urethra, infecting the bladder or spreading further into the upper urinary tract. The shorter urethra in females makes them more susceptible to UTIs. Uncircumcised infants are another high-risk group because they harbor increased numbers of bacteria in the periurethral area. Racial and genetic differences in rates of UTI may be explained by differences in blood group antigens on the surface of uroepithelial cells, which affect bacterial adherence. In young infants, infection may be caused by hematogenous spread rather than ascending infection.

Epidemiology

UTIs are the most common serious bacterial infections affecting infants and young children. UTI has been increasingly recognized as an important occult cause of fever in young children. Rates of UTI vary widely with respect to age, gender, race, and other factors. Screening studies performed in emergency departments suggest an overall prevalence of UTI of 3% to 5% in febrile children <2 years of age. The prevalence is higher in Caucasian girls, uncircumcised boys, and children without another source of fever. The peak incidence of UTI occurs in the first year of life for all children, with a second peak occurring among female adolescents. After infancy, females are far more likely than males to have a UTI.

Etiology

The bacterial pathogens associated with UTI are summarized in Table 43-1. Almost all clinically significant UTIs are caused by a single bacterial species. The gram-negative Enterobacteriaceae family is responsible for most uncomplicated UTIs. *Escherichia coli* causes more than 80% of acute infections. Gram-positive organisms account for a minority of uncomplicated UTIs (approximately 5% to 10%). *Staphylococcus saprophyticus* in particular

TABLE 43-1
The Etiology of Bacterial Urinary Tract Infections

Common	Less Common	Rare
Gram-negative organisms		
Escherichia coli	*Pseudomonas* spp.	*Corynebacterium*
Klebsiella spp.	*Citrobacter* spp.	*urealyticum*
Proteus mirabilis	*Staphylococcus*	*Ureaplasma*
Enterobacter spp.	*aureus*	*urealyticum*
Serratia spp.		*Mycoplasma*
Gram-positive organisms		*hominis*
Staphylococcus saprophyticus		
Group B streptococci		
Enterococcus spp.		

tends to infect sexually active adolescent females. Organisms such as *Proteus*, *Enterobacter*, *Citrobacter*, and *Klebsiella* spp. are often cultured in cases of recurrent UTI, particularly in children with urinary anomalies. Children who are hospitalized, immunocompromised, or who have indwelling catheters or undergo frequent bladder instrumentation are at risk for a UTI caused by *Pseudomonas* spp.

ACUTE MANAGEMENT AND WORKUP

The acute management and workup of the patient with UTI helps to distinguish the few patients with urosepsis who need aggressive management from the majority of patients who can be managed safely as outpatients. Because UTI is often an occult diagnosis in febrile young infants, the acute management and workup often addresses a broad range of diagnoses. The goal is to rapidly identify and treat the cause of fever.

The First 15 Minutes

Determine whether the child needs an immediate intervention or whether it is safe to proceed with your history and physical examination. Look closely at the vital signs. Most patients will be febrile and therefore tachycardic. **Look for tachycardia that is out of proportion to fever or is not resolving with fever control.** Because of a smaller ventricular muscle mass, children with sepsis rely on increasing their heart rate to maintain their cardiac output rather than increasing their stroke volume. Do not wait for hypotension, because this is a very late finding in septic children. The child with severe tachycardia, poor perfusion, or a depressed mental status needs immediate resuscitation.

The First Few Hours

A good history and thorough physical exam combined with the appropriate laboratory studies is often strongly suggestive of UTI. This should be performed rapidly so that the proper antibiotics can be administered promptly. In most cases of UTI or pyelonephritis, there is no role for diagnostic imaging in the acute setting.

History

The historical features consistent with UTI vary widely with the age of the child. The overwhelming majority of infants with UTI present with isolated fever. They may also exhibit other nonspecific signs such as lethargy, irritability, and poor feeding. In contrast, the older child or adolescent's presentation will vary depending on the site of the infection. Children with cystitis often present with the classic symptoms noted in adults, such as dysuria, hematuria, and urinary urgency and frequency. They are often afebrile. Those with pyelonephritis often have these lower urinary tract symptoms in addition to fever, chills, nausea, vomiting, and abdominal or flank pain. Be suspicious of secondary enuresis in a child; this could be the presentation of a UTI. Although parents sometimes report malodorous urine, this is not a reliable indicator of UTI. Any of the following historical features should be noted: chronic constipation, dysfunctional voiding, prior UTIs, recent antibiotic use, a history of vesicoureteral reflux or urinary abnormalities, and previous undiagnosed febrile illnesses.

Physical Examination

Infants commonly present with isolated fever in the context of an otherwise normal physical exam. Jaundice has also been associated with UTI in neonates. The older child may exhibit suprapubic and flank tenderness. A genitourinary exam should be performed and the circumcision status should be noted in males. Because constipation can lead to urinary stasis and infection, hard stool may be palpable on exam.

Labs and Tests to Consider

Urine testing alone is required to make the diagnosis of UTI. In some cases, however, the urinary tract can be colonized with bacteria in the absence of clinical symptomatology. As such, serum laboratory testing may help to distinguish this *asymptomatic bacteriuria* from acute infections. Elevated inflammatory markers are suggestive of infection as opposed to benign colonization of the urinary tract. Although C-reactive protein (CRP) is the most sensitive for pyelonephritis, neither CRP nor white blood cell count nor erythrocyte sedimentation rate (ESR) is specific for upper tract infection as opposed to lower tract infection. Consider a basic metabolic panel to assess the creatinine level when there is a concern for pyelonephritis. A blood culture should be obtained in young infants with UTI because they have a higher risk of bacteremia and should be obtained in anyone who appears very ill.

Key Diagnostic Labs and Tests

The gold standard for the diagnosis of UTI is a positive urine culture, but these results are unavailable for 24 to 48 hours. As such, several rapid diagnostic tests, which vary in terms of their sensitivity and specificity, are commonly used. Patients with suspected UTI should have a urinalysis (UA) and culture obtained either by bladder catheterization in the non-toilet-trained child or the midstream clean-catch method in the older child or adolescent. Suprapubic aspiration can also be performed in young children and has extremely low rates of contamination because it bypasses the distal urethra. Most practitioners however, are far more comfortable with transurethral bladder catheterization. The use of a sterile bag affixed to the perineum is an unacceptable means of collection for urine culture. While it may be used for screening for UTI, rapid screening tests fail to diagnosis pediatric UTI in

10% to 25% of cases. As such, a culture should always be sent when UTI is suspected, so the child often still requires catheterization.

In general, UTI can be diagnosed when there is growth of $>10^2$ colony-forming units (CFU) per milliliter of a single pathogen on suprapubic aspirate, $>10^4$ CFU per milliliter on a catheterized specimen, and $>10^5$ CFU per milliliter on a clean-catch specimen. In cases with equivocal results, the clinical picture often dictates whether treatment is initiated, and a repeat culture may be necessary.

Typically, however, treatment is initiated based upon the results of rapid screening tests. Multiple screening tests are available; traditional UA in which white blood cells are examined by microscopy on a centrifuged specimen; enhanced urinalysis, which uses a hemocytometer cell count and Gram stain on an unspun specimen; and basic dipstick testing for leukocyte esterase (LE) and nitrites. Having ≥10 white blood cells on any specimen, a positive Gram stain, or positive LE or nitrites is indicative but not diagnostic of UTI. While the enhanced UA and positive Gram stains are highly sensitive and specific for UTI, the bedside dipstick test performs almost as well and is the most affordable and readily available option.

CLINICAL PEARL

On urinary dipstick, the nitrite test detects the conversion of nitrate to nitrite by bacteria. Urine must be in the bladder for several hours for this conversion to occur. Therefore, in toilet-trained children with a UTI, nitrites are most likely to be detected in an early-morning urinalysis.

One of the more difficult clinical decisions is which of the many febrile infants encountered requires screening for UTI. Gorelick and Shaw (see "Suggested Readings") developed a clinical decision rule to identify febrile young girls <2 years of age who are particularly at risk for UTI. They recommended screening for UTI when two or more of the following features are present: age <1 year, high fever (≥39°C [102.2°F]), fever for ≥2 days, Caucasian race, and absence of another fever source. Likewise, males with risk factors such as being ≤6 months of age, being uncircumcised, or lacking an alternative fever source also deserve consideration for urine screening.

Our case patient had all of the above risk factors; her mild upper respiratory symptoms do not constitute a definitive source. Clearly she required urine testing. Her initial laboratory results included a peripheral white blood cell count of 18,000/UL with 4% bands and 70% segmented neutrophils. Her basic metabolic panel was normal. Inflammatory markers and blood culture were not performed. Her dipstick UA was positive for LE and negative for nitrites. Formal microscopy showed 10 to 25 white blood cells per high-power field. These findings were consistent with the initial diagnosis of pyelonephritis, and therapy was initiated. Two days later, her urine culture from a catheterized specimen grew >100,000 CFU of *E. coli*.

Imaging

No imaging is required for the *diagnosis* of UTI, but imaging of the urinary system is currently the standard of care for young children with UTIs. A renal ultrasound is helpful for detecting anatomic abnormalities such as hydronephrosis, ureteroceles, and duplications of the collecting system and can be performed at any time after the diagnosis of a febrile UTI. In the patient who fails to improve on appropriate antibiotic therapy, a renal ultrasound can also detect a renal abscess. A voiding cystourethrogram (VCUG), in which the bladder is catheterized and filled with contrast, is a dynamic study that can identify vesicoureteral reflux during voiding. Although some authors have claimed that both of these studies seldom change patient management, the American Academy of Pediatrics continues to recommend a renal ultrasound and VCUG at the "the earliest convenient time" for children <2 years of age following their first UTI. The renal scan, which uses radionuclide-labeled dimercaptosuccinic acid (DMSA), can be used as an adjunctive study to demonstrate pyelonephritis and renal scarring.

Treatment

Antibiotic therapy should be based on urine culture sensitivity testing. Empiric therapy for the first UTI should cover the most common pathogens implicated in pediatric UTIs, which are typically sensitive to many antimicrobials. Options for empiric therapy are included in Table 43-2; the best

TABLE 43-2
Empiric Treatment Options for Febrile UTI

Inpatient	Outpatient
Ampicillin	Amoxicillin
Gentamicin	Amoxicillin-clavulanate
Cefazolin	Cotrimoxazole
Ceftriaxone	Cephalexin
Cefotaxime	Cefixime
	Ceftibuten
	Cefdinir
	Sulfisoxazole

choice for a particular patient often depends on local resistance patterns and issues of compliance. In children with pyelonephritis who require intravenous antibiotics, it is reasonable to begin with two antibiotics, such as ampicillin and gentamicin, and to narrow coverage once sensitivities are known. Children who are immunocompromised, have indwelling catheters, or have a history of recurrent UTIs should be started on broad-spectrum antibiotics that cover the pathogens cultured from past infections. The typical duration of antibiotic therapy in children is 7 to 14 days, with younger children typically receiving 14 days of therapy.

Admission Criteria and Level-of-Care Criteria

Absolute admission criteria include children with signs of urosepsis, age <2 months, or suspected renal abscess. Admission should be considered for young infants (<6 months) and those with underlying complex medical conditions, failed outpatient therapy, dehydration, emesis, or an unreliable social situation. The vast majority of patients with UTI who require admission can be managed on the general pediatric floor; patients with urosepsis, however, require admission to the intensive care unit.

EXTENDED IN-HOSPITAL MANAGEMENT

Children with pyelonephritis typically do not require prolonged hospitalization unless they have preexisting comorbidities or urosepsis. Children are typically hospitalized until they have defervesced and culture sensitivities are known. In a child with UTI, the failure to improve while receiving antibiotics should prompt a search for a renal abscess or an underlying urologic anomaly. Patients who are following the more typical course may obtain a follow-up renal ultrasound or VCUG before or shortly after hospital discharge.

Our patient was hospitalized for intravenous antibiotics because she was ill-appearing and vomiting. She was started on ampicillin and gentamicin and rapidly defervesced within 48 hours. Her urine sensitivity testing showed that her *E. coli* was susceptible to ampicillin, amoxicillin, and cephalexin, as well as several other antibiotics. She was switched to oral amoxicillin and discharged home to follow up with her primary care provider. She had a normal renal ultrasound and was scheduled for an outpatient VCUG.

DISPOSITION

Discharge Goals

Children may be safely discharged when they have demonstrated clinical improvement, are well hydrated, and can tolerate oral antibiotics. Typically they are no longer febrile at this point. Labs need not be followed, but if they are, note a downward trend in the white blood cell count and CRP. If an initial blood culture was obtained and was positive, then clearance of bacteremia on repeat culture should be documented. There is no need for a repeat urine culture or "test of cure" prior to discharge in a patient who has improved clinically; urine cultures are almost always negative after 24 hours of antibiotic therapy.

Outpatient Care

After hospital discharge, patients should see their pediatrician within the next few days. Although it has not been clearly demonstrated that prophylactic antibiotics in fact prevent UTI recurrence, the current practice is to place children on antibiotic prophylaxis once they finish their treatment doses of antibiotics, at least until their VCUG has been obtained. Children who have recurrent UTIs, anatomic anomalies, or severe vesicoureteral reflux (e.g., grade 3 or 4) need to see a pediatric urologist. The few patients who are ill at their follow-up visit, with recurrence of high fevers, have likely failed their outpatient antibiotics and may require readmission, repeat urine testing, and imaging to rule out an abscess. Once children have had one UTI, their pediatrician should consider repeat urine testing in the setting of future febrile illnesses.

WHAT YOU NEED TO REMEMBER

- Consider UTI in a young girl or young uncircumcised male with fever.
- Do not waste time with bagged specimens; if you suspect UTI, catheterize.
- Rapid tests miss a lot of pediatric UTIs. Always send a culture.

SUGGESTED READINGS

American Academy of Pediatrics. Practice parameter: the diagnosis, treatment, and evaluation of the initial urinary tract infection in febrile infants and young children. Committee on Quality Improvement. Subcommittee on Urinary Tract Infection. *Pediatrics* 1999;103(4 Pt 1):843–852.

Gorelick MH, Shaw KN. Clinical decision rule to identify febrile young girls at risk for urinary tract infection. *Arch Pediatr Adolesc Med* 2000;154(4):386–390.

Hoberman A, Charron M, Hickey RW, et al. Imaging studies after a first febrile urinary tract infection in young children. *N Engl J Med* 2003;348(3):195–202.

Hoberman A, Wald ER, Hickey RW, et al. Oral versus initial intravenous therapy for urinary tract infections in young febrile children. *Pediatrics* 1999;104(1 Pt 1):79–86.

McGillivray D, Mok E, Mulrooney E, Kramer MS. A head-to-head comparison: "clean-void" bag versus catheter urinalysis in the diagnosis of urinary tract infection in young children. *J Pediatr* 2005;147(4):451–456.

Williams GJ, Wei L, Lee A, et al. Long-term antibiotics for preventing recurrent urinary tract infection in children. *Cochrane Database Syst Rev* 2006;3:CD001534.

Zamir G, Sakran W, Horowitz Y, et al. Urinary tract infection: is there a need for routine renal ultrasonography? *Arch Dis Child* 2004;89(5):466–468.

Zorc JJ, Kiddoo DA, Shaw KN. Diagnosis and management of pediatric urinary tract infections. *Clin Microbiol Rev* 2005;18(2):417–422.

Ventricular Shunt Infections and Malfunction

JESSICA HART

THE PATIENT ENCOUNTER

A 6-month-old male who underwent ventriculoperitoneal shunt placement at 4 months of age for hydrocephalus presented to the emergency department with an increase in head size, downward deviation of his eyes (setting-sun sign), and poor feeding. Before shunt placement, his head circumference was 53 cm; after shunt placement, it reduced to 43 cm. At present admission, it measures 47 cm with a tense anterior fontanelle and prominent scalp veins. Local examination revealed a noncompressible, firm swelling at the cranial entry point of ventricular catheter over the burr hole site. The infant was febrile to 39.2°C (102.6°F) and responsive only to painful stimuli. He also had bradycardia despite the fever, hypertension, and depressed respirations.

OVERVIEW

Definition

Cerebrospinal fluid (CSF), or ventricular, shunts are the predominant mode of therapy for children with hydrocephalus. Common causes of hydrocephalus in children include intraventricular hemorrhage, congenital cyst, and tumor. Myelomeningocele and meningocele are also associated with hydrocephalus. Most shunts are inserted in the perinatal period. The shunts divert CSF away from the ventricles, preventing increases in intracranial pressure that would otherwise lead to neurologic sequelae. The typical CSF shunt has a proximal portion that enters the CSF space, an intermediate reservoir that lies outside the skull but underneath the skin, and a distal portion that terminates in either the peritoneal (ventriculoperitoneal [VP] shunt), vascular (ventriculoatrial [VA] shunt), or pleural space.

Pathophysiology

Staphylococcal species (i.e., coagulase-negative *Staphylococcus* and *Staphylococcus aureus*), account for almost two-thirds of all shunt infections. The remaining infections are produced by a wide variety of organisms, including gram-negative bacilli. Gram-negative organisms (i.e., *Escherichia coli*, *Klebsiella pneumoniae*, *Pseudomonas aeruginosa*) tend to have a delayed onset, suggesting inoculation after surgery. *Propionibacterium acnes* is isolated more often in a recent series of VP shunt infections; this bacterium generally causes low-grade, indolent infections. *Candida* species should be considered in premature infants and other immunocompromised patients as well as in those receiving parenteral nutrition or prolonged corticosteroid therapy.

Epidemiology

Infection develops in 5% to 15% of all CSF shunts; most infections occur within 6 months of shunt placement. Factors associated with CSF shunt infections include a recent shunt insertion, premature birth, young age, neuroendoscope use during shunt insertion, prior shunt infection, and a hospital stay >3 days at the time of shunt insertion. Insertion of a VP shunt in a premature neonate (age <3 months) has been associated with a nearly five-fold increase in the risk of shunt infection. Patients <1 year of age also have a substantially higher risk of shunt infection than those >1 year of age at the time of shunt placement. The insertion of a shunt after a previous shunt infection is associated with a fourfold increase in the risk of shunt infection.

Etiology

There are four common mechanisms of shunt infection: (i) local inoculation of bacteria at the time of surgery; (ii) a breakdown of the skin overlying the shunt, with subsequent bacterial entry; (iii) hematogenous shunt inoculation; and (iv) retrograde infection from the distal end of the shunt. The most common mechanism of infection, local inoculation of bacteria at the time of surgery, usually manifests itself within several weeks of the operation. Bacterial entry following the breakdown of skin overlying the shunt may occur if the incision fails to heal properly or if the patient disrupts the healing process by scratching the open wound. Children who are relatively immobile, such as those with severe neurologic disability, may develop an overlying decubitus ulcer, which gives bacteria direct access to the shunt. Rarely, accessing the shunt by needle puncture introduces colonizing skin bacteria into the shunt system. Children with shunts in their vascular systems (e.g., ventriculoatrial shunts) are continually at risk of infection from bacteremia, with retrograde spread to the ventricles. Finally, retrograde infection from the distal end of the shunt as a consequence of viscus (e.g., bowel, gallbladder) perforation may lead to distal catheter contamination.

ACUTE MANAGEMENT AND WORKUP

The acute management and workup helps identify those patients with severe or life-threatening illness who require emergent neurosurgical evaluation or more intensive inpatient management. A common dilemma facing physicians evaluating patients with VP shunts is that signs or symptoms thought to be associated with shunt malfunction may overlap with common childhood illnesses.

The First 15 Minutes

As with any patient presenting in an acute setting, it is essential to take an initial survey and focus on the ABCs (airway, breathing, and circulation). If these are stable, it is important to then assess the patient's mental status (or "D" for disability). Patients with an altered mental status, such as unresponsiveness or decreased responsiveness, suggest severe illness (such as meningitis or increased intracranial pressure) that requires immediate management.

> ## CLINICAL PEARL
>
> *With severe intracranial hypertension caused by shunt malfunction in the context of infection, Cushing's triad may be noted. Cushing's triad classically involves systemic hypertension, bradycardia, and respiratory depression; this response usually occurs when brainstem perfusion is compromised by elevated intracranial pressure.*

The First Few Hours

A good history, a thorough physical exam, and the appropriate use of labs and imaging are essential to managing and treating children with VP shunt malfunctions or infections. The use of consulting services, especially neurosurgery, can also be integral in the workup and management of these patients.

History

Historical information obtained from the patients or their caregivers should include indications for shunt placement, the postoperative course, and the history of shunt infection or malfunction. In obtaining the patient's pertinent history, make sure to secure the following important information:

- Indications for insertion
- Dates of insertion and revision
- The type of valve and reservoir
- Medications and allergies
- History of prior shunt infections (organisms and therapy)
- History of shunt malfunction (cause and correction)

A patient with a ventricular shunt requires a review of the symptoms and signs associated with increased intracranial pressure and central nervous system infection. In a child <1 year of age, the symptoms are usually nonspecific and may include lethargy, irritability, vomiting, diminished appetite or anorexia, disordered sleep patterns, and fever. Older children more commonly present with headache, lethargy, nausea and vomiting, and a decreased level of consciousness. Diplopia or other oculomotor disturbances, ataxia, seizures, and visual loss occur less commonly. In many cases, the symptoms may be subtle and may alternate with symptom-free periods.

Physical Examination

In infants, the physical examination should include a measurement of head circumference and an assessment of the size and softness of the anterior fontanelle. The skull and scalp should be palpated and inspected for signs of fluid accumulation or soft-tissue infection, such as erythema and tenderness to palpation. Characteristics of the burr hole(s) should be noted and all incision sites on the skull, neck, chest, and abdomen should be inspected. Attention should be directed toward swelling and fluctuation, which may represent CSF or a purulent fluid collection.

The extracranial portions of the shunt system should be examined to assess for shunt patency. Digital compression of the valve is an integral part of shunt examination. Shunt pumping is easy to perform, does not require special equipment, and can support the diagnosis of overt shunt malfunction.

A complete neurologic exam should also be performed, including cranial nerve assessment and funduscopy to detect papilledema or optic atrophy, which suggest elevated intracranial pressure. The neck should be palpated to detect cervical and posterior auricular adenopathy, which occurs with infections of the shunt insertion site.

The child in the case presentation was critically ill and had manifestations of Cushing's triad, which suggested shunt obstruction. The high fever suggested concomitant shunt infection.

Labs and Tests to Consider

Diagnosis of a CSF shunt infection requires either isolation of a pathogen from ventricular fluid, lumbar CSF, or blood (for VA shunts) or the presence of CSF pleocytosis (usually defined as >50 white blood cells [WBCs] per cubic millimeter in the context of a CSF shunt) in combination with either shunt malfunction or one or more of the signs or symptoms described in the previous section. Neuroimaging studies are also considered an essential part of the initial workup to evaluate for possible shunt malfunctions.

Key Diagnostic Labs and Tests

Key diagnostic laboratory evaluations and tests include CSF studies, shunt series, a computed tomography (CT) scan of the head, and blood culture. Depending on the situation, magnetic resonance imaging (MRI) of the brain or abdominal imaging may also be indicated.

Cerebrospinal Fluid Studies

The CSF should be sent for cell count, glucose, protein, Gram's stain, and aerobic and anaerobic bacterial culture. A CSF fungal culture should also be performed in premature infants and in children with other immunocompromising conditions. A mild CSF pleocytosis, a low CSF glucose level (hypoglycorrhachia), and an elevated CSF protein level are usually present in cases of ventricular infection. CSF white blood cell counts typically range from 100 to 2,500/mm³ in VP shunt infections, although normal CSF parameters (including a normal CSF white blood cell count) have been reported in 17% to 35% of children with VP shunt infections. CSF pleocytosis alone is not diagnostic of infection. Mild-to-moderate pleocytosis (20 to 500 WBCs/mm³) also occurs as a consequence of inflammation after surgery or inflammation associated with a foreign body (i.e., a shunt). Furthermore, infections caused by indolent organisms such as *Propionibacterium. acnes* may fail to induce a vigorous inflammatory response.

Ideally, fluid from the *reservoir* should be obtained by percutaneous aspiration under sterile conditions. Shunt drainage should be performed by a neurosurgeon or a clinician with experience in performing this procedure. Bacteria are identified by a Gram stain of CSF obtained from the reservoir in up to 80% of cases, although the likelihood of a positive Gram stain depends on the causative organism. *S. aureus* and aerobic gram-negative rods such as *E. coli* typically have positive Gram stain results, while *P. acnes*, coagulase-negative staphylococci, and *viridans* group streptococci are positive in <40% of cases. Therefore, a negative Gram stain does not exclude the diagnosis of shunt infection.

Other Laboratory Studies

Blood should be obtained for culture from patients evaluated for suspected shunt infection. Although a negative peripheral blood culture does not rule out a shunt infection, a positive blood culture often influences the choice of antimicrobial therapy. Blood culture results are usually negative in cases of VP infection but positive in VA shunt infection.

Imaging

Neuroimaging studies—including x-rays of the skull, neck, chest, and abdomen (the "shunt series") and computed tomography—should be performed as part of the evaluation of a child with a suspected CSF shunt infection or malfunction. Specific abnormalities that can be visualized on the shunt series include disconnection of the distal catheter, retraction of the distal catheter tip, and discontinuity near the proximal shunt bulb. Routine performance of shunt series has a low overall yield but on rare occasions detects abnormalities that are missed by CT. Both CT and magnetic resonance imaging (MRI) of the head will detect increased ventricular size, a finding that suggests either increased intracranial pressure or hydrocephalus ex vacuo (increased ventricle size reflects shrinkage of brain parenchyma rather than increased intracranial pressure). Ventriculitis and meningitis can be visualized on CT and MRI as enhancement of the ventricular ependymal lining or cerebrocortical sulci. In rare cases, subdural empyema or brain abscess may be the first indication of shunt infection. Radiologic imaging of other areas should be considered depending on the location of the distal catheter tip. CT or ultrasound of the abdomen may identify abdominal peritoneal pseudocysts at the distal portion of a VP shunt. Chest radiography detects pleural effusions associated with ventriculopleural shunt infection.

The child in the case presentation had an emergent ventriculostomy performed. The shunt was externalized and a temporary external reservoir was placed to drain the CSF. Examination of the CSF revealed 750 WBCs/mm^3 and gram-positive bacteria on Gram stain. *S. aureus* was isolated from CSF culture.

Treatment

A child with a ventricular shunt infection should be managed in consultation with neurosurgical and infectious disease specialists. Optimal management of a CSF shunt infection includes intravenous antibiotics and removal of all components of the infected shunt, with placement of a temporary external ventricular drain (EVD) until the CSF is sterile. The EVD facilitates resolution of the ventriculitis and permits continued monitoring of CSF parameters.

Admission Criteria and Level-of-Care Criteria

All patients with shunt infections should be admitted for the administration of intravenous antibiotics. Consider admission to an intensive care unit for patients with altered mental status, evidence of sepsis, or elevated intracranial pressure. Patients with shunt malfunctions without signs of infections are often admitted for repair of the shunt with neurosurgical consult.

EXTENDED IN-HOSPITAL MANAGEMENT

Until an organism is isolated, patients should be treated with empiric antibiotic therapy that covers the range of potentially causative pathogens. Reasonable options include vancomycin in combination with ceftazidime, cefepime, or meropenem.

Situations that may warrant additional measures include cases of delayed ventricular fluid sterilization (>3 days) and cases where the patient cannot safely undergo surgical catheter removal. First, intraventricular antibiotic administration should be considered. No antibiotic has been approved by the U.S. Food and Drug Administration for intraventricular use. However, commonly used intraventricular antibiotics include vancomycin, gentamicin, tobramycin, and amikacin. Penicillin and cephalosporins should *not* be instilled directly into the ventricles because intraventricular administration of these antibiotics has been associated with increased neurotoxicity, including seizures. Second, rifampin has excellent CSF penetration and should be administered orally (in addition to an intravenous antistaphylococcal agent such as vancomycin) when the infection is caused by susceptible staphylococci.

Third, neuroimaging should be performed to diagnose an intracranial abscess or empyema.

The duration of therapy depends on the organism isolated. Coagulase-negative staphylococcal infections require 5 to 7 days of negative cultures prior to shunt reinsertion, while *S. aureus* and gram-negative infections require longer therapy prior to shunt replacement. If the shunt was not initially removed, therapy should be continued for an even longer period of time, although the optimal duration in such cases is not known.

In cases of distal shunt infection, some neurosurgeons prefer to externalize only the distal portion of the shunt. This strategy still maintains CSF flow while offering the ability to perform frequent ventricular fluid sampling without subjecting the patient to a more extensive surgical procedure. However, early infection of the proximal portion of the shunt may be obscured by antibiotic treatment and may become active after the discontinuation of therapy.

DISPOSITION

Discharge Goals

Consider discharge when patients are clinically improved. If blood or CSF cultures were initially positive, repeated blood and CSF cultures (usually about three negative cultures) should document clearance of the infection. If the shunt was externalized or removed, reinsertion should be performed prior to discharge.

Outpatient Care

Shunt infections are typically cared for in the inpatient setting. After discharge, patients will require close follow-up with their pediatrician and neurosurgeon. Parents should be instructed to seek immediate medical attention should symptoms of shunt infection recur.

WHAT YOU NEED TO REMEMBER

- Staphylococcal species, especially coagulase-negative *Staphylococcus* and *S. aureus*, account for almost two-thirds of all shunt infections.
- Most infections occur within 6 months of shunt placement; the insertion of a shunt after a previous shunt infection is associated with a fourfold increase in the risk of shunt infection.
- Symptoms of shunt infection include lethargy, headache, vomiting, and a full fontanel.
- Optimal management of a CSF shunt infection includes intravenous antibiotics and removal of all components of the infected shunt.

SUGGESTED READINGS

Anderson EJ, Yogev R. A rational approach to the management of ventricular shunt infections. *Pediatr Infect Dis J* 2005;24(6):557–558.

Hart JK, Shah SS. Cerebrospinal fluid shunt infections. In: Shah SS(ed). Pediatric practice: Infectious diseases. McGraw-Hill Medical: New York, NY 2009:751–759.

McGirt MJ, Zaas A, Fuchs HE, et al. Risk factors for pediatric ventriculoperitoneal shunt infection and predictors of infectious pathogens. *Clin Infect Dis* 2003;36(7):858–862.

Odio C, McCracken GH Jr, Nelson JD. CSF shunt infections in pediatrics. A seven-year experience. *Am J Dis Child* 1984;138(12):1103–1108.

Pople IK, Bayston R, Hayward RD. Infection of cerebrospinal fluid shunts in infants: a study of etiological factors. *J Neurosurg* 1992;77(1):29–36.

Ring JC, Cates KL, Belani KK, et al. Rifampin for CSF shunt infections caused by coagulase-negative staphylococci. *J Pediatr* 1979;95(2):317–319.

Ronan A, Hogg GG, Klug GL. Cerebrospinal fluid shunt infections in children. *Pediatr Infect Dis J* 1995;14(9):782–786.

Schreffler RT, Schreffler AJ, Wittler RR. Treatment of cerebrospinal fluid shunt infections: a decision analysis. *Pediatr Infect Dis J* 2002;21(7):632–636.

Zorc JJ, Krugman SD, Ogborn J, Benson J. Radiographic evaluation for suspected cerebrospinal fluid shunt obstruction. *Pediatr Emerg Care* 2002;18(5):337–340.

Reference Ranges for Vital Signs in Childhood

TABLE A-1
Range of Normal Values for Respiratory Rate and Heart Rate in Childhood

Age	Respiratory Rate (per minute)	Heart Rate (per minute)
Neonate	35–66	93–154
1 month	34–64	121–182
3 months	32–61	106–186
6 months	30–56	109–169
12 months	27–49	89–151
5 years	16–31	65–133
10–18 years	12–20	60–120

TABLE A-2
Range of Blood Pressure Values for Children of Average Height[a]

Age		BP Percentile	Value or Range[b]
Neonate (term)	Systolic	5th	63
		50th	78
		95th	92
	Diastolic	5th	30
		50th	45
		95th	60
1–5 years	Systolic	50th	85–95
		95th	103–112
	Diastolic	50th	37–53
		95th	56–72
6–10 years	Systolic	50th	96–102
		95th	114–119
	Diastolic	50th	55–61
		95th	74–80
11–18 years	Systolic	50th	104–118
		95th	121–136
	Diastolic	50th	61–67
		95th	80–87

BP = blood pressure

[a]Please consult alternate sources for a more precise classification of normal blood pressure because the values vary slightly by gender, age, and height.

[b]By convention, the inflatable bladder width of an appropriate size cuff covers at least 40% of the arm circumference at a point midway between the olecranon and the acromion (for more information, consult the American Heart Association or search their website at www.americanheart.org).

Data derived in part from (1) American Academy of Pediatrics. The fourth report on the diagnosis, evaluation, and treatment of high blood pressure in children and adolescents. *Pediatrics* 2004;114:555–576; (2) Zubrow AB et al. Determinants of blood pressure in infants admitted to neonatal intensive care units: a prospective, multicenter study. *J Perinatol* 1995;15:470–479; and (3) Rusconi F et al. Reference values for respiratory rate in the first 3 years of life. *Pediatrics* 1994;94:350–355.

Childhood Immunization Schedule

The childhood immunization schedule is updated annually. The most recent recommendations are published by the Centers for Disease Control and Prevention: http://www.cdc.gov/vaccines/recs/schedules/child-schedule.htm.

Index

Page numbers followed by f indicate figure; those followed by t indicate table.